FIFTH EDITION

CASE FILES®
Psychiatry

Eugene C. Toy, MD
Assistant Dean for Education
Professor and Vice Chair of Medical
Education
Department of Obstetrics and Gynecology
University of Texas Medical School at
Houston
Houston, Texas

Debra Klamen, MD, MHPE
Associate Dean of Education and
Curriculum
Professor and Chair, Department of
Medical Education
Professor, Department of Psychiatry
Southern Illinois University School of
Medicine
Springfield, Illinois

Mc
Graw
Hill
Education

New York   Chicago   San Francisco   Athens   London   Madrid
Mexico City   Milan   New Delhi   Singapore   Sydney   Toronto

Case Files®: Psychiatry, Fifth Edition

Copyright © 2016 by McGraw-Hill Education. All rights reserved. Printed in the United States of America. Except as permitted under the United States Copyright Act of 1976, no part of this publication may be reproduced or distributed in any form or by any means, or stored in a data base or retrieval system, without the prior written permission of the publisher.

Previous editions copyright © 2012, 2009, 2007, and 2004 by The McGraw-Hill Companies, Inc.

Case Files® is a registered trademark of McGraw-Hill Education Global Holdings, LLC. All rights reserved.

3 4 5 6 7 8 9 10   LCR   20 19 18 17 16

ISBN 978-0-07-183532-9
MHID 0-07-183532-6

This book was set in Goudy by Cenveo® Publisher Services.
The editors were Catherine A. Johnson and Cindy Yoo.
The production supervisor was Catherine H. Saggese.
Project management was provided by Raghavi Khullar, Cenveo Publisher Services.
RR Donnelley was printer and binder.

This book is printed on acid-free paper.

Library of Congress Cataloging-in-Publication Data

Toy, Eugene C., author.
   Case files. Psychiatry / Eugene C. Toy, Debra Klamen.—Fifth edition.
      p. ; cm.
   Psychiatry
   Includes index.
   ISBN 978-0-07-183532-9 (pbk.)—ISBN 0-07-183532-6
   I. Klamen, Debra L., author.   II. Title.   III. Title: Psychiatry.
   [DNLM: 1. Mental Disorders—Case Reports.   2. Mental Disorders—Problems and Exercises.
3. Psychology, Clinical—Case Reports.   4. Psychology, Clinical—Problems and Exercises.   WM 18.2]
   RC465
   616.89—dc23   2015008831

McGraw-Hill Education books are available at special quantity discounts to use as premiums and sales promotions or for use in corporate training programs. To contact a representative, please visit the Contact Us pages at www.mhprofessional.com.

In loving memory of my grandparents, Lew Yook Toy and Manway Toy, who courageously pioneered our family's legacy in this great country. They gave us through their example and uncompromising standards the foundation of hard work, honesty, generosity, and the pursuit of education.

– ECT

To my wonderful husband, Phil, who loves me and supports me in all things. To my mother, Bonnie Klamen, and to my late father, Sam Klamen, who were and are always there. Thank you also to my best friends and coaches, Kate Fleming-Kuhn and Martin Kuhn, for proving once again that persistence and hard work pay off.

– DLK

CONTENTS

Staci Becker, RN, MS
Nurse Educator
Adjunct Instructor
Department of Medical Education
Southern Illinois University School of Medicine
Springfield, Illinois
Depressive Disorder
Persistent Depressive Disorder
Acute Stress Disorder
Somatic Symptom Disorder with Predominant Pain
Factitious Disorder
Dependent Personality Disorder
Schizotypal Personality Disorder
Narcissistic Personality Disorder
Paranoid Personality Disorder
Borderline Personality Disorder

Sean M. Blitzstein, MD
Director, Psychiatry Clerkship
Clinical Associate Professor of Psychiatry
University of Illinois at Chicago
Chicago, Illinois
Anxiety Disorder Due to Another Medical Condition
Panic Disorder versus Medication-Induced Anxiety Disorder
Specific Phobia
Posttraumatic Stress Disorder
Conversion Disorder (Functional Neurological Symptom Disorder)
Opioid Withdrawal
Alcohol Use Disorder
Stimulant (Cocaine) Intoxication and Stimulant (Cocaine) Use Disorder
Tobacco Use Disorder
Medication-Induced Acute Dystonia (Extrapyramidal Symptoms)

Amber C. May, MD
Resident, Physician
Department of Psychiatry
University of Illinois College of Medicine
Chicago, Illinois
Schizophrenia
Psychosis Caused by Another Medical Condition
Cyclothymic Disorder
Premenstrual Dysphoric Disorder
General Anxiety Disorder
Anxiety Disorder Due to Another Medical Condition
Dissociative Identity Disorder
Enuresis, Nocturnal Type
Delirium
Major Vascular Neurocognitive Disorder (Vascular Dementia)

Philip Pan, MD
Psychiatrist
Memorial Physician Services
Springfield, Illinois
Substance/Medication-Induced Depressive Disorder (Cocaine)
Adjustment Disorder
Phencyclidine Intoxication
Alcohol Withdrawal
Benzodiazepine Withdrawal
Amphetamine Intoxication
Schizoid Personality Disorder
Antisocial Personality Disorder
Avoidant Personality Disorder
Malingering

Stephen M. Soltys, MD
Professor and Chair
Department of Psychiatry
Southern Illinois University School of Medicine
Springfield, Illinois
Mild Intellectual Disability
Attention Deficit Hyperactivity Disorder
Tourette Disorder
Bipolar Disorder (Child)
Major Depressive Disorder with Psychotic Features
Separation Anxiety Disorder
Bulimia Nervosa
Insomnia Disorder
Gender Dysphoria
Illness Anxiety Disorder

Thomas E. Wright, MD
Assistant Clinical Professor of Psychiatry
University of Illinois College of Medicine
Chief Medical Officer, Rosecrance Health Network
Rockford, Illinois
Obsessive-Compulsive Personality Disorder
Histrionic Personality Disorder
Fetishistic Disorder
Conduct Disorder
Nonrapid Eye Movement Sleep Arousal Disorder, Sleep Terror Type
Anorexia Nervosa
Autism Spectrum Disorder
Schizoaffective Disorder
Social Anxiety Disorder
Obsessive-Compulsive Disorder (Child)

We appreciate all the kind remarks and suggestions from the many medical students over the past 3 years. Your positive reception has been an incredible encouragement, especially in light of the short life of the Case Files® series. In this fifth edition of *Case Files®: Psychiatry*, the basic format the cases have been retained, but we have made dramatic improvements in the overall order and structure of the book. Improvements were made in streamlining many of the chapters and completely updating the content to reflect new *DSM-5* criteria. Also, numerous clinical cases were rewritten to be representative of more typical patient presentations rather than the "flamboyant" presentation. We grouped the cases in the same order as they may be found in the *DSM-5* categories in the book. For example, neurodevelopmental disorders such as intellectual disability and attention deficit hyperactivity disorder come first, and the personality and paraphilic disorders come last. This will allow for the ability to "compare and contrast" related disorders side by side, something that has been requested by our medical student readers. The case listing and the index will allow a student to quickly reference similar cases for the sake of comparison as well. The multiple choice questions have been carefully reviewed and rewritten to ensure that they comply with the National Board and USMLE Step 2 CK format. There have been additional review questions added to the book, and a useful Case Correlation feature has been added as well. New psychiatric medications have been introduced too. By using this fifth edition, we hope that the reader will continue to enjoy learning psychiatry through the simulated clinical cases. It is certainly a privilege to be a teacher for so many students, and it is with humility that we present this edition.

The Authors

ACKNOWLEDGMENTS

The curriculum from which the ideas for this series evolved was inspired by two talented, forthright students, Philbert Yau and Chuck Rosipal, who have since graduated from medical school. It has been a great joy to work with Debra Klamen, a brilliant psychiatrist, educator, and lover of horses, and with all the excellent contributors. I appreciate McGraw-Hill's belief in the concept of teaching through clinical cases. I am greatly indebted to my editor, Catherine Johnson, whose exuberance, experience, and vision helped shape this series and to the incomparable Cindy Yoo, Development Editor. I am also grateful to Catherine Saggese for her excellent production expertise. I appreciate the outstanding work of Raghavi Khullar, Project Manager for this book. At Southern Illinois University, I thank Dr Kevin Dorsey for his help and support in completing this project. At the University of Texas Medical School at Houston, I appreciate the support of Dr. Patricia Butler, Vice Dean of Education, and Dr. Sean Blackwell, my chairman for their commitment to education. I am grateful to Linda Berg-strom for her sage advice and support. Without my esteemed colleagues, Drs Konrad Harms, Priti Schachel, Russ Edwards and Gizelle Brooks-Carter, this book could not have been written. Most of all, I appreciate my loving wife, Terri, and my four wonderful children, Andy, Michael, Allison, and Christina, for their patience and understanding.

Eugene C. Toy

Mastering the cognitive knowledge within a field such as psychiatry is a formidable task. It is even more difficult to draw on that knowledge, procure and filter through the clinical data, develop a differential diagnosis, and finally form a rational treatment plan. To gain these skills, the student often learns best by directly interviewing patients, guided and instructed by experienced teachers and inspired toward self-directed, diligent reading. Clearly, there is no replacement for education at the patient's side. Unfortunately, clinical situations usually do not encompass the breadth of the specialty. Perhaps the best alternative is to prepare carefully crafted cases designed to simulate the clinical approach and decision making. In an attempt to achieve this goal, we have constructed a collection of clinical vignettes to teach diagnostic or therapeutic approaches relevant to psychiatry. Most important, the explanations for the cases emphasize mechanisms and underlying principles rather than merely rote questions and answers.

This book is organized for versatility: to allow the student "in a rush" to read the scenarios quickly and check the corresponding answers, as well as to provide more detailed information for the student who wants thought-provoking explanations. The answers are arranged from simple to complex: a summary of the pertinent points, the bare answers, an analysis of the case, an approach to the topic, case correlations allowing for easily accessible comparisons among similar cases, and a comprehension test at the end for reinforcement and emphasis, and a list of resources for further reading. A listing of cases is included in Section III to aid students who desire to test their knowledge of a certain area or to review a topic, including the basic definitions. Several MCQs are included at the end of each scenario to reinforce concepts or introduce related topics, and a "Summary" review section allows readers to test their comprehensive knowledge of the material.

HOW TO GET THE MOST OUT OF THIS BOOK

Each case is designed to simulate a patient encounter by using open-ended questions. At times, the patient's complaint differs from the issue of greatest concern, and sometimes extraneous information is given. The answers are organized into four different parts.

PART I

1. A **Summary:** The salient aspects of the case are identified, filtering out extraneous information. The student should formulate a summary of the case before looking at the answers. A comparison with the summation appearing in the answer will help improve the student's ability to focus on the important data while appropriately discarding irrelevant information, a fundamental skill required in clinical problem solving.
2. A **Straightforward Answer** to each open-ended question.
3. An **Analysis of the Case** consisting of two parts:

a. **Objectives:** A listing of the two or three main principles that are crucial for a practitioner in treating the patient. Again, the student is challenged to make "educated guesses" about the objectives of the case on initial review of the case scenario, which helps sharpen his or her clinical and analytical skills.

b. **Considerations:** A discussion of the relevant points and a brief approach to the specific patient.

PART II

An Approach to the Disease Process consisting of two distinct parts:

a. **Definitions:** Terminology pertinent to the disease process.

b. **Clinical Approach:** A discussion of the approach to the clinical problem in general, including tables and figures.

c. **Case Correlation:** A handy reference to other cases in the book that may present similarly.

PART III

Comprehension Questions: Each case contains several multiple-choice questions that reinforce the material presented or introduce new and related concepts. Questions about material not found in the text are explained in the answers.

PART IV

Clinical Pearls: A listing of several clinically important points that are reiterated as a summation of the text and allow for easy review, such as before an examination, and is fully updated for *DSM-5*.

How to Approach Clinical Problems

Part 1. Approach to the Patient

It is a difficult transition from reading about patients with psychiatric disorders, and reading the diagnostic criteria from the *Diagnostic and Statistical Manual of Mental Disorders, 5th edition* (DSM-5), to actually developing a psychiatric diagnosis for a patient. It requires the physician to understand the criteria and be able to sensitively elicit symptoms and signs from patients, some of whom have difficulty providing a clear history. The clinician must then put together the pieces of a puzzle in order to find the single best diagnosis for the patient. This process can require further information from the patient's family, additions to the medical and psychiatric history, careful observation of the patient, a physical examination, selected laboratory tests, and other diagnostic studies. Establishing rapport and a good therapeutic alliance with patients is critical to both their diagnosis and their treatment.

CLINICAL PEARL

▶ A patient's history is the single most important tool in establishing a diagnosis. Developing good rapport with patients is key to effective interviewing and thorough data gathering. Both the content (what the patient *says and does not say*) and the manner in which it is expressed (body language, topic shifting) are important.

HISTORY

1. **Basic information:**
   a. Data such as name, age, marital status, gender, occupation, and language(s) spoken other than English if applicable is included while identifying information. Ethnic background and religion can also be included if they are pertinent.
   b. It is helpful to include the circumstances of the interview because they provide information about potentially important patient characteristics that can be relevant to the diagnosis, the prognosis, or compliance. Circumstances include where the interview was conducted (emergency setting, outpatient office, in leather restraints) and whether the episode reported was the first occurrence for the patient.
   c. Sources of the information obtained and their reliability should be mentioned at the beginning of the psychiatric history.

2. **Chief complaint:** The chief complaint should be written exactly as the patient states it, no matter how bizarre. For example, "The space aliens are attacking outside my garage so I came in for help." Putting the statement in quotes lets readers know it is a verbatim transcription of what the patient actually said, rather than the writer's words. Other individuals accompanying the patient can

then add their versions of why the patient is presenting currently, but the chief complaint stated in the patient's words helps with the initial formulation of a differential diagnosis. For example, if a patient comes in with a chief complaint about aliens, as just noted, one would immediately begin to consider diagnoses that have psychosis as a component and conduct the interview accordingly.

CLINICAL PEARLS

▶ When recording a chief complaint in the patient's own words, put quotation marks around the patient's statements to indicate that they are indeed the patient's words, not the writer's.

▶ A 45-year-old woman comes to the emergency department with the chief complaint, "I know everyone is going to try to hurt me."

---

3. **History of present illness (HPI):** This information is **probably the most useful part of the history** in terms of **making a psychiatric diagnosis.** It should contain a **comprehensive, chronological picture** of the circumstances leading up to the encounter with the physician. It is important to include details such as when symptoms first appeared, in what order, and at what level of severity, as this information is critical in making the correct diagnosis. Relationships between psychological stressors and the appearance of psychiatric and/or physical symptoms should be carefully outlined. Both pertinent positives (the patient complained of auditory hallucinations) and pertinent negatives (the patient reports no history of trauma) should be included in the HPI. In addition, details of the history such as the use of drugs or alcohol, which are normally listed in the social history, should be put in the HPI if they are thought to make a significant contribution to the presenting symptoms.

4. **Psychiatric history:** The patient's previous encounters with psychiatrists and other mental health therapists should be listed in reverse chronological order, with the most recent encounters listed first. Past psychiatric hospitalizations, the treatment received, and the length of stay should be recorded. Other details, like whether or not the patient has received psychotherapy, of what kind, and for how long, are also important. Any pharmacotherapy received by the patient should be recorded, and details such as dosage, response, length of time on the drug, and compliance with the medication should be included. Any treatments with electroconvulsive therapy (ECT) should be noted as well, including the number of sessions and the associated effects.

5. **Medical history:** Any medical illnesses should be listed in this category along with the date of diagnosis. Hospitalizations and surgeries should also be included with their dates. Episodes of **head trauma, seizures, neurologic illnesses** or **tumors**, and positive assays for **human immunodeficiency virus (HIV)** are all pertinent to the psychiatric history. If it is felt that some aspect of the

medical history may be directly pertinent to the current chief complaint, it should be mentioned in the HPI.

6. **Medications:** A list of medications including their doses and their duration of use should be obtained. All medications, including over-the-counter, herbal, and prescribed, are relevant and should be delineated.

7. **Allergies:** A list of agents causing allergic reactions, including medications and environmental agents (dust, henna, etc), should be obtained. For each, it is important to describe what reaction actually occurred, such as a skin rash or difficulty breathing. (Many patients who have a dystonic reaction to a medication consider it an allergy, although it is actually a side effect of the medication.)

8. **Family history:** A brief statement about the patient's family history of psychiatric as well as medical disorders should be included. Listing each family member, his or her age, and medical or psychiatric disorders is generally the easiest, clearest way to do this.

9. **Social history:**

   a. The **prenatal and perinatal history** of the patient is probably relevant for all young children brought to a psychiatrist. It can also be relevant in older children and/or adults if it involves birth defects or injuries.

   b. A **childhood history** is important when evaluating a child and can be important in evaluating an adult if it involves episodes of trauma, long-standing personal patterns, or problems with education. For a child, issues such as age of and/or difficulty in toilet training, behavioral problems, social relationships, cognitive and motor development, and emotional and physical problems should all be included.

   c. Occupational history, including military history.

   d. Marital and relationship history.

   e. Education history.

   f. Religion.

   g. Social history, including the nature of friendships and interests.

   h. Drug and alcohol history. Both the quantity of substance(s) used and the duration of their use should be documented.

   i. Current living situation.

10. **Review of systems:** A systematic review should be performed with emphasis on common side effects of medications and common symptoms that might be associated with the chief complaint. For example, patients taking typical antipsychotic agents (such as haloperidol) might be asked about dry mouth, dry eyes, constipation, and urinary hesitancy. Patients with presumed panic disorder might be questioned about cardiac symptoms such as palpitations and chest pain or neurologic symptoms such as numbness and tingling.

Mental Status Examination

The **mental status examination** comprises the **sum total** of the **physician's observations** of the patient at the time of the interview. Of note is that this examination can change from hour to hour, whereas the patient's history remains stable. The mental status examination includes impressions of the patient's **general appearance, mood, speech, actions, and thoughts.** Even a mute or uncooperative patient reveals a large amount of clinical information during the mental status examination.

> ## CLINICAL PEARL
>
> ▶ The mental status examination provides a snapshot of the patient's symptoms at the time of the interview. It can differ from the patient's history, which is what has happened to the patient **up until the time** of the interview. For example, if a patient has thought about suicide for the past 3 weeks but during the interview says that he or she is not feeling suicidal, his or her **history** is considered **positive for suicidal ideation** although the **thought content section** of the **mental status examination** is said to be **negative** for (current) suicidal ideation.

1. **General description:**
    a. **Appearance:** A description of the patient's overall appearance should be recorded, including posture, poise, grooming, hygiene, and clothing. Signs of anxiety and other mood states should also be noted, such as wringing of hands, tense posture, clenched fists, or a wrinkled forehead.
    b. **Behavior and psychomotor activity:** Any bizarre posturing, abnormal movements, agitation, rigidity, or other physical characteristics should be described.
    c. **Attitude toward examiner:** The patient's attitude should be noted using terms such as "friendly," "hostile," "evasive," "guarded," or any of a host of descriptive adjectives.

2. **Mood and affect:**
    a. **Mood:** The emotion (anger, depression, emptiness, guilt, etc.) that underlies a person's perception of the world. Although mood can often be inferred throughout the course of an interview, it is best to ask the patient directly, "How has your mood been?" Mood should be **quantified wherever possible**—a **scale from 1 to 10** is often used. For example, a person rates his or her depression as 3 on a scale of 1 to 10 where 10 is the happiest he or she has ever felt.
    b. **Affect:** The person's emotional responsiveness during the examination as inferred from his or her expressions and behavior. In addition to the affect noted, the **range (variation) of the affect** during the interview, as well as its **congruency** with (consistency with) the stated mood, should be noted.

A **labile affect** denotes a patient whose emotional responsiveness varies greatly (and often quickly) within the interview period. A **blunted** or **constricted** affect means that there is little variation in facial expression or use of hands; a **flat affect** is even further reduced in range.

3. **Speech:** The physical characteristics of the patient's speech should be described. Notations as to the **rate, tone, volume, and rhythm** should be made. Impairments of speech, such as stuttering, should also be noted.

4. **Perception:** Hallucinations and illusions reported by the patient should be listed. The sensory system involved (tactile, gustatory, auditory, visual, or olfactory) as well as the content of the hallucination (eg, "It smells like burning rubber," "I hear two voices calling me bad names.") Should be indicated. Of note is that whereas some clinicians use perception as a separate category, others combine this section with the thought content portion of the write-up/ presentation.

5. **Thought process:** Thought process refers to the *form* of thinking or *how* a patient thinks. It does not refer specifically to *what* a person thinks, which is more appropriate to the thought content. In order of most logical to least logical, thought process can be described as **logical/coherent, circumstantial, tangential, flight of ideas, loose associations, and word salad/incoherence.** Neologisms, punning, or thought blocking also should be mentioned here.

6. **Thought content:** The actual thought content section should include **delusions (fixed, false beliefs), paranoia (a form of delusion), preoccupations, obsessions and compulsions, phobias, ideas of reference, poverty of content, and suicidal and homicidal ideation.** Patients with suicidal or homicidal ideation should be asked whether, in addition to the presence of the ideation, they have a *plan* for carrying out the suicidal or homicidal act as well as about their *intent* to do so.

7. **Sensorium and cognition:** This portion of the mental status examination assesses **organic brain function, intelligence, capacity for abstract thought,** and **levels of insight and judgment.** The basic tests of sensorium and cognition are performed on every patient. Those whom the clinician suspects are suffering from an organic brain disorder can be tested with further cognitive tests beyond the scope of the basic mental status examination.

   a. **Consciousness:** Common descriptors of levels of consciousness include "alert," "somnolent," "stuporous," and "clouded consciousness."

   b. **Orientation and memory:** The classic test of orientation is to discern the patient's ability to locate himself or herself in relation to person, place, and/ or time. Any impairment usually occurs in this order as well (ie, a sense of time is usually impaired before a sense of place or person). Memory is divided into four areas: immediate, recent, recent past, and remote. **Immediate memory** is tested by asking a patient to **repeat numbers** after the examiner, in both forward and backward orders. **Recent memory** is tested by asking a patient **what he or she ate for dinner the previous night** and asking if he or she remembers the examiner's name from the beginning of the interview. **Recent past memory** is tested by asking about news items publicized in the past several months, and **remote memory** is assessed by asking patients about their childhood. Note that information must be verified to be sure of its accuracy because confabulation (making up false answers when memory is impaired) can occur.

c. **Concentration and attention: Subtracting serial 7s from 100** is a common way of testing concentration. Patients who are unable to do this because of educational deficiencies can be asked to subtract serial 3s from 100. Attention is tested by asking a patient to spell the word "world" forward and backward. The patient can also be asked to name five words that begin with a given letter.

d. **Reading and writing:** The patient should be instructed to read a given sentence and then do what the sentence asks, for example, "Turn this paper over when you have finished reading." The patient should also be asked to write a sentence. Examiners should be aware that illiteracy might impact a patient's ability to follow instructions during this part of the examination.

e. **Visuospatial ability:** The patient is typically asked to **copy the face of a clock** and fill in the numbers and hands so that the clock shows the correct time. Images with **interlocking shapes or angles** can also be used—the patient is asked to copy them.

f. **Abstract thought:** Abstract thinking is the ability to deal with concepts. Can patients distinguish the similarities and differences between two given objects? Can patients understand and articulate the meaning of simple proverbs? (Be aware that patients who are immigrants and/or have learned English as a second language can have problems with proverbs for this reason rather than because of a mental status disturbance.)

g. **Information and intelligence:** Answers to questions related to a general fund of knowledge (presidents of the United States, mayors of the city in which the mental status examination is conducted), vocabulary, and the ability to solve problems are all factored in together to come up with an estimate of intelligence. A patient's educational status should of course be taken into account as well.

h. **Judgment:** During the course of the interview, the examiner should be able to get a good idea of the patient's ability to understand the likely outcomes of his or her behavior and whether or not this behavior can be influenced by knowledge of these outcomes. Having the patient predict what he or she would do in an imaginary scenario can sometimes help with this assessment. For example, what would the patient do if he or she found a stamped envelope lying on the ground?

i. **Insight:** Insight is the degree to which a patient understands the nature and extent of his or her own illness. Patients can express a complete denial of their illnesses or progressive levels of insight into knowing that there is something wrong within them that needs to be addressed.

> CLINICAL PEARL

▶ Nearly the entire mental status examination can be performed by careful observation of the patient while obtaining a detailed, complete history. Only a few additional questions need to be addressed to the patient directly, for example, those regarding the presence of suicidal ideation and specific cognitive examination questions.

Physical Examination

The physical examination can be an important component of the assessment of a patient with a presumed psychiatric illness. Many physical illnesses masquerade as psychiatric disorders and vice versa. For example, a patient with **hypothyroidism** can first present to a psychiatrist with symptoms of **major depression.** Thus, an examiner should be alert to all of a patient's signs and symptoms, physical and mental, and be prepared to perform a physical examination, especially in an emergency department setting. Some patients can be too agitated or paranoid to undergo parts of the physical examination, but when possible, all elements should be completed.

1. **General appearance:** Cachectic versus well nourished, anxious versus calm, alert versus obtunded.

2. **Vital signs:** Temperature, blood pressure, heart rate, respiratory rate, and weight.

3. **Head and neck examination:** Evidence of trauma, tumors, facial edema, goiter (indicating hyper- or hypothyroidism), and carotid bruits should be sought. Cervical and supraclavicular nodes should be palpated.

4. **Breast examination:** Inspection for symmetry, skin or nipple retraction with the patient's hands on hips (to accentuate the pectoral muscles), and with arms raised. With the patient supine, the breasts should then be palpated systematically to assess for masses. The nipple should be examined for discharge, and the axillary and supraclavicular regions for adenopathy.

5. **Cardiac examination:** The point of maximal impulse should be ascertained, and the heart auscultated at the apex of the heart as well as at the base. Heart sounds, murmurs, and clicks should be characterized.

6. **Pulmonary examination:** The lung fields should be examined systematically and thoroughly. Wheezes, rales, rhonchi, and bronchial breath sounds should be recorded.

7. **Abdominal examination:** The abdomen should be inspected for scars, distension, masses or organomegaly (ie, spleen or liver), and discoloration. Auscultation of bowel sounds should be accomplished to identify normal versus high-pitched and hyperactive versus hypoactive sounds. The abdomen should be percussed for the presence of shifting dullness (indicating ascites), and palpated to assess liver span and the presence or absence of masses.

8. **Back and spine examination:** The back should be assessed for symmetry, tenderness, or masses. Costovertebral angle tenderness should be documented.

9. **Pelvic and/or rectal examination:** Although these examinations are not often done in the emergent setting of psychiatric illness, it is important to realize that many patients with a psychiatric illness do not see their physicians regularly and that these important preventive maintenance procedures are often neglected. Patients should be reminded of the need for these examinations.

10. **Extremities and skin:** The presence of tenderness, bruising, edema, and cyanosis should be recorded.

11. **Neurologic examination:** Patients require a thorough assessment, including evaluation of the cranial nerves, strength, sensation, gaits, and reflexes.

Laboratory Tests

Compared to other medical practitioners, psychiatrists depend more on the patient's signs and symptoms and the clinician's examination than on laboratory tests. There are no definitive assays for bipolar disorder, schizophrenia, or major depression. However, assays can be used to identify potential medical problems appearing as psychiatric disturbances, as well as to look for substances such as lysergic acid diethylamide (LSD) or cocaine in a patient's system. Laboratory tests are also useful in long-term monitoring of medications such as lithium and valproic acid.

I. Screening tests
   A. A complete blood count (CBC) to assess for anemia and thrombocytopenia
   B. Renal function tests
   C. Liver function tests
   D. Thyroid function tests
   E. Laboratory studies including determinations of chloride, sodium, potassium, bicarbonate, serum urea nitrogen, creatinine, and blood sugar levels
   F. Urine toxicology or serum toxicology tests when drug use is suspected

II. Tests related to psychotropic drugs
   A. **Lithium:** A white blood cell (WBC), serum electrolyte determination, **thyroid and renal function tests (specific gravity, blood urea nitrogen [BUN], and creatinine),** fasting blood glucose determination, **pregnancy test,** and an **electrocardiogram (ECG)** are recommended before treatment and yearly thereafter (every 6 months for thyroid stimulating hormone [TSH] and creatinine levels). **Lithium levels** should also be monitored at least every 3 months once the patient has been stabilized on the medication.
   B. **Clozapine:** Because of the risk of developing **agranulocytosis,** patients taking this medication should have their WBC and differential count measured

at the onset of treatment, weekly during treatment for the first 6 months, every other week during chronic treatment, and for 4 weeks after discontinuation of treatment.

C. **Tricyclic and tetracyclic antidepressants:** An **ECG** should be obtained before a patient begins treatment with these medications.

D. **Carbamazepine:** A pretreatment CBC should be obtained to assess for **agranulocytosis.** A CBC should be drawn every 2 weeks for the first 2 months of treatment, and thereafter, once every 3 months. Platelet, reticulocyte, and serum iron levels should also be determined and all these tests performed yearly thereafter. Liver function tests should be performed initially, every month for the first 2 months of treatment, and every 3 months thereafter. Carbamazepine levels should be monitored this often as well. Serum electrolytes and an ECG should be done before treatment and yearly thereafter as well.

E. **Valproate:** Valproate levels should be monitored every 6 to 12 months, along with liver function tests. Because this drug is teratogenic, pregnancy tests should be drawn before initiating this drug.

III. Psychometric testing

A. **Structured clinical diagnostic assessments**

1. Tests based on structured or semistructured interviews designed to produce numerical scores.

2. Scales useful in determining the severity of an illness and in monitoring the patient's recovery.

3. Examples: **Beck Rating Scale for Depression, Hamilton Anxiety Rating Scale, Brief Psychiatric Rating Scale,** and Structured Clinical Interview for DSM-5 Dissociative Disorders (SCID-5).

B. **Psychological testing of intelligence and personality**

1. Tests designed to measure aspects of the patient's intelligence, ability to process information, and personality.

2. Tests generally **administered by psychologists** trained to administer and interpret them.

3. Such tests play a relatively small role in the diagnosis of psychiatric illness: The psychiatric interview and other observable signs and symptoms play a much larger role. These tests are therefore reserved for special situations.

4. Objective tests generally consisting of pencil-and-paper examinations based on specific questions. They yield numerical scores and are statistically analyzed.

a. **Minnesota Multiphasic Personality Inventory:** This self-report inventory is widely used and has been thoroughly researched. It assesses personality using an objective approach.

b. **Projective tests:** These tests present stimuli that are not immediately obvious. The **ambiguity of the situation forces patients to project their**

own needs into the test situation. Therefore, there are no right or wrong answers.

    i. **Rorschach test:** This projective test is used to assess personality. A series of 10 inkblots are presented to the patient, and the psychologist keeps a verbatim record of the patient's responses to each one. The test brings the patient's thinking and association patterns into focus. In skilled hands, it is helpful in bringing out defense mechanisms, subtle thought disorders, and pertinent patient psychodynamics.

    ii. **Thematic Apperception Test (TAT):** This test also assesses personality but does so by presenting patients with selections from 30 pictures and 1 blank card. The patient is required to create a story about each picture presented. Generally, the TAT is most useful for investigating personal motivation (eg, why a patient does what he or she does) than it is in making a diagnosis.

    iii. **Sentence completion test:** A projective test in which the patient is given part of a sentence and asked to complete it. It taps the unconscious associations of the patient to locate areas of functioning in which the interviewer is interested, for example, "My greatest fear is...."

  c. **Intelligence tests:** These tests are used to establish the degree of mental retardation in situations where this is the question. The Wechsler Adult Intelligence Scale is the test most widely used in clinical practice today.

  d. **Neuropsychologic tests:** The aim of these tests is to compare the patient being tested with "normal" people of similar background and age. They are used to identify cognitive deficits, assess the toxic effects of substances, evaluate the effects of treatment, and identify learning disorders.

    i. **Wisconsin Card Sorting Test:** This test assesses abstract reasoning and flexibility in problem solving by asking the patient to sort a variety of cards according to principles established by the rater but not known to the sorter. Abnormal responses are seen in patients with damaged frontal lobes and in some patients with schizophrenia.

    ii. **Wechsler Memory Scale:** This is the most widely used battery of tests for adults. It tests rote memory, visual memory, orientation, and counting backward, among other dimensions. It is sensitive to amnestic conditions such as Korsakoff syndrome.

    iii. **Bender Visual-Motor Gestalt Test:** A test of visuomotor coordination. Patients are asked to copy nine separate designs onto unlined paper. They are then asked to reproduce the designs from memory. This test is used as a screening device for signs of organic dysfunction.

IV. Further diagnostic tests

    A. Additional psychiatric diagnostic interviews (eg, the Diagnostic Interview Schedule for Children)

    B. Interviews conducted by a social worker with family members, friends, or neighbors

    C. Electroencephalogram to rule in or rule out a seizure disorder

    D. Computed tomography scan to assess intracranial masses

    E. Magnetic resonance imaging to assess intracranial masses or any other neurologic abnormality

    F. Tests to confirm other medical conditions

Part 2. Approach to Clinical Problem-Solving

A clinician typically undertakes four distinct steps to solve most clinical problems in a systematic fashion:

1. Making a diagnosis

2. Assessing the severity of the disease

3. Rendering treatment based on the disease

4. Following the patient's response to the treatment

Making a Diagnosis

A diagnosis is made by careful evaluation of the database, analysis of the information, assessment of the risk factors, and development of a list of possibilities (the differential diagnosis). The process involves knowing which pieces of information are meaningful and which can be discarded. Experience and knowledge help the physician "key in" on the most important possibilities. A good clinician also knows how to ask the same question in several different ways and to use different terminology. For example, patients at times can deny having been treated for bipolar disorder but answer affirmatively when asked if they have been hospitalized for mania. A diagnosis can be reached by systematically reading about each possible disease. The patient's presentation is then matched up against each of the possibilities, and each disorder is moved higher up or lower down on the list as a potential etiology based on the prevalence of the disease, the patient's presentation, and other clues. The patient's risk factors can also influence the probability of a diagnosis.

    Usually, a long list of possible diagnoses can be pared down to the two or three most likely ones based on a careful delineation of the signs and symptoms displayed by the patient, as well as on the time course of the illness. For example, a patient with a history of depressive symptoms, including problems with concentration, sleep, appetite, *and* symptoms of psychosis that started *after* the mood disturbances may have major depression with psychotic features, whereas a patient with a psychosis that started *before* the mood symptoms may have schizoaffective disorder.

> CLINICAL PEARL
>
> ▶ The first step in clinical problem solving is **making a diagnosis.**

Assessing the Severity of the Disease

After ascertaining the diagnosis, the next step is to characterize the severity of the disease process; in other words, describe "how bad" it is. With a malignancy, this is done formally by staging the cancer. With some infections, such as syphilis, staging depends on the duration and extent of the infection and follows its natural history (ie, primary syphilis, secondary syphilis, latent period, and tertiary/neurosyphilis). Some major mental illnesses, such as schizophrenia, can be characterized as acute, chronic, or residual, whereas the same clinical picture, occurring with less than 6-month duration, is termed schizophreniform disorder. Other notations frequently used in describing psychiatric illnesses include "mild," "moderate," "severe," "in partial remission," and "in full remission."

> CLINICAL PEARL
>
> ▶ The second step in clinical problem solving is to **establish the severity or subcategory of the disease.** This categorization usually has prognostic or treatment significance.

Selecting Treatment Based on Disease

Many illnesses are stratified according to severity because prognosis and treatment often vary based on these factors. If neither the prognosis nor the treatment is influenced by the stage of the disease process, there is no reason to subcategorize a disease as mild or severe. For example, some patients with **suicidal ideation but no intent or plan** can be **treated as outpatients,** but other patients who report **intent and a specific plan must be immediately hospitalized** and even committed involuntarily if necessary.

> CLINICAL PEARL
>
> ▶ The third step in clinical problem solving requires that, for most conditions, **the treatment be tailored** to the extent or severity of the disease.

Following the Response to Treatment

The final step in the approach to disease is to follow the patient's response to the therapy. The measure of response should be recorded and monitored. Some responses are clinical, such as improvement (or lack of improvement) in the level of depression, anxiety, or paranoia. Obviously, the student must work on becoming skilled in eliciting the relevant data in an unbiased, standardized manner. Other responses can be followed by laboratory tests, such as a urine toxicology screening for a cocaine abuser or a determination of lithium level for a bipolar patient. The student must be prepared to know what to do if the measured marker does not respond according to what is expected. Is the next step to reconsider the diagnosis, to repeat the test, or to confront the patient about the findings?

CLINICAL PEARL

▶ The fourth step in clinical problem solving is to **monitor treatment response or efficacy,** which can be measured in different ways. It can be based on symptoms (the patient feels better) or on a laboratory or some other test (a urine toxicology screening).

Part 3. Approach to the *Diagnostic and Statistical Manual of Mental Disorders*

The *Diagnostic and Statistical Manual of Mental Disorders*, currently in its 5th edition, text revision (DSM-5), is published by the American Psychiatric Association. It is the official psychiatric coding system used in the United States. The DSM-5 describes mental disorders and only rarely attempts to account for how these disturbances come about. Specified diagnostic criteria are presented for each disorder and include a list of features that must be present for the diagnosis to be made. The DSM-5 also systematically discusses each disorder in terms of its associated descriptors such as age, gender, prevalence, incidence, and risk; course; complications; predisposing factors; familial pattern; and differential diagnosis.

The DSM-5 **no longer** uses a five-axis system that evaluates patients along several dimensions, as was done in the previous DSM-IV-TR. In order to help readers make the change to DSM-5, a brief discussion of the DSM-IV-TR axes will be given, immediately followed by a comparison to the new DSM-5 methodology.

In *DSM-IV-TR*, Axes I and II made up the entire classification of mental disorders. The five-axis diagnosis usually appeared at the end of a write-up in the assessment section.

Axis I: Clinical disorders and other disorders that were the focus of clinical attention such as schizophrenia, major depression.

Axis II: Personality disorders and mental retardation only.

Axis III: Physical disorders and other general medical conditions. The physical condition could be causing the psychiatric one (eg, delirium, coded on axis I, caused by renal failure, coded on axis III), be the result of a mental disorder (eg, alcoholic cirrhosis, coded on axis III, secondary to alcohol dependence, coded on axis I), or be unrelated to the mental disorder (eg, chronic diabetes mellitus).

DSM-5 changes: DSM-5 has gone to a nonaxial documentation of diagnosis (formerly Axes I, II, and III). This is in keeping with the idea that mental disorders are related to physical or biological factors or processes, and that general medical conditions are related to behavioral and/or psychosocial factors or processes. In the documentation of mental disorders, physicians should now document other pertinent medical disorders as part of the diagnosis too. In DSM-5, the new notations of diagnosis (medical and psychiatric), with separate notations for psychosocial and contextual factors, and for disability (functioning), should all be included at the end of a write-up in the assessment section.

Axis IV: This axis was used to code the **psychosocial problems** contributing to the patient's psychiatric problem. Information about these stressors can be helpful when it is time to develop treatment plans for the patient. Problems could include those involving the primary support group, educational problems, job problems, housing problems, economic problems, problems with access to health care, or problems related to the legal system/crime.

DSM-5 changes: DSM-5 now recommends that a selected set of the ICD-9-CM V codes and the new Z codes contained in ICD-10-CM be used to document psychosocial and environmental problems that may affect the patient's diagnosis, treatment, and prognosis. (Axis IV will no longer be used per se, though the important information that it used to convey will be kept as above.)

Axis V: This axis was used to provide a **global assessment of functioning** (GAF). The scale was based on a continuum of health and illness, using a 100-point scale on which 100 was the highest level of functioning. People who had high GAF values before an episode of illness often had a better prognosis than those whose functioning was at a lower-level premorbidly.

DSM-5 changes: DSM-5 recommends that the GAF be dropped, because of questionable psychometrics and a general lack of clarity. Instead it is suggested that clinicians use the WHO Disability Assessment Schedule (WHODAS) to provide a global measure of disability.

Part 4. Approach to Reading

The clinical problem-oriented approach to reading is different from the classic "systematic" researching of a disease. Patients rarely present with symptoms that permit a clear diagnosis; hence, the student must become skilled in applying textbook information in the clinical setting. Furthermore, a reader retains more information when reading with a purpose. In other words, the student should read with the goal of answering specific questions. There are several fundamental questions that facilitate **clinical thinking:**

1. What is the most likely diagnosis?

2. What should the next step be?

3. What is the most likely mechanism for this process?

4. What are the risk factors for this condition?

5. What complications are associated with this disease process?

6. What is the best therapy?

7. How can you confirm the diagnosis?

Note that Questions 3 and 4 are probably used less in the field of psychiatry than in other specialties, such as medicine, where the pathophysiology and risk factors of a particular disease process are known. Likewise, confirmation of a diagnosis (Question 7) is less often made by further laboratory tests or other diagnostic studies but can be achieved by carefully obtaining additional history from family, colleagues, and so on. The preceding questions should, however, be kept in mind for all patients.

CLINICAL PEARL

> ▶ Reading with the purpose of answering the seven fundamental clinical questions improves retention of information and facilitates the application of book knowledge to clinical knowledge.

What is the Most Likely Diagnosis?

The method of establishing a diagnosis was covered in the previous section. One way to attack this problem is to develop standard "approaches" to common clinical situations. It is helpful to understand the most common presentation of a variety of illnesses, for example, a common presentation of major depression. (Clinical Pearls appear at the end of each case.)

The clinical scenario might be the following:

A 36-year-old woman presents to her physician with the chief complaint of a depressed mood and difficulty sleeping. What is the most likely diagnosis?

With no other information to go on, the student notes the depressed mood and the vegetative symptom of insomnia. Using the "common presentation" information, the student might make an educated guess that the patient has a **major depressive disorder.**

However, what if the scenario also includes the following?

She states that she has been depressed and has had trouble sleeping since she was raped 2 weeks ago.

Then the student would use the clinical pearl: A diagnosis of acute stress disorder should be considered in a patient with a depressed mood, insomnia, and a history of recent trauma.

CLINICAL PEARLS

▶ A common presentation of major depression is depressed mood and the vegetative symptom of insomnia. These symptoms, however, are common in instances of trauma and bereavement as well, and so these details must be investigated in reference to the patient.

▶ If mood changes and insomnia are secondary to a recent emotional and/ or physical trauma, the clinician should consider a diagnosis of acute stress disorder.

What Should the Next Step Be?

This question is difficult because *the next step* has many possibilities: The answer can be to obtain more diagnostic information, rate the severity of the illness, or introduce therapy. It is often a more challenging question than what is the most likely diagnosis because there can be insufficient information to make a diagnosis and the next step can be to pursue more diagnostic information. Another possibility is that there is enough information for a probable diagnosis and that the next step is to assess the severity of the disease. Finally, the most appropriate answer can be to start treatment. Hence, based on clinical data, a judgment needs to be rendered regarding how far along one is in the following process:

(1) **Make a diagnosis** → (2) **Stage the severity of the disease** → (3) **Treat based on the severity of the disease** → (4) **Follow the response**

Frequently, students are taught to "regurgitate" information that someone has written about a particular disease but are not skilled in describing the next step. This ability is learned optimally at the bedside, in a supportive environment, with freedom to make educated guesses, and with constructive feedback. A sample scenario describes a student's thought process as follows:

1. **Make a diagnosis:** "Based on the information I have, I believe that Ms Smith has major depression because she has a depressed mood, problems with concentration, anhedonia, insomnia, loss of appetite, anergia, and an unintentional weight loss of 10 lb in 3 weeks."

2. **Stage the severity of the disease:** "I don't believe that this is severe disease because the patient does not have suicidal ideation or any psychotic symptoms. I don't think the patient needs to be hospitalized at this time either."

3. **Treat based on the severity of the disease:** "Therefore, my next step is to treat her with a selective serotonin reuptake inhibitor (SSRI) such as paroxetine."

4. **Follow the response:** "I want to follow the treatment by assessing her depressed mood (I will ask her to rate her mood on a scale of 1 to 10 weekly),

her insomnia (I will ask her to keep a sleep log), and her appetite (I will weigh her weekly)."

In a similar case, when the clinical presentation is unclear, perhaps the best next step should be diagnostic in nature, such as a thyroid function test to rule out hypothyroidism.

> ### CLINICAL PEARL
>
> ▶ Usually, the vague query, "What is the next step?" is the most difficult question because the answer can be diagnostic, involve staging, or be therapeutic.

What is the Likely Mechanism for this Process?

This question goes further than making the diagnosis and also requires the student to understand the underlying mechanism of the process. For example, a clinical scenario can describe a 26-year-old man who develops a sudden onset of blindness 3 days after being told of his mother's death. The student must first diagnose a conversion disorder, which can occur after an emotionally traumatic event, once physical explanations for blindness have been ruled out. Then the student must understand that there is a psychodynamic explanation for the particular nature of the symptoms as they have arisen. The mechanism for the conversion disorder, blindness in this scenario, is the patient's fear (and guilt) about never "seeing" his mother again. Although many mechanisms of disease are not well understood in psychiatry at the present time, it is anticipated that they will be further elucidated as the fields of neuropsychiatry and neuroimaging continue to grow.

What are the Risk Factors for this Process?

Understanding the risk factors helps a practitioner establish a diagnosis and determine how to interpret tests. For example, understanding the risk factor analysis can help in treating a 56-year-old man who presents to a physician with a chief complaint of loss of memory. If the man does not have a family history of (and thus a risk for) Huntington chorea, an autosomally transmitted disease, the workup for memory loss would not likely include an examination of his genotype. Thus, the presence of risk factors helps categorize the likelihood of a disease process.

> ### CLINICAL PEARL
>
> ▶ When patients are at high risk for a disease based on risk factors, additional specific testing can be indicated.

What are the Complications of this Process?

Clinicians must be cognizant of the complications of a disease so that they understand how to follow and monitor the patient. Sometimes the student has to make a diagnosis from clinical clues and then apply the knowledge of the consequences of the pathologic process. For example, a woman who presents with a depressed mood, anhedonia, anergia, loss of concentration, insomnia, and weight loss is first diagnosed as having major depression. A complication of this process includes psychosis or suicidal ideation. Therefore, understanding the types of consequences helps the clinician to become aware of the dangers to the patient. Not recognizing these possibilities might lead the clinician to miss asking about psychotic symptoms (and treating them) or to overlook a potentially fatal suicidal ideation.

What is the Best Therapy?

To answer this question, the clinician needs to make the correct diagnosis, assess the severity of the condition, and weigh the situation to determine the appropriate intervention. For the student, knowing exact doses is not as important as understanding the best medication, route of delivery, mechanism of action, and possible complications. It is important for the student to be able to verbalize the diagnosis and the rationale for the therapy. A common error is for a student to *jump to a treatment* by making a random guess; as a result, he or she receives *correct or incorrect* feedback. In fact, the student's guess can be correct, but for the wrong reason; conversely, the answer can be a reasonable one with only one small error in thinking but can simply be labeled "wrong." Instead, the student should verbalize the steps so that feedback can be given at every reasoning point.

For example, if the question is what is the best therapy for a 24-year-old woman with an elated mood, lack of a need for sleep, excessive buying behavior, hypersexuality, and psychomotor agitation, the incorrect manner of responding is for the student to blurt out "a mood stabilizer." Rather, the student's reasoning should resemble the following: "The most common cause of these kinds of symptoms is mania, which would make the diagnosis bipolar disorder. There was no mention of a general medical condition (such as hyperthyroidism) or a substance abuse problem (such as cocaine use) that would account for these symptoms. Therefore, the best treatment for this patient with probable bipolar disorder would be lithium or valproic acid (after the final diagnosis is made)."

CLINICAL PEARL

▶ Therapy should be logically based on the severity of disease. There is no need to hospitalize all patients with major depression, but it can be lifesaving to do so if suicidal ideation with intent and plan is present.

How Can You Confirm the Diagnosis?

In the previous scenario, the 24-year-old woman is likely to have bipolar disorder, manic phase. Confirmation can be achieved by obtaining an additional history of manic or depressive episodes from the patient and/or from family members and friends who have observed her behavior over a period of time. Further information about the presence of other symptoms common in mania can also be helpful, as is ruling out any general medical conditions or substance abuse problems. The student should strive to know the limitations of various diagnostic tests and the manifestations of disease.

Summary

1. There is no replacement for a meticulously constructed history and physical examination.

2. There are four steps in the clinical approach to a patient: making a diagnosis, assessing the severity of the disease, treating based on the severity of the disease, and following the response to treatment.

3. There are seven questions that help bridge the gap between the textbook and the clinical arena.

4. The DSM-5 has moved to a nonaxial system to delineate patient presentations/disorders. These include the diagnosis (formerly Axes I, II, and III), an assessment of psychosocial and environmental/contextual stressors (formerly Axis IV), and a global assessment of disability (formerly Axis V) using the WHODAS.

REFERENCES

American Psychiatric Association. *Diagnostic and Statistical Manual of Mental Disorders.* 5th ed. Washington, DC: American Psychiatric Publishing; 2013.

Black BW, Andreasen NC. *Introductory Textbook of Psychiatry.* 6th ed. Washington, DC: American Psychiatric Publishing; 2014:164-170.

Hales RE, Yudofsky SC, Roberts LW. *The American Psychiatric Publishing Textbook of Psychiatry.* 6th ed. Washington, DC: American Psychiatric Publishing; 2014.

Higgins ES, George MS. *The Neuroscience of Clinical Psychiatry.* 2nd ed. Philadelphia, PA: Lippincott Williams & Wilkins; 2013.

Sadock BJ, Sadock VA, Ruiz P. *Kaplan and Sadock's Synopsis of Psychiatry: Behavioral Sciences/Clinical Psychiatry.* 11th ed. Baltimore, MD: Lippincott Williams & Wilkins; 2014.

Stern TA, Herman JB, Gorrindo T. *Massachusetts General Hospital Psychiatry.* 3rd ed. Boston, MA: MGH Psychiatry Academy Publishing; 2012.

Psychiatric Therapeutics

Part 1. Psychotherapy

Although there are literally hundreds of types of psychotherapy, psychological or "talking therapy" treatments fall into four broad categories: (1) individual psychotherapy, (2) behavior modification, (3) cognitive therapies, and (4) social therapies.

I. **Individual psychotherapy:** Varies according to the time frame used (psychotherapy can be either brief or protracted). It can be *supportive, directive, and reality-oriented* versus *expressive, exploratory, and oriented toward a discussion of unconscious material.*

 A. **Supportive psychotherapy**

  1. Goals: Form a **close alliance with the patient,** help the patient **define current problems,** consider and implement possible problem solutions, and "shore up" the patient's current ego defenses.

  2. Indicated in the treatment of **adjustment disorders, acute emotional crises,** and when a long-lasting "cure" is not expected but **improved functioning** is hoped for (as in the case of chronic schizophrenia).

 B. **Insight-oriented psychotherapy**

  1. Goals: Form an alliance with the patient, recognize **transference/countertransference feelings** as they occur, and **uncover unconscious wishes and defenses** that have caused the patient to behave in a maladaptive manner.

  2. Indicated in the treatment of **anxiety, depression in all of its forms, somatoform and dissociative disorders, personality disorders, neuroses, and trauma.** It should be noted that although psychotherapy can be indicated for all these disorders, the degrees of patient insight and motivation for undergoing treatment are critical to its success.

II. **Behavior modification/therapy:** Includes a group of loosely related therapies that work according to the principles of learning. A short list of examples of these therapies follows:

 A. **Systematic desensitization:** Exposing the patient to increasingly anxiety-provoking stimuli and at the same time teaching him or her to relax. This therapy is used in the treatment of phobias and in preventing compulsions.

 B. **Substitution:** Replacing an undesirable behavior (smoking) with a desirable one (chewing gum).

 C. **Hypnosis:** Induction of an advanced state of relaxation or a "trance" during which suggestions can be made. Hypnosis works in selected patients in the management of pain, the resolution of conversion disorders, and relaxation training.

III. **Cognitive therapy**

 A. Focuses on the cognitive responses that are the primary targets for intervention.

B. Used in changing maladaptive behavior occurring as a result of cognitive responses.

C. The most common use for this form of therapy is in the **treatment of major depression,** where the **self-defeating attitudes (called automatic thoughts)** that are so common are identified, challenged, and **replaced with more realistic thoughts.**

IV. **Social therapies:** These therapies use the principles of supportive and individual or **marital therapy,** but occur in groups of similar patients, a family, or a couple.

Part 2. Psychopharmacotherapy

Medications can be subdivided into **antidepressants,** including miscellaneous and mood-stabilizing agents, **antipsychotic** medications, and **anxiolytic/hypnotic** medications. Tables II–1 through II–9 summarize the characteristics of these agents. Many of these medications affect neurotransmitters (Figure II–1). The main neurotransmitters are monoamines (norepinephrine, dopamine, serotonin, acetylcholine, histamine), amino acids (gamma-aminobutyric acid [GABA]), and glutamic acid.

I. **Antidepressants:** Antidepressants can be placed in four main categories.

A. **Tricyclics and heterocyclics** once represented the first line of treatment. These drugs work by **increasing the level of monoamines in the synapse by reducing the reuptake of norepinephrine and serotonin.** Although they are quite effective, they are dangerous in overdose because they have a rather narrow therapeutic to toxic range, **causing fatal cardiac arrhythmias (Table II–1).**

B. **Selective serotonin reuptake inhibitors (SSRIs) and selective serotonin-norepinephrine reuptake inhibitors (SSNRIs) are the most commonly used antidepressants today. Major side effects include gastrointestinal disturbances and sexual dysfunction (Table II–2).**

C. **Monoamine oxidase inhibitors (MAOIs) are not commonly used** because a **tyramine-free diet (no red wine or aged cheese) must be followed or a hypertensive crisis can result.** These agents can be more helpful in depression with atypical features (overeating, oversleeping, irritability) (Table II–3).

D. Miscellaneous medications (Table II–4).

II. **Mood stabilizers:** These medications are used to treat mania and include agents such as lithium, valproic acid, and carbamazepine. **Lithium** has many adverse effects including **tremor, polyuria/diabetes insipidus, acne, hypothyroidism, cardiac dysrhythmias, weight gain, edema, and leukocytosis.** Lithium is cleared through the **kidneys** and must be used carefully in older patients and in those with renal insufficiency. **Valproic acid is teratogenic** and must be used with caution in women of childbearing age (Table II–5).

Table II–1 • TRICYCLIC/TETRACYCLIC MEDICATIONS				
Name[a]	Class of Compound[b]	Side Effects	Comments	Half-Life (h)
All tricyclics and tetracyclics		Anticholinergic: dry mouth, blurry vision, urinary retention, constipation, sedation, orthostatic hypotension (alpha-adrenergic blockade), tachycardia, prolongation of QT interval, weight gain (antihistamine-1 effect)	Concern about a risk of falling in elderly patients	6-30
Amitriptyline (Elavil)	Tertiary amine		Highly anticholinergic, very sedating	20
Doxepin (Adapin, Sinequan, Silenor)	Tertiary amine		Highly anticholinergic, very sedating	16
Imipramine (Tofranil)	Tertiary amine		Highly anticholinergic	20
Clomipramine (Anafranil)	Tertiary amine		Highly anticholinergic, very sedating obsessive-compulsive disorder (OCD) responds specifically to clomipramine, may also be useful in those with depression with marked obsessive features	21
Trimipramine (Surmontil)	Tertiary amine		Highly anticholinergic, very sedating	22
Desipramine (Norpramin)	Secondary amine		Least anticholinergic, not sedating	24
Nortriptyline (Pamelor, Aventyl)	Secondary amine		Less anticholinergic	12
Protriptyline (Vivactil)	Secondary amine	Psychomotor stimulation	Less anticholinergic, not sedating	6
Amoxapine (Asendin, Asendas)	Tetracyclic	**May cause extrapyramidal syndrome and NMS (metabolite of loxapine)**	Less anticholinergic	30

[a]Proprietary names are given in parentheses.
[b]Secondary amines and tetracyclic compounds tend to have fewer anticholinergic and sedating effects.

Table II–2 • SELECTIVE SEROTONIN REUPTAKE INHIBITORS

Name	Half-Life	Side Effects	Comments
Nearly all selective serotonin reuptake inhibitors (SSRIs) and selective serotonin-norepinephrine reuptake inhibitors (SSNRIs)		Agitation, akathisia, anxiety, panic, insomnia, diarrhea, gastrointestinal distress, headache, sexual dysfunction: delayed ejaculation or impotence (male); anorgasmia (female); **may increase risk of suicidal thoughts and behaviors in children, adolescents, and young adults**	**To avoid fatal serotonin syndrome,[b] no SSRI or SSNRI should be combined with a monoamine oxidase inhibitor (MAOI), and an SSRI should be discontinued at least 5 wk before starting an MAOI**
Fluoxetine (Prozac)	1-3 d		SSRI; used in the treatment of obsessive-compulsive disorder (OCD)
Sertraline (Zoloft)	25 h		SSRI; cause **diarrhea** more commonly than others; used in the treatment of OCD
Paroxetine (Paxil)	24 h		SSRI; mildly **anticholinergic;** used in the treatment of OCD
Fluvoxamine (Luvox)	15 h		SSRI; **nausea and vomiting more common;** used in the treatment of OCD
Citalopram (Celexa)	35 h		SSRI; **possibly fewer sexual side effects**
Escitalopram (Lexapro)	27-30 h		SSRI
Venlafaxine (Effexor)	3.5 h (active metabolite 9 h)	Anxiety, may increase blood pressure at higher doses, headache, insomnia, sweating	SNRI; also used to treat generalized anxiety disorder (GAD) and social anxiety
Levomilnacipran (Fetzima)	12 h	Blood pressure increases, nausea/vomiting, sweating, constipation, erectile dysfunction	SNRI
Desvenlafaxine (Pristiq)	24 h		SNRI
Duloxetine (Cymbalta)	12 h		SSNRI; also used for the treatment of GAD and painful diabetic neuropathy.

[a]*Proprietary names are given in parentheses.*
[b]*Serotonin syndrome is characterized by (in order of appearance) diarrhea, restlessness, extreme agitation, hyperreflexia, autonomic instability, myoclonus, seizures, hyperthermia, rigidity, delirium, coma, and death.*

Table II–3 • MONOAMINE OXIDASE INHIBITORS

Name[a]	Half-Life (h)	Side Effects	Comments
Phenelzine (Nardil)	4-5	Orthostatic hypotension, somnolence, weight gain	**All cheese, fermented or aged foods, wine, and liver should be avoided. Should not be coadministered with SSRIs;** should never be coadministered with drugs that increase intrasynaptic levels of amine neurotransmitters.
Isocarboxazid (Marplan)	2.5	Orthostatic hypotension, somnolence, weight gain	**All cheese, fermented or aged foods, wine, and liver should be avoided. Should not be coadministered with SSRIs;** should never be coadministered with drugs that increase intrasynaptic levels of amine neurotransmitters.
Selegiline (Eldepryl) (Emsam)	2	Orthostatic hypotension, somnolence, weight gain, irritation at site of patch	**All cheese, fermented or aged foods, wine, and liver should be avoided. Should not be coadministered with SSRIs;** should never be coadministered with drugs that increase intrasynaptic levels of amine neurotransmitters. A transdermal delivery system is available for use in depression; also used to treat parkinsonism.
Tranylcypromine (Parnate)	2-3	Orthostatic hypotension, somnolence, weight gain	**All cheese, fermented or aged foods, wine, and liver should be avoided. Should never be coadministered with SSRIs;** should never be coadministered with drugs that increase intrasynaptic levels of amine neurotransmitters.

[a]*Proprietary names are given in parentheses.*

Table II–4 • MISCELLANEOUS ANTIDEPRESSANT MEDICATIONS				
Name[a]	Mechanism of Action	Half-Life (h)	Side Effects	Comments
Nefazodone (Serzone)	Serotonin-2 antagonist and serotonin reuptake inhibitor	2-4	Sedation, hepatotoxicity	Decreased sexual dysfunction occurs with this drug
Trazodone (Desyrel)	Serotonin-2 antagonist and serotonin reuptake inhibitor	10-15	**Priapism: prolonged erection may lead to impotence,** ortho-static hypotension, sedation	Can be used in lower doses to manage sleep problems, should be avoided with mono-amine oxidase inhibitors
Mirtazapine (Remeron)	Noradrenergic and specific serotonin antagonist	20-40	Weight gain, sedation	No interference with sexual function, no nausea or diarrhea
Bupropion (Wellbutrin)	Norepinephrine and dopamine reuptake inhibitor	14	Gastrointestinal: nausea, anorexia; risk of seizures at higher doses, less sexual dysfunction	Used for smoking cessa-tion; contraindicated in patients with an eating disorder or a seizure disorder
Vortioxetine (Brintellix)	Serotonin modula-tor and stimulator	66	Constipation, nausea/vomiting, diarrhea, sexual dysfunction	
Vilazodone (Viibryd)	5-HT_{1A} receptor partial agonist, serotonergic reup-take inhibitor	25	Diarrhea, nausea, headache	Also used for general-ized anxiety disorder and obsessive compul-sive disorder

[a]*Proprietary names are given in parentheses.*

III. **Antipsychotic agents**

  A. **First-generation antipsychotics (typical antipsychotics)**

  1. These medications work by **blocking central dopamine receptors.** They are most effective in reducing the positive symptoms of schizophrenia, including hallucinations and delusions.

  2. Side effects (Table II–6) include the following:

   a. **Central nervous system effects:**

    i. **Extrapyramidal symptoms (EPS):** Parkinsonian syndrome, acute dystonias, and akathisia.

    ii. **Tardive dyskinesias: Late onset** of choreiform and athetoid movements of the trunk, extremities, or mouth.

    iii. **Sedation.**

    iv. **Neuroleptic malignant syndrome (NMS):** Can occur at any time with an antipsychotic agent, typically movement disorder

Table II-5 • MOOD STABILIZERS

Name[a]	Mechanism of Action	Half-Life (h)	Side Effects	Testing	Comments
Lithium	Inhibits adenylate cyclase enzyme	24	Nausea, tremor, hypothyroidism, cardiac dysrhythmias, diarrhea. **Diabetes insipidus:** thirst, urination, weight gain, acne. At toxic levels, significant alterations in consciousness, seizures, coma, and death may occur.	A white blood cell (WBC), serum electrolyte determination, **thyroid and renal function tests (specific gravity, blood urea nitrogen [BUN], and creatinine)**, fasting blood glucose determination, **pregnancy test,** and an **electrocardiogram (ECG)** are recommended before treatment and yearly thereafter (every 6 mo for a thyroid-stimulating hormone [TSH] and creatinine). **Lithium levels** should also be monitored at least every 3 mo once the patient has been stabilized on the medication.	Propranolol may help with tremor; benign increase in WBC count seen
Valproic acid, valproate (Depakene)	Opens chloride channels, unknown	8	Thrombocytopenia, pancreatitis, weight gain, hair loss, gastrointestinal distress, cognitive dulling, **neural tube defects in pregnancy.**	Complete blood count (CBC), liver function tests, pancreatic enzyme levels, serum human chorionic gonadotropin (hCG) level in childbearing women.	
Divalproex Sodium (Depakote)	Opens chloride channels, unknown	6-16	Thrombocytopenia, pancreatitis, weight gain, hair loss, gastrointestinal distress, cognitive dulling, **neural tube defects in pregnancy.**	CBC, liver function tests, pancreatic enzyme levels, serum hCG level in childbearing women.	

Drug	Mechanism	Level	Side effects	Monitoring	Comments
Carbamazepine (Tegretol)	Inhibits kindling, inhibits repetitive firing of action potentials by inactivating sodium channels	18-55	Nausea, vomiting, slurred speech, dizziness, drowsiness, low WBC count, high liver function tests, cognitive slowing, may cause craniofacial defects in newborn.	A pretreatment CBC should be obtained to assess for **agranulocytosis**. A CBC should be drawn every 2 wk for the first 2 mo of treatment, and thereafter, once every 3 mo. Platelet, reticulocyte, and serum iron levels should also be determined and all these tests performed yearly thereafter. Liver function tests should be performed initially, every month for the first 2 mo of treatment, and every 3 mo thereafter. Carbamazepine levels should be monitored this often as well. Serum electrolytes and an ECG should be done before treatment and yearly thereafter as well.	Potent inducer of P450 system
Lamotrigine (Lamictal)		15	Leukopenia, rash, hepatic failure nausea, vomiting, diarrhea, somnolence, dizziness.	CBC with platelet count every 6-12 mo.	Alternative choice, may have acute antidepressant effect; dose must be increased slowly to avoid rash
Gabapentin (Neurontin)		5-9	Somnolence, dizziness, ataxia, fatigue, leukopenia, weight gain.		No drug interactions, rash can be fatal
Topiramate (Topamax)	Exact mechanism is unknown	19-23	Psychomotor slowing, memory problems, fatigue.		Many drug-drug interactions

Table II–6 • FIRST-GENERATION ANTIPSYCHOTIC AGENTS			
Name[a]	Half-Life (h)	Potency	Comments
Chlorpromazine (Thorazine)	24	Low	Sedation and orthostatic hypotension are very common
Haloperidol (Haldol)	24	High	**Extrapyramidal syndrome very common;** available in a long-acting intramuscular depot
Thioridazine (Mellaril)	24	Low	Higher incidence of cardiac disturbances, **retinitis pigmentosa**
Mesoridazine (Serentil)	30	Low	Cardiac arrhythmias (torsade de pointes)
Molindone (Lidone, Moban)	12	Medium	
Fluphenazine (Prolixin)	18	High	Available in a long-acting intramuscular depot
Trifluoperazine (Stelazine)	18	High	
Thiothixene (Navane)	34	High	
Perphenazine (Etrafon, Trilafon)	12	High	
Loxapine (Loxitane)	8	Medium	
Pimozide (Orap)	55	High	

[a]*Proprietary names are given in parentheses.*

(muscle rigidity, dystonia, agitation) and autonomic symptoms (high fever, sweating, tachycardia, hypertension). Treatment is mostly supportive (hydration and cooling) but can include medication with dantrolene and/or bromocriptine.

b. **Anticholinergic effects.**

c. **Cardiovascular effects.**

   i. **Alpha-adrenergic blockade,** which causes **orthostatic hypotension.**

   ii. **Cardiac rhythm disturbances,** especially prolongation of the **QT interval.**

d. **Endocrine effects:** Decreasing the amount of dopamine in the pituitary gland leads to increased **prolactin levels,** which can cause gynecomastia and **galactorrhea** as well as sexual dysfunction.

e. **Weight gain.**

B. **Second-generation antipsychotics (atypical antipsychotics):** These medications are more commonly used than first-generation antipsychotics because they are **less likely to produce EPS, tardive dyskinesia, and NMS.** However, many have significant side effects (Table II–7) of their own that limit their use (eg, **clozapine can cause fatal agranulocytosis**). There is also new concern that the atypical antipsychotics can increase the risk of Type 2 diabetes. The two of most concern are Zyprexa (olanzapine) and Clozaril (clozapine).

Table II-7 • SECOND-GENERATION ANTIPSYCHOTIC AGENTS

Name[a]	Site of Action	Half-Life (h)	Side Effects	Comments
Clozapine (Clozaril)	Serotonin-dopamine antagonist	5-15	**Agranulocytosis,** anticholinergic side effects, weight gain, sedation, neuroleptic malignant syndrome	Complete blood count and differential counts required weekly or for the first 6 mo and biweekly thereafter
Risperidone (Risperdal)	Serotonin-dopamine antagonist	3 in fast metabolizers, 120 in poor metabolizers	Extrapyramidal withdrawal syndrome in high doses, postural hypotension, increased prolactin; weight gain, sedation, decreased concentration	Present in breast milk
Olanzapine (Zyprexa)	Serotonin-dopamine antagonist	31	Increased prolactin, orthostatic hypotension, anticholinergic side effects, weight gain, **somnolence**	Alanine amino-transferase levels as drug affects the liver
Quetiapine (Seroquel)	Serotonin-dopamine antagonist	7	Orthostatic hypotension, somnolence, transient increase in weight	Slit lamp eye examination at baseline and every 6 mo for those at risk for developing cataracts
Ziprasidone (Geodon, Zeldox)	Serotonin-dopamine antagonist	7	Dose-related **QT interval prolongation,** postural hypotension, sedation	Present in breast milk; baseline potassium and magnesium measurements
Aripiprazole (Abilify)	Partial agonist at dopamine and serotonin-1A receptors and antagonist at postsynaptic serotonin-2A receptors	75	Headache, nausea, anxiety, insomnia, somnolence	Nonsedating; no increased risk of weight gain or diabetes
Lurasidone (Latuda)	Mechanism of action unknown; central dopamine Type 2 (D) and serotonin Type 2 (5HT$_{2A}$) receptor antagonism?	18	Nausea/vomiting, dyspepsia, somnolence	Increased mortality in elderly patients with dementia-related psychosis
Paliperidone (Invega)	Dopamine antagonist	23	Headache, tachycardia, somnolence	Increased mortality in elderly with dementia-related psychosis; comes in 1 mo injectable form

[a]Proprietary names are given in parentheses.

Table II–8 • BENZODIAZEPINES

Name	Proprietary Name	Half-Life (Including Metabolites) (h)
Diazepam	Valium	20-70
Lorazepam	Ativan	10-70
Clonazepam	Klonopin	19-50
Alprazolam	Xanax	8-15
Chlordiazepoxide	Librium	24-48
Oxazepam	Serax	5-15
Temazepam	Restoril	8-12
Midazolam	Versed	1.5-3.5
Triazolam	Halcion	1.5-5

Table II–9 • OTHER ANXIOLYTICS/SEDATIVE-HYPNOTICS

Name[a]	Indication	Half-Life (h)	Side Effects	Comments
Buspirone (BuSpar)	Generalized anxiety	5-11	Headache, gastrointestinal distress, dizziness	Less useful in patients who have used benzodiazepines; should not be used with monoamine oxidase inhibitors
Zolpidem (Ambien)	For insomnia	2-4	Headache, drowsiness, dizziness, nausea, diarrhea	Increased effect with alcohol or selective serotonin reuptake inhibitors
Zaleplon (Sonata)	For insomnia	1	Headache, peripheral edema, amnesia, dizziness, rash, nausea, tremor	
Ramelteon (Rozerem)	For insomnia	1-2.6	Headache, galactorrhea	Melatonin receptor agonist, no affinity for GABA receptor complex
Eszopiclone (Lunesta)	For insomnia	6	Anxiety, decrease in sexual desire; dry mouth; unpleasant taste	Stopping the drug suddenly may cause anxiety, unusual dreams, stomach and muscle cramps, nausea, vomiting, sweating, and shakiness

[a]*Proprietary names are given in parentheses.*

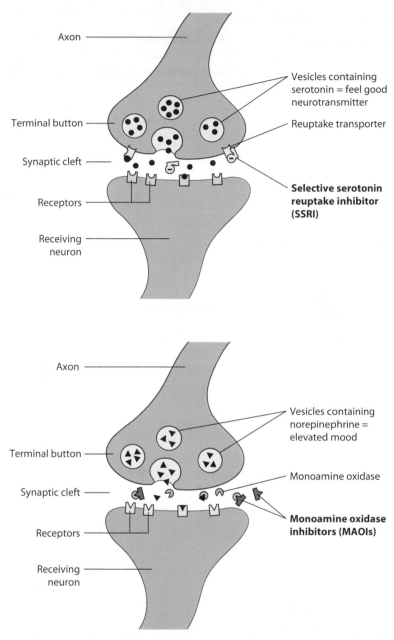

Figure II–1. Neurotransmitters in the neuronal synapse. Selective serotonin reuptake inhibitors (SSRIs) block the reuptake of serotonin by the presynaptic neuron (top), allowing more serotonin to be available at the postsynaptic receptor. Monoamine oxidase inhibitors (MAOIs) block the ability of this enzyme to inactivate monoamines such as norepinephrine in the synaptic cleft (bottom), allowing more neurotransmitter to bind to the postsynaptic receptor.

IV. **Anxiolytics and sedative/hypnotics**

   A. **Benzodiazepines:** These drugs work by binding to sites on GABA receptors. They are effective in anxiety and sleep disorders and in reducing anxiety and agitation in other disorders such as acute psychosis. They are generally safe in overdose if used alone. They are metabolized mainly in the liver. Their side effects include sedation, behavioral disinhibition (especially in the young or the elderly), psychomotor impairment, cognitive impairment, confusion, and ataxia. They are **addictive,** and after prolonged use, **withdrawal can cause seizures and death.** Shorter-acting benzodiazepines carry a higher risk for dependency, although they carry less risk of a "hangover" after use. Table II–8 lists commonly used benzodiazepines. Table II–9 lists other anxiolytics.

 V. Drugs used to treat the **side effects** of other psychotropic medications

   A. **Anticholinergic agents** used to **treat dystonias** (caused by the use of antipsychotic medication) include benztropine, biperiden, diphenhydramine, and trihexyphenidyl.

   B. Medications used to treat **akathisias** (restlessness caused by the use of antipsychotic medication) include **propranolol and benzodiazepines.**

   C. Medications used to treat parkinsonian side effects (caused by the use of antipsychotic medication) include **amantadine and levodopa.**

VI. **Stimulants:** These drugs exert their effects through a number of different pharmacological mechanisms, the most prominent of which include facilitation of norepinephrine (noradrenaline) and/or dopamine activity. They are used to increase attention and alertness in a variety of conditions, including attention-deficit hyperactivity disorder (ADHD). Table II–10 lists commonly prescribed stimulants.

Table II–10 • STIMULANTS

Name[a]	Indication	Half-Life (h)	Side Effects	Comments
Dextroam- phetamine and amphetamine (Adderall)	Attention- deficit hyperac- tivity disorder (ADHD)	10	Nervousness, restless- ness, and difficulty falling asleep or stay- ing asleep	May slow children's growth or weight gain; may be addictive
Modafinil (Provigil, Alertec, Modavigil)	Narcolepsy, excessive day- time sleepiness	15	Dizziness, insomnia, diarrhea	Increases the release of mono- amines and elevates hypotha- lamic histamine levels
Dextroamphet- amine (Dex- edrine)	ADHD, narcolepsy	2-3	Nervousness, restless- ness, and difficulty falling asleep or stay- ing asleep	May be addictive
Methylpheni- date (Ritalin, Concerta)	ADHD, narcolepsy	2-3	Nervousness, restless- ness, and difficulty falling asleep or stay- ing asleep	May be addictive
Methylphenidate (liquid) (Quil- livant XR)	ADHD	5.6	Decreased appetite, weight loss, trouble falling asleep, nervousness	May be addictive
Dexmethylphe- nidate (Focalin)	ADHD	4 (7 for XR)	Decreased appetite, weight loss, trouble falling asleep, nervousness	May be addictive
Lisdexamfet- amine (Vyvanse)	ADHD	10-13	Decreased appetite, weight loss, trouble falling asleep, nervousness	May be addictive
Atomoxetine (Strattera)	ADHD	5.2	Nausea, dry mouth, appetite loss, insom- nia, fatigue, headache, cough	A selective- norepinephrine reuptake inhibitor (SNRI) No abuse potential

[a]*Proprietary names are given in parentheses.*

COMPREHENSION QUESTIONS

II.1   A 43-year-old woman with a long history of schizophrenia complains of a loss of night vision. Which of the following medications is most likely responsible?

A. Haloperidol

B. Thioridazine

C. Risperidone

D. Chlorpromazine

E. Clozapine

II.2   A 28-year-old man with a history of a psychiatric admission 6 months previously is seen in the emergency department with a painful erection, which he says has persisted for 18 hours. Which of the following is the best next step?

A. Epinephrine injection into the penis

B. Follow-up in 12 hours

C. Oral benzodiazepines and careful observation

D. Magnetic resonance imaging of the lumbosacral spine

E. IM injection of benztropine

II.3   A 57-year-old woman complains of feeling dizzy when she gets up in the morning and when standing. She takes imipramine each evening for depression. Which of the following is the most likely cause of her symptoms?

A. Hypovolemia from decreased appetite

B. Hypoglycemia

C. Diabetes insipidus

D. Alpha-adrenergic blockade

E. Dehydration

II.4   A 34-year-old man is seen in the emergency department with a headache, dizziness, and blood pressure of 210/150 mm Hg. He has no medical problems, states that he feels fine, and says that last night he even had a nice meal with wine. Which of the following medications is he most likely taking?

A. Bupropion

B. Lithium

C. Amitriptyline

D. Phenelzine

E. Fluoxetine

II.5 A 22-year-old college student with a history of depression is being treated with sertraline. He enjoys drinking beer on the weekends. Which of the following side effects is most likely to occur?

A. Alcohol potentiation

B. Alcohol withdrawal

C. Sexual dysfunction

D. Diabetes insipidus

E. Serotonin syndrome

II.6 Because of the side effects of his original antidepressant, the college student in Question II.5 is switched to another agent. He comes to the emergency department several days later with muscle spasms, confusion, fever, tachycardia, and hypertension. Which of the following is the most likely cause?

A. Serotonin syndrome

B. Cocaine intoxication

C. Meningitis

D. Alcohol withdrawal (delirium tremens)

E. Neuroleptic malignant syndrome (NMS)

II.7 A 17-year-old adolescent suffers from bulimia nervosa and is very depressed. She is also suffering from insomnia and apathy. Which of the following medications should be avoided?

A. Fluoxetine

B. Trazodone

C. Imipramine

D. Bupropion

E. Amitriptyline

II.8 A 32-year-old woman has been taking medication (the name of which she does not remember) for her psychiatric condition. She complains of excessive thirst and urinating "all the time." Which of the following is the most likely diagnosis?

A. Bipolar disorder

B. Major depression

C. Panic disorder

D. Schizophrenia

E. Social phobia

II.9 A 29-year-old man who "hears voices" at times complains of fever and chills. His temperature is 102°F (38.9°C) with no findings of infection. His white blood cell count is 800 cells/mm³. Which of the following medications is most likely responsible?

A. Haloperidol

B. Risperidone

C. Clozapine

D. Thioridazine

E. Fluphenazine

II.10 A 38-year-old woman is admitted to the hospital for an elective hysterectomy. On hospital day 3, she experiences auditory and visual hallucinations, has tremors, and is agitated. Which of the following would be the best therapy?

A. Selective serotonin reuptake inhibitor (SSRI)

B. Propranolol

C. Imipramine

D. Benzodiazepine

E. Atypical antipsychotic

II.11 A 35-year-old African American woman with bipolar disorder delivers a male newborn who has spina bifida. Which of the following is the most likely etiology?

A. Advanced maternal age

B. Mood-stabilizing medication

C. Folate excess

D. Ethnicity

E. Maternal malnutrition

II.12 A 39-year-old man tries to commit suicide by taking an overdose of amitriptyline tablets. He is rushed to the emergency room where resuscitation is attempted but fails. Which of the following is most likely to be noted during the attempted resuscitation or the autopsy?

A. Massive coronary artery occlusion

B. Aortic valve stenosis

C. Electrocardiographic conduction abnormalities

D. Cardiac tamponade

E. Massive pulmonary embolism

Match the following therapies (A-F) to the clinical scenarios listed (Questions II.13-II.18).

- A. Benztropine
- B. Propranolol
- C. Amantadine
- D. Dantrolene
- E. Dialysis
- F. Flumazenil
- G. Methylphenidate
- H. Modafinil

II.13 A 25-year-old man with bipolar disorder took too many pills, had two seizures, and is now in a coma.

II.14 A 38-year-old schizophrenic woman feels restless and cannot sit still; her physician states that this behavior is caused by her medication.

II.15 A 32-year-old woman with panic disorder and anxiety took an overdose of diazepam and is taken to the emergency department with somnolence and hypoventilation.

II.16 A 30-year-old man being treated for schizophrenia complains of tremor and a slow gait.

II.17 A 14-year-old adolescent boy being treated for ADHD complains of not being able to go to sleep at night.

II.18 A 56-year-old man on the night shift complains of excessive daytime sleepiness.

ANSWERS

II.1   **B.** High doses of thioridazine are associated with irreversible pigmentation of the retina, leading initially to symptoms of night vision difficulty and ultimately to blindness.

II.2   **A.** This priapism is most likely caused by trazodone. One treatment is epinephrine injected into the corpus of the penis.

II.3   **D.** The mechanism for orthostatic hypotension caused by tricyclic/heterocyclic antidepressants is alpha-adrenergic blockade.

II.4   **D.** This patient probably experienced a hypertensive crisis induced by an interaction between the wine and phenelzine, an MAOI.

II.5   **C.** Sexual dysfunction is a very common side effect of SSRI medications.

II.6   **A.** This patient was likely switched from an SSRI, sertraline, to an MAOI, such as phenelzine. Because both agents increase serotonin levels, 5 weeks should elapse between discontinuation of one medication and initiation of the other. The danger is very serious serotonin syndrome, which has features similar to those of NMS.

II.7   **D.** Seizure disorders and eating disorders are contraindications for bupropion because of its possible lowering of the seizure threshold and its anorectic effects.

II.8   **A.** This patient has symptoms of diabetes insipidus, a side effect of lithium used in the treatment of bipolar disease.

II.9   **C.** This individual has neutropenic fever as a result of agranulocytosis, a side effect of the atypical antipsychotic agent clozapine.

II.10   **D.** This woman is probably experiencing either alcohol or benzodiazepine withdrawal; in either case, benzodiazepines would be the treatment.

II.11   **B.** This woman was likely taking valproic acid, a mood stabilizer used in treating bipolar disorder, which increases the risk for teratogenicity (eg, a neural tube defect).

II.12   **C.** A tricyclic antidepressant overdose can lead to increased QT intervals and ultimately to cardiac dysrhythmias.

II.13   **E.** Dialysis is used to treat lithium toxicity when it is severe and life threatening, such as causing seizures or coma.

II.14   **B.** Akathisia (restlessness) can be treated with propranolol.

II.15   **F.** A benzodiazepine overdose can be treated with flumazenil, which is a benzodiazepine antagonist.

II.16   **C.** The parkinsonian-like symptoms of neuroleptic agents are treated with amantadine or levodopa.

II.17   **G.** Methylphenidate, a common treatment for ADHD, has a common side effect—insomnia. For this reason, it is rarely prescribed for patients to take in the late afternoon or early evening.

II.18   **H.** Modafinil may be used for the treatment of excessive daytime sleepiness in shift workers.

CLINICAL PEARLS

▶ In general, the side effects of tricyclic/heterocyclic antidepressant agents are anticholinergic effects, sedation, orthostatic hypotension, cardiac rhythm disturbances, and weight gain.

▶ Usually, tricyclic/heterocyclic antidepressants do not cause EPS. An exception to this rule is amoxapine, which is a metabolite of the antipsychotic loxapine.

▶ Selective serotonin reuptake inhibitors are the most commonly used medications for depression but should not be used in conjunction with MAOIs. One medication should be discontinued for at least 5 weeks before the other is initiated to avoid serotonin syndrome.

▶ Serotonin syndrome is characterized by **(in order of appearance) diarrhea, restlessness, extreme agitation, hyperreflexia, autonomic instability, myoclonus, seizures, hyperthermia, rigidity, delirium, coma, and death.**

► The most common side effects of SSRIs are gastrointestinal disturbance and sexual dysfunction.

► Individuals taking MAOIs should avoid aged cheese, red wine, liver, and smoked foods (tyramine) or an acute hypertensive crisis can ensue.

► Trazodone can lead to priapism; a prolonged painful erection that is trazodone induced is considered an emergency and is treated with an intracorporeal injection of epinephrine or drainage of blood from the penis.

► Bupropion is used for smoking cessation but must be avoided in patients with eating disorders or seizures.

► Lithium has numerous side effects, including tremor, polyuria/diabetes insipidus, acne, hypothyroidism, cardiac dysrhythmias, weight gain, edema, and leukocytosis.

► Lithium is cleared through the kidneys and must be used with caution in older patients and in those with renal insufficiency.

► Valproic acid can be teratogenic and must not be used in women of childbearing age (switch to another mood stabilizer).

► Antipsychotic agents produce many adverse effects, including EPS, sedation, and orthostatic hypotension.

► Neuroleptic malignant syndrome can be caused at any time by an antipsychotic agent. It typically includes a movement disorder (muscle rigidity, dystonia, agitation) and autonomic symptoms (high fever, sweating, tachycardia, hypertension). White blood cell (WBC) and creatine phosphokinase (CPK) levels are both typically high.

► Clozapine can cause fatal agranulocytosis, and thus frequent leukocyte-count monitoring is mandatory.

► Benzodiazepine withdrawal resembles alcohol withdrawal and can be fatal.

REFERENCES

Hales RE, Yudofsky SC, Roberts LW. *The American Psychiatric Publishing Textbook of Psychiatry*. 6th ed. Washington, DC: American Psychiatric Publishing; 2014.

Higgins ES, George MS. *The Neuroscience of Clinical Psychiatry*. 2nd ed. Philadelphia, PA: Lippincott Williams & Wilkins; 2013.

Stern TA, Herman JB, Gorrindo T. *Massachusetts General Hospital Psychiatry*. 3rd ed. Boston, MA: MGH Psychiatry Academy Publishing; 2012.

Listing of Cases

Listing by Case Number

Listing by Disorder (Alphabetical)

Listing by DSM-5 Categories

Listing by Case Number

Listing by Disorder (Alphabetical)

Listing by DSM-5 Categories

Clinical Cases

An 8-year-old boy is brought to a psychiatrist by his parents because he is having increasing difficulty keeping up academically with his classmates. His parents report that he has always been a slow learner but that they were not really aware of how significant their son's difficulties were until this year, when their other child, a 5-year-old girl, started school. Their daughter is progressing much more quickly and easily than their 8-year-old son did. His teacher says that their son is pleasant but is behind the class in the acquisition of skills in all areas. In preschool, the teacher reported that he had a tendency to hit others, but he does this much less often now. He gets along with other children well, although he seems to enjoy the company of his younger sibling's friends over his same-age peers.

The parents report that their son met all his developmental milestones at the low end of the normally expected range, but their pediatrician told them not to be concerned. He has never had any significant medical illnesses. He had an uneventful prenatal period and birth.

▶ What is the most likely diagnosis?
▶ What are the next diagnostic steps?
▶ What is the role of the psychiatrist in the care of this patient?

ANSWERS TO CASE 1:

Mild Intellectual Disability (Formerly Mental Retardation)

Summary: An 8-year-old boy is brought to a psychiatrist because he is a "slow learner" and has fallen behind his peers in class. He has a history of being aggressive to some degree in preschool, although he seems to have "grown out" of this behavior. His parents do not report any significant current or past medical conditions. He has a younger sister who is doing well and surpasses him in academic and social skills.

- **Most likely diagnosis:** Mild intellectual disability

- **Diagnostic steps:** Some form of individualized intelligence testing is required in addition to an assessment of the patient's current adaptive functioning. It can be necessary to supplement intelligence testing with other educational testing to ensure that the patient does not have learning disabilities that inhibit his performance on the intelligence tests, thus producing a lower intelligence quotient (IQ) score than would otherwise occur.

- **Role of the psychiatrist:** The psychiatrist plays a number of critical roles in the treatment of those with intellectual disabilities. The first is ensuring a complete evaluation (including karyotyping when appropriate) has occurred to ensure that any syndrome associated with intellectual disability is detected and appropriate interventions (ie, dietary, hormonal replacement) occur. Second, 35% to 40% of people with intellectual disability have another psychiatric disorder. The psychiatrist must make sure the symptoms of any psychiatric disorder are diagnosed and that these symptoms are not misattributed to the intellectual disability. The psychiatrist must then provide adequate treatment. Finally, if there are no acute symptoms requiring medication management, a child psychiatrist typically serves in a coordinating role to ensure that the need for services by other mental health professionals is properly coordinated.

ANALYSIS

Objectives

1. Understand the diagnostic criteria for intellectual disability (Table 1–1).

2. Understand the role of the psychiatrist in the treatment of mental retardation.

Considerations

An 8-year-old boy is brought to a psychiatrist because his parents have noticed that he has global deficits in both social and educational skills. They became more aware of their son's deficits after he entered school. The couple now has a younger daughter who surpasses her older brother in skill acquisition and development. When intelligence testing is completed, the child will likely score in the mildly deficient range. On adaptive testing, he will likely score in the deficient range as well.

Table 1–1 • *DSM-5* DIAGNOSTIC CRITERIA FOR INTELLECTUAL DISABILITY (INTELLECTUAL DEVELOPMENTAL DISORDER, FORMERLY MENTAL RETARDATION)
A. Deficits in reasoning, problem solving, planning, abstract thinking, judgment, academic learning, and experiential learning confirmed by clinical assessment and individualized, standardized intelligence testing.
B. And concurrent deficits in adaptive functioning that limit functioning in key areas of daily life like communication, social participation and independent living, and result in the individual failing to meet developmental and societal standards for personal independence and social responsibility without social supports in multiple environments.
C. With onset during the developmental period.

APPROACH TO:

Intellectual Disability

DEFINITIONS

ADAPTIVE FUNCTIONING TESTS: Psychological assessments that measure social, communication, daily living, and community functioning skills. A collateral source who knows the patient well is required to answer questions needed to complete the assessment. Some of these skills can be measured with the Vineland Social Maturity Scale, a test commonly used.

DOWN SYNDROME: Trisomy 21, which is associated with hypotonia, language and motor developmental delay, and typical facial features. It is the most common cause of moderate to severe intellectual disability in the United States.

FRAGILE X SYNDROME: The second most common cause of intellectual disability in the United States, resulting from a mutation at the $Xq27.3$ locus. Males generally have moderate to severe intellectual disability, while female carriers are less severely affected.

INTELLIGENCE TESTS: Psychological assessments that measure intellectual capacity. The results of these tests vary based on educational attainment. The most commonly used tests include the Wechsler scales (the Wechsler Preschool and Primary Scale of Intelligence, the Wechsler Intelligence Scale for Children, and the Wechsler Adult Intelligence Scale) and the Stanford-Binet Scale.

CLINICAL APPROACH

The prevalence of intellectual disability is approximately 1% of the population, with males being more affected than females. There are a multitude of etiologies, including genetics, prenatal infections and toxins, prematurity, and acquired conditions. In one-third of individuals, no cause can be identified. Down syndrome, fragile X syndrome, and phenylketonuria (PKU) are common etiologies for moderate to severe intellectual disability. Mild intellectual disability is often associated with a familial pattern. A diagnosis of this disorder requires a diminished capacity for cognitive functioning measured by an objective intelligence test, as well as a diminished capacity for adaptive functioning in multiple environments (refer to Table 1–2 for

Table 1–2 • DEGREES OF INTELLECTUAL DISABILITY (FORMERLY MENTAL RETARDATION)			
Severity of Retardation	Conceptual Domain	Social Domain	Practical Domain
Mild	While potentially having no deficits in preschool, by school age has difficulty learning academics without greater support. As adult uses concrete thinking to approach problems with deficits in abstract thinking, executive functioning, and memory.	Immature in social interactions, language use more concrete, difficulty regulating emotion, poor understanding of risk with immature social judgment and at risk of being manipulated because of gullibility.	While potentially able to keep up age appropriate personal care, needs help with complex daily living tasks, requires support to be able to engage in recreation, works jobs not needing conceptual skill, needs help with legal and health care decisions.
Moderate	Even before school, language and motor skills are delayed, academics in school are markedly limited and even as adult does not progress beyond elementary level, needs daily assistance as adult to complete simple day-to-day tasks.	Marked delays in social and communicative behavior, speech is much less complex but still primary tool for communication, can have satisfying relationships but understands social cues inaccurately. Caretakers must assist with life decisions with high social support needed for future work success.	Can care for personal needs but requires extended teaching and reminders. On-going supports are needed after extended teaching of household tasks. May work at limited jobs with ongoing support. Maladaptive behavior in a significant minority.
Severe	Very limited conceptual skill. Little understanding of written language, numbers, quantity, time, or money. Caretakers extensively needed for problem-solving support.	Spoken language limited in vocabulary and grammar. Focuses on the immediate needs of the moment. Understands simple speech or basic sign language. Relationships with family and familiar others may be source of pleasure.	Requires extensive support for all activities of daily living and supervision at all times. Cannot make any responsible decision and needs supervision for any household or work tasks which must be very basic in nature. Maladaptive behavior present in a significant minority.
Profound	Can conceptualize the physical world but not symbolic processes. May use objects in goal-directed fashion. May be able to match or sort object but often cannot use objects functionally.	May understand a few simple words or gestures. Largely expresses self through nonverbal, nonsymbolic behavior. Many enjoy contact with known family members and familiar others. Impairments may prevent many social activities.	Dependent on others for all activities of daily living. Can perform only the most basic actions with objects. May enjoy activities but only with the immediate support of others. Maladaptive behavior present in a significant minority.

degrees of impairment in a patient's ability to conceptualize, socialize, and practically function on a day-to-day basis). The causes of intellectual disability are as numerous as are the treatments. General causes include genetic prenatal problems such as chromosomal abnormalities or mutations, prenatal causes related to an external source such as toxins or infections, and postnatal causes such as anoxia, infection, or deprivation experienced by an infant after birth.

DIFFERENTIAL DIAGNOSIS

Specific communication or learning disorders must be differentiated from intellectual disability, which is associated with greater global functional impairment. Patients with pervasive development disorder frequently have uneven areas of deficit, particularly regarding social interaction skills. Onset must be before the age of 18. If the impairment is noted after the age of 18 years, dementia and its various causes should be considered.

Therapeutic Approach

There are several principles behind the treatment of intellectual disability. The first is the concept of **prevention.** Whenever possible, potential causes of intellectual disability should be minimized: **Women should abstain from drinking alcohol during pregnancy,** should receive **appropriate immunizations before becoming pregnant, and should get proper nutrition including folic acid and other vitamin supplements.** The next specific treatment involves the minimization of causes wherever possible. The best example of this is **diet restrictions for babies born with PKU.** Although the genetic problem cannot be corrected, the environmental exposure that allows this problem to be manifested can be controlled. The next level of treatment involves interventions designed to lessen the impact of intellectual disability early in a child's life. These might include early education, speech therapy, occupational therapy, family support, and respite care.

Appropriate medical care should also be provided, as medical problems can complicate the progress of a child with intellectual disability. Finally, clinicians should realize that depression, anxiety, psychosis, and conduct disorders are common in the intellectual disability population but often go undetected. The reason for this is that these comorbid disorders often present with behavioral disturbance or aggression that is attributed to the patient having an intellectual disability rather than being seen as a symptom of the underlying psychiatric disorder. Any significant change in behavior in a patient suffering from intellectual disability should result in a careful examination with information from multiple sources to tease out the presence of any psychiatric or general medical illness. Specific treatments for these disorders in this population do not usually differ from treatments for those in the general population.

In individuals with moderate to profound intellectual disability, it is important to remember that medical conditions causing pain can result in aggressive or self-destructive behavior in an individual with limited means of communicating. Whenever evaluating a patient with an intellectual disability for aggressive or self-destructive behavior, a complete physical examination and medical reassessment is indicated rather than immediately proceeding with psychotropic medication.

> **CASE CORRELATION**
>
> - See also Case 2 and Case 47. Intellectual disability is common in patients with autism spectrum disorders. Appropriate assessment of intellectual functioning in autism spectrum disorders is essential. Intellectual disability is characterized as a neurodevelopmental disorder, distinct from neurocognitive disorders, which are characterized by the loss of cognitive functioning.

COMPREHENSION QUESTIONS

1.1 Patients with which level(s) of intellectual capacity are capable of holding jobs?

  A.   All levels.

  B.   Mild only.

  C.   Moderate and mild.

  D.   Severe, moderate, and mild.

  E.   Individuals with intellectual disability are unable to hold jobs.

1.2 Which of the following is the most common cause of intellectual disability?

  A.   Fragile X syndrome

  B.   Genetic deficits

  C.   Idiopathic or unknown

  D.   In utero exposure to toxins

  E.   Lead intoxication

1.3 An 18-year-old boy has benefited from training in social and occupational skills but has been unable to progress beyond the second-grade level in academic subjects. He needs supervision and guidance when under mild social or economic stress. Which level of intellectual disability is being described?

  A.   Mild

  B.   Moderate

  C.   Severe

  D.   Profound

  E.   Borderline level of intellectual functioning

ANSWERS

1.1 **B.** Although persons with all degrees of intellectual disability can require some support to function in the community, those with a mild intellectual disability are able to hold a job. Individuals with moderate intellectual disability are often able to manage small amounts of money and make change. Persons with severe and profound intellectual disability have limited abilities to manage themselves and have difficulty learning these skills.

1.2 **C.** Although each of the conditions listed is associated with intellectual disability, the largest percentage continues to be attributed to idiopathic causes.

1.3 **B.** This description refers to a person with moderate intellectual disability. Refer to Table 1–2 for descriptions of the various degrees and functionality of persons with intellectual disability.

CLINICAL PEARLS

▶ Two pieces of information are needed to make a diagnosis of intellectual disability: Evidence of deficits in intellectual functioning both clinically and via standardized testing AND evidence of deficits in adaptive functioning.

▶ **In individuals with moderate to profound intellectual disability, it is important to remember that medical conditions causing pain can result in aggressive or self-destructive behavior in an individual with limited means of communicating.**

▶ The impairment associated with intellectual disability is global and fairly consistent across all areas of functioning.

REFERENCES

Ervin DA, Hennen B, Merrick J, Morad M. Healthcare for persons with intellectual and developmental disability in the community. *Frontiers in Public Health*. 2014;2(83);1-8.

Ervin DA, Williams A, Merrisk J. Primary care: mental and behavioral health and persons with intellectual and developmental disabilities. *Frontiers in Public Health*. 2014;2(76):1-5.

Sadock BJ, Sadock VA, Ruiz P. *Kaplan and Sadock's Synopsis of Psychiatry: Behavioral Sciences/Clinical Psychiatry*. 11th ed. Baltimore, MD: Lippincott Williams & Wilkins; 2014

A 2½-year-old boy is brought to a pediatrician by his parents for his regular yearly examination. He is the couple's only child. The parents relate a normal medical history with a single episode of otitis media. They recently placed their son in day care for 2 half-days a week. However, he has not adjusted well, crying and having tantrums during the first hour of school. Then he usually quiets down, but he does not interact with the rest of the children. The teacher cannot seem to make him follow directions and notes that he does not look at her when she is near him and attempting to interact with him.

On further discussion with the parents, the pediatrician finds that the patient has only a limited vocabulary of perhaps 10 words. He does not use these words in any greater length than two words in a row and often uses them inappropriately. He did not speak his first clear word until 6 to 9 months. The patient does not interact well with other children but does not seem upset by them. His favorite toys are often used inappropriately—he performs single, repetitive movements with them for what seems like hours on end. The pediatrician picks the child up to help him onto the examination table and notices that he seems quite stiff, pushing himself away from the examiner with his hands. Although his hearing and eyesight appear to be intact, the child does not respond to requests by the pediatrician and does not make eye contact. All other gross neurologic and physical features are within normal limits.

▶ What is the most likely diagnosis?
▶ What is the most likely prognosis for this condition?

ANSWERS TO CASE 2:

Autism Spectrum Disorder

Summary: A 2½-year-old child is brought to a pediatrician for his yearly physical examination. His history reveals various behavioral issues, including poor interaction with peers and family, delayed language development, repetitive movements, and difficulty accepting change. The child stiffens physically when touched, does not respond to the examiner, and does not make eye contact.

- **Most likely diagnosis:** Autism spectrum disorder (ASD).

- **Prognosis:** The child will likely experience a number of developmental delays, but with intensive treatment at home and at school, he could achieve near-normal or normal development. Language development is the most important indicator of future developmental potential in ASD children.

ANALYSIS

Objectives

1. Recognize ASD based on symptom presentations.

2. Understand the unique symptomatic aspects of ASD.

3. Understand the importance of early treatment.

Considerations

The patient's presentation and history are typical of a child with ASD. The symptoms of ASD often go unrecognized until the child is placed in an environment with other children of a similar age. This lack of recognition of the problem is especially likely to occur in a family with no other children, where it is not possible to compare developmental milestones. The patient displays typical symptoms: difficulty with social reciprocity, poor peer interaction, poor language development, and repetitive and odd play. His language development is poor for his age. A normal 2½-year-old child should have a much larger vocabulary—hundreds of words—and should easily be able to use several words in a sentence. A normal child's comprehension of words should be even better than his ability to use them. The presence of ASD does not necessarily indicate mental retardation, but a large percentage of autistic individuals have this disorder. There are new DSM specifiers to indicate the level of patients' intellectual or language impairments. The parents have come for help relatively early in the course of the illness. Intensive behavioral and educational interventions will be necessary to help accelerate the child's development.

APPROACH TO:
Autism Spectrum Disorder

DEFINITIONS

ASPERGER DISORDER: This is old terminology for a type of ASD that describes individuals who display social impairment and restricted interests and behavior (stereotyped behavior) but have normal language and cognitive skills.

MENTAL RETARDATION: A classification of cognitive functioning involving both a low intelligence quotient (IQ) and an impairment in adaptive functioning.

RETT DISORDER: This is old terminology for a type of ASD that describes individuals who show a type of childhood developmental disorder of unknown etiology in which the patient develops progressive encephalopathy, loss of speech capacity, gait problems, stereotyped movements, microcephaly, and poor social interaction skills. The child must have shown normal development in early infancy, and only females are affected.

SOCIAL RECIPROCITY: The ability to read and to exhibit verbal and nonverbal behaviors because of interacting with others.

STEREOTYPED BEHAVIORS: Purposeless, repetitive movements and behaviors such as spinning toys, toe walking, or hand flapping.

CLINICAL APPROACH

Boys are more often affected by ASD than girls by a three- to fivefold increased prevalence. Typically, the disorder is noticed by the parents of an affected child before 3 years of age and is characterized by developmental delay, aloofness, and stereotypical behavior. The etiology of ASD is unknown, but a genetic etiology is likely. Family studies show a markedly increased incidence in monozygotic twins and a low risk in dizygotic twins. Elevated serum serotonin levels can be a clue to the neurochemical abnormality. Approximately 40% of children with autistic disorder are mentally retarded; however, some demonstrate unusual or extremely precocious abilities, the so-called islets of precocity. One such talent is the ability to perform extraordinary mathematical calculations although the child is cognitively impaired in other ways.

Much research has been dedicated to brain abnormalities and possible causes of ASD. **Magnetic resonance imaging** (MRI) studies have shown that patients with autism demonstrate evidence of increased cortical thickness that may relate to abnormalities in cortical connectivity. Functional magnetic resonance imaging (fMRI) studies have shown less activation of the prefrontal regions indicating a dysfunction of the frontostriatal networks in patients with autism spectrum disorders. Other studies have demonstrated abnormalities in glutamate/glutamine physiology, particularly in the limbic areas. Certainly it should be said that autism and its related conditions are complex entities with multiple dimensions of etiology.

There has been some controversy regarding the role of childhood vaccinations in the development of ASD. However, researchers and clinicians in the field have reviewed and tested this hypothesis exhaustively. A large meta-analysis of almost 15 million children looked at vaccine efficacy and safety. The generally accepted conclusion is that there is **no association between childhood vaccinations** (or their preserving agents) in the development of autism.

Diagnostic Criteria

Patients demonstrate a qualitative impairment in social interaction skills, manifested by symptoms such as **a marked impairment in nonverbal behaviors, a failure to develop appropriate peer relationships, or a lack of social reciprocity.** There are also qualitative impairments in their ability to communicate, manifested by a delay in learning or a failure to learn spoken language. Patients exhibit **repetitive and stereotyped patterns of behavior,** including inflexible adherence to rules or stereotyped motor mannerisms. They can also be persistently preoccupied with parts of objects.

DIFFERENTIAL DIAGNOSIS

In *DSM-5* the previous diagnoses of autistic disorder, Rett disorder, childhood disintegrative disorder, Asperger disorder, and pervasive developmental disorder not otherwise specified have been consolidated into the term **autistic spectrum disorder (ASD).**

These were changed to ASDs because of research showing these categories were not as discrete and independent as once thought. The differences in presentation are now differentiated by severity specifiers. These severity specifiers include social communication impairments and repetitive patterns of behavior. ASD children often function within the mentally retarded range; however, unlike ASD children, mentally retarded children generally do not exhibit restricted activities and interests or impairments in communication and social skills. Although a child with schizophrenia can exhibit poor social functioning and affective withdrawal, the onset of childhood schizophrenia usually occurs later, there is a family history of schizophrenia, and the child is less impaired in the area of intellectual functioning. Children with obsessive-compulsive disorder (OCD) can display stereotypical behavior or perform rituals, but they have a more normal course of development otherwise. They also do not exhibit impairment in social interaction or communication.

TREATMENT

ASD, perhaps more than any other childhood psychiatric disorder, requires a well-rounded, multisystemic treatment approach: **family education, behavior shaping, speech therapy, occupational therapy, and educational planning.** Care should be taken to coordinate these activities across school and home settings. Parental support and training are essential to a successful outcome. Applied behavioral analysis can be helpful in autistic patients, especially those with limited verbal skills. This treatment involves an intensive behavioral program that works best if started early in the course of the illness. The goals of this treatment are to teach the child a variety of **basic skills,** such as attending to adults, language use, and how to interact with peers, all of which can increase the child's ability to be more successful in educational as well as social settings.

There are recent studies indicating a role for the neuropeptide, oxytocin in the etiology and treatment of ASD. These studies have shown a likely benefit for the use of oxytocin in improving nonverbal communication behaviors.

No specific medications are used in treating the core symptoms of ASD, although some recent studies using low-dose Risperdal (risperidone) show some promise. In addition, recent studies have shown that the use of aripiprazole may also be of benefit with the irritability symptoms of ASD. Other psychiatric disorders such as attention deficit hyperactivity disorder (ADHD), OCD, behavior disorders, and psychotic disorders can be present in children with ASD. These conditions should be targeted and treated if the symptoms meet the diagnostic criteria for that particular illness. Proper recognition and treatment of comorbid psychiatric disorders can have a significant impact on the overall outcome for children with autism.

CASE CORRELATION

- See also Case 1 and Case 3. Intellectual disability is common in patients with autism spectrum disorders, and appropriate assessment of intellectual functioning is essential. Abnormalities of attention are common in patients with autism spectrum disorder, but an additional diagnosis of ADHD would only be given in those cases where attentional difficulties or hyperactivity exceeds that seen in those with comparable mental age.

COMPREHENSION QUESTIONS

2.1 Which medication has shown some mild benefit for the irritability symptoms of autistic spectrum disorders?

A. Fluoxetine

B. Aripiprazole

C. Haldol

D. Clonidine

E. Methylphenidate

2.2 A 4-year-old boy who is an only child starts preschool. His parents are quite nervous about this and describe themselves as protective and overinvolved. However, they are looking forward to seeing him more involved with school, as he has had little peer interaction prior to this because he has never shown much of an interest in interacting with others. He has never used many words which the parents attribute to his isolation. They tell the teacher he has always done best with a strict schedule and doesn't tolerate changes well. He has always seemed to have a very narrow repertory of play—focusing primarily on spinning objects such as tops and balls. He comes to the classroom for the first time, runs right to these toys, and does not say goodbye to his mother, nor even acknowledge she is leaving. Other children attempt to play with him but his response is to either ignore them or get angry at their advances. His focus on spinning objects in play might be considered what type of behavior often seen with ASD?

A. Rigidity

B. Stereotyped behavior

C. Lack of social reciprocity

D. Poor language development

E. Obsessional thinking

2.3 In the patient from Question 2.2, what statement might best describe the etiology of his disorder?

A. MMR vaccination has been shown to be a major factor in the development of autism.

B. A cold unyielding mother and absent father is the most significant factor leading to ASD.

C. A deficit in oxytocin.

D. A complex heritable and in utero environmental influence.

E. Brain trauma at birth.

2.4 What is the reason that many other previously distinct disorders were grouped in ASDs by *DSM-5*?

A. *DSM-5* has attempted to rid diagnoses of proper names.

B. The previous names did not translate easily across cultures.

C. The disorders were not as discrete and independent as previously thought.

D. The other disorders previously considered part of this group have been made new discrete disorders.

E. ICD-10 required this.

ANSWERS

2.1 **B.** Aripiprazole has been shown to be clinically useful for irritability symptoms such as tantrums or self-injurious behaviors.

2.2 **B.** Stereotyped or repetitive motor movements, part of criterion B for ASD.

2.3 **D.** The etiology of ASD is not known. There is a large heritable component and some indication of in utero environmental influences. Vaccinations have been shown time and again to not contribute to the formation of ASD.

2.4 **C.** Clinicians and researchers found that the separate diagnoses were not discrete as once thought and they were difficult to distinguish within the group.

CLINICAL PEARLS

▶ Language development is the best predictor of future outcome in autistic disorder.

▶ Mental retardation is often but not always associated with autism.

▶ In cases where early autism is suspected, a full medical workup should always be scheduled to rule out hearing or vision difficulties that can result in poor language development.

▶ It is unlikely that thimerosal-containing vaccinations are the cause of autism spectrum diseases.

REFERENCES

de Los Reyes EC. Autism and immunizations: separating fact from fiction. *Arch Neurol.* Apr 2010; 67(4):490-492.

Demicheli V, Rivetti A, Debalini MG, Di Pietrantonj C. Vaccines for measles, mumps and rubella in children. *Cochrane Database Syst Rev.* February 15, 2012;2:CD004407. doi: 10.1002/14651858. CD004407.pub3.

Findling RL, Mankoski R, Timko K, et al. A randomized controlled trial investigating the safety and efficacy of aripiprazole in the long-term maintenance treatment of pediatric patients with irritability associated with autistic disorder. *J Clin Psychiatry.* January 2014;75(1):22-30. doi: 10.4088/JCP.13m8500.

Hardan AY, Muddasani S, Vemulapalli M, Keshavan MS, Minshew NJ. An MRI study of increased cortical thickness in autism. *Am J Psychiatry.* 2006;163(7):1290-1292.

Page LA, Daly E, Schmitz N, et al. In vivo 1H-magnetic resonance spectroscopy study of amygdala-hippocampal and parietal regions in autism. *Am J Psychiatry.* 2006;163(12):2189-2192.

Sadock BJ, Sadock VA, Ruiz P. *Kaplan and Sadock's Synopsis of Psychiatry: Behavioral Sciences/Clinical Psychiatry.* 11th ed. Baltimore, MD: Lippincott Williams & Wilkins; 2014.

Silk TJ, Rinehart N, Bradshaw JL, et al. Visuospatial processing and the function of prefrontal-parietal networks in autism spectrum disorders: a functional MRI study. *Am J Psychiatry.* 2006;163(8): 1440-1443.

Watanabe T, Abe O, Kuwabara H, et al. Mitigation of sociocommunicational deficits of autism through oxytocin-induced recovery of medial prefrontal activity: a randomized trial. *JAMA Psychiatry.* February 2014;71(2):166-75. doi: 10.1001/jamapsychiatry.2013.3181.

A 7-year-old girl is brought to her pediatrician on the suggestion of her second-grade teacher. The patient has been back in school for 3 weeks following a summer break. According to the teacher, the patient has found it very difficult to complete her classroom tasks since returning to school. The child is seldom disruptive but cannot finish assignments in the allotted time although her classmates do so without difficulty. She also makes careless mistakes in her work. Although she is still passing her classes, her grades have dropped, and she seems to daydream a great deal in class. The teacher reports that it takes several repetitions of the instructions for the patient to complete a task (eg, in an art class). The patient enjoys physical education and does well in that class. The child indicates that when it appears to others that she is not paying attention she is thinking about other things. Teachers report that her attention wanders constantly and they have to call her name or wave to get her immediate attention. There have been no episodes where she stares blankly or is briefly nonresponsive.

Although her parents have noticed some of the same behaviors at home, they have not been particularly concerned because they have found ways to work around them. If they monitor the child and her work directly, she can complete her homework, but they must continually check her work for careless mistakes. She does seem to know the right answer when it is pointed out. The parents also report that the patient does not get ready for school in the mornings without moment-by-moment monitoring. Her bedroom is in shambles, and she loses things all the time. The parents describe their daughter as a happy child who enjoys playing with her siblings and friends. They note that she does not like school, except for the physical education classes.

▶ What is the most likely diagnosis?
▶ What are the recommended treatments for this disorder?

ANSWERS TO CASE 3:
Attention Deficit Hyperactivity Disorder

Summary: A 7-year-old girl has been referred to a psychiatrist by her teacher because she displays inattention, distractibility, and poor concentration and because her poor academic performance has resulted in problems with her grades. Her parents describe difficulty in following directions, disorganization, and forgetfulness. She does not have any symptoms of depression, psychosis, or developmental problems.

- **Most likely diagnosis:** Attention deficit hyperactivity disorder (ADHD), predominantly inattentive presentation.

- **Recommended treatments:** Use of a psychostimulant or atomoxetine along with behavioral parenting training and classroom behavior modification programs.

ANALYSIS

Objectives

1. Discern a diagnosis of attention deficit disorder based on the symptoms presented.

2. Understand the differences between the subtypes of attention deficit disorder.

3. Understand the best treatment choices for this condition.

Considerations

This patient's history is fairly typical of attention deficit disorder, predominantly inattentive presentation (vs predominantly hyperactive/impulsive presentation). She shows numerous traits consistent with this disorder, including inattention, making careless mistakes, difficulty paying attention, difficulty following instructions, difficulty organizing tasks, and forgetfulness (Table 3–1). This disorder is seen more commonly in girls than in boys. The patient does not have significant hyperactive symptoms, as do patients with the hyperactive/impulsive and the combined types; specifically, she does not display behaviors such as squirming, leaving her seat, running or climbing, talking excessively, or constantly being "on the go."

Current American Academy of Child and Adolescent Psychiatry (AACAP) practice guidelines suggest that the patient be treated with either a stimulant or atomoxetine. Stimulants have the advantage of more rapid onset and greater treatment effect size than atomoxetine. Atomoxetine is often considered as the first-line medication for treating ADHD in individuals or families with substance abuse problems (it is not an abusable controlled substance), individuals with tics (does not cause or worsen tics as stimulants do), or patients with comorbid anxiety disorders.

If the patient does not respond to stimulants or atomoxetine, then other alternatives include the use of clonidine and guanfacine as second-line choices. Bupropion and imipramine would be third-tier choices. Low-dose clonidine or guanfacine

Table 3–1 • DIAGNOSTIC CRITERIA FOR ATTENTION DEFICIT HYPERACTIVITY DISORDER
The patient exhibits six or more symptoms of inattention or hyperactivity/impulsivity. There is evidence that these symptoms were present before the age of 12 years. The impairment is present in more than one setting (school, work, or home). There is clinically significant impairment. Inattention symptoms include: <ul><li>Making careless mistakes</li><li>Having difficulty focusing one's attention</li><li>Often seeming not to listen</li><li>Often failing to follow directions</li><li>Having difficulty in organizing tasks</li><li>Avoiding tasks requiring sustained mental effort</li><li>Often losing things</li><li>Often becoming distracted by other stimuli</li><li>Being forgetful</li></ul> Hyperactivity symptoms include: <ul><li>Fidgeting or squirming</li><li>Often leaving one's seat</li><li>Running or climbing excessively and inappropriately</li><li>Difficulty playing quietly</li><li>Often being "on the go"</li><li>Talking excessively</li></ul> Impulsivity symptoms include: <ul><li>Often blurting out on answer before a question is completed</li><li>Difficulty waiting for one's turn</li><li>Often interrupting others</li></ul>

is also often used in ADHD patients to help with sleep disturbances or agitated behavior after they are on a stable dose of stimulant or other ADHD medication.

Therapy alone is seldom effective. Usually, once medication has controlled symptoms, behavioral parenting training to teach parents how to adapt their parenting style to the child's special needs is helpful along with classroom behavioral modification approaches.

APPROACH TO:
Attention Deficit Hyperactivity Disorder

DEFINITIONS

DISTRACTIBILITY: Inability to focus attention for age-appropriate periods of time.

HYPERACTIVITY: Excessive activity significantly above the level expected for the setting and the individual's developmental stage.

IMPULSIVITY: Taking action without appropriate thought and consideration which often leads to a dangerous situation.

CLINICAL APPROACH

Attention deficit hyperactivity disorder is defined as a **persistent pattern of inattention and/or hyperactivity/impulsivity** that is more frequent or severe than expected for a given level of development. Symptoms must be present for **at least 6 months,** begin before age 12, and be observed in more than one setting (eg, home and school). It is important to remember that sometimes in homes that do not have a lot of structure, the parents can sometimes not realize that the patient's attention span is poor or that the child is unusually hyperactive or impulsive. In such cases, it is critical to contact other observers besides the school (day cares, after-school programs, baby-sitters) to confirm the pervasiveness of the ADHD symptoms. The incidence is 3% to 5% of prepubertal children, and boys are affected with the hyperactive-impulsive type more often than girls. The inattentive type is characterized by failure to pay attention to details, failure to focus attention when performing tasks, failure to follow through with instructions, impaired ability to organize tasks, misplacing items, becoming easily distracted by external stimuli, and forgetfulness during the performance of daily activities. Hyperactivity is manifested by increased fidgeting of the hands and feet, inability to stay seated in a classroom setting, being unduly noisy during playtime activities, and a persistent pattern of increased motor activity not significantly modified by social context. Impulsivity is characterized by the blurting out of answers, difficulty waiting in line or for one's turn, interrupting, and talking excessively without an appropriate response to a given social situation.

Although the exact etiology of ADHD is not yet clear, the body of evidence suggests it is a disorder involving decreased dopaminergic and noradrenergic tracts in several areas of the prefrontal cortex. The dorsal anterior cingulate gyrus is involved in selecting what an individual focuses on while the dorsolateral prefrontal cortex is involved with sustaining attention on a topic as well as various executive functions. Both appear involved in ADHD. Impairment in the prefrontal motor cortex appears to account for the hyperactivity. Decreased activity in the orbitofrontal cortex is involved with impulsive actions. The symptom presentation of any particular child with ADHD will be dependent on the relative impairment in each of these portions of the prefrontal cortex.

DIFFERENTIAL DIAGNOSIS

The presence of oppositional defiant disorder (ODD) or conduct disorder in a child or youth with ADHD is relatively common. It is important to remember that medication can do only three things: (1) help the child sit still—if the child wants to sit still, (2) help the child to focus his or her attention—if the child wants to pay attention, and (3) help the child to think before he or she acts—but will not affect whether the child makes a good decision or not. Failing to recognize the presence of ODD or conduct disorder in a child with ADHD results in many physicians trying to medicate away purposeful disruptive behavior.

Patients with ADHD often have learning disabilities, and a thorough evaluation should be conducted for every child suspected of having this disorder once optimal treatment of ADHD symptoms has occurred. Patients with bipolar disorder, early onset, can have symptoms of restlessness and distractibility, but their symptoms also have an affective component. **Lead intoxication** can lead to hyperactivity, and the presence of this disorder should be ruled out by determining the lead level in the blood of the child at the initial evaluation.

Patients with petit mal seizures may report poor attention. However, with careful questioning, clinicians can usually get a history of brief periods where the patient is unaware of what is happening around him- or herself, often describing brief periods when there is lost time (absences). In the case of inattentive ADHD, patients will report having their minds occupied with something else during such periods. Parents and teacher should be asked about staring spells when the child is unresponsive even when directly spoken to face-to-face, suggesting petit mal seizures. If there are still questions regarding petit mal seizures after taking a history, an electroencephalogram (EEG) should be obtained.

ADHD, especially if occurring with oppositional defiant disorder, may be mistaken for childhood bipolar disorder. See Case 8 for a full discussion of this issue.

TREATMENT

Approximately 70% to 80% of all children with ADHD will respond to stimulant medications, either methylphenidate or amphetamine preparations. Adverse effects typically include decreased appetite (sometimes with subsequent slowed growth rate), initial insomnia, irritability, dysphoria, and headache. Occasionally, the stimulants are associated with the development of **tics** or worsening of tics in those with tic disorders. Stimulants have, as a group, a very rapid onset of action, and typically their therapeutic effects wear off by the end of the day.

Atomoxetine is a potent selective inhibitor of the presynaptic norepinephrine transporter and is an effective alternative to the stimulants in controlling ADHD symptoms. It is not a stimulant or a controlled substance. It tends to have a more gradual onset of action over a period of 2 to 3 weeks and, once working, seems to have a 24-hour length of action. Many patients sleep well with the medication and occasionally complain of sedation. Atomoxetine is not likely to cause tics.

Both stimulants and atomoxetine can decrease the patient's appetite, so monitoring height and weight for a medication-related reduction in growth rate is essential. Clonidine and guanfacine improve sleep and appetite while impacting ADHD symptoms and can be used together with a stimulant or as monotherapy.

Bupropion and imipramine have studies indicating efficacy in the treatment of ADHD. **In the case of imipramine, blood levels and electrocardiograms (ECGs) should be followed because of QT prolongation.** Bupropion is contraindicated in individuals with seizure disorder. Bupropion can also exacerbate tics because of its dopaminergic action.

Behavioral parent training and classroom behavior modification are often effective approaches, whereas the efficacy of other types of psychotherapy remains to be convincingly demonstrated.

> ## CASE CORRELATION
>
> - See also Case 8 and Case 18. ADHD and anxiety disorders both present
>   with symptoms of inattention, but those with ADHD are inattentive because
>   of their attraction to external stimuli, or interest and focus on pleasurable
>   behaviors, while those with anxiety are internally focused, ruminative, and
>   worried. Those with bipolar disorder might have increased psychomotor
>   activity, poor concentration, and increased impulsivity, but they will also have
>   elevated mood, grandiosity, and a decreased need for sleep.

COMPREHENSION QUESTIONS

3.1 A 9-year-old boy is referred to a psychiatrist because of poor school performance. He has been tested for learning disabilities but none are present, and
has an IQ in the high normal range. The teacher reports that it is hard to hold
his attention. In addition, he appears hyperactive and fidgety at school, which
disrupts the class. However, he does not purposefully go out of his way to
disobey the teacher. His parents have noticed no difficulties at home, but his
soccer coach has noticed attention problems during practice, and his Sunday
school teacher has trouble teaching him because of distractibility. Which of the
following is the most likely diagnosis for this patient?

A. ADHD, combined type

B. ADHD, predominantly hyperactive type

C. ADHD, predominantly inattentive type

D. Oppositional defiant disorder

E. No diagnosis, because the ADHD symptoms must be reported in the
home

3.2 A 6-year-old boy with an early, ongoing history of distractibility, hyperactivity,
and impulsivity is diagnosed with ADHD. He is treated with methylphenidate. Three weeks later he is brought in, and his inattention and hyperactivity
are much better. The mother also notes that he has a small bald spot from
where he has begun repeatedly rubbing his head. You periodically observe him
to suddenly raise his hand to the spot, rub back and forth once, and put his
hand down. There is no rash but the area is hairless. The most likely diagnosis
is which of the following?

A. Alopecia secondary to stimulant

B. Drug allergy with contact dermatitis

C. Stimulant-induced complex motor tic

D. Scabies

E. Attention-seeking behavior

3.3 Atomoxetine is a relatively new drug used for the treatment of ADHD. Which of the following represents the advantage of using atomoxetine over Ritalin?

A. Atomoxetine has a shorter half-life.

B. Atomoxetine is available in a generic form that is less costly than Ritalin.

C. Atomoxetine appears to have less of a potential for abuse than does Ritalin.

D. Atomoxetine's effects begin working immediately to reduce symptoms of ADHD.

E. Atomoxetine can be taken on an empty stomach.

ANSWERS

3.1 **A.** Attention deficit disorder, combined type. The diagnostic criteria for ADHD require that the symptoms be present in more than one setting, usually at home and at school. However, this child seems to have evidence of symptoms observed at school, church, and soccer. The child has prominent distractibility and hyperactivity.

3.2 **C.** This is a classic complex motor tic. Alopecia is spontaneous hair loss and an unlikely side effect of a stimulant. This is not the presentation of scabies or a drug allergy. Tics are stereotyped movements as compared to attention-seeking behavior which tends to be more diverse in the motor movements. Atomoxetine will not promote tics, while methylphenidate and amphetamine salts will do so. Bupropion can stimulate dopamine and worsen tics as well.

3.3 **C.** Atomoxetine appears to have a lower potential for abuse than Ritalin. Initial use can produce a feeling of sleepiness and grogginess, and the drug does not appear to exhibit its effects for up to 3 weeks. It is not recommended to take atomoxetine on an empty stomach, as side effects of the drug include nausea and vomiting. Atomoxetine is not currently available in a generic form. Advantages of this drug are that it affords 24-hour control of ADHD symptoms (ie, it has a longer half-life than Ritalin) and it has less potential for abuse.

CLINICAL PEARLS

▶ There are three primary subtypes of ADHD (inattentive type, hyperactive-impulsive type, and combined type), all of which have different presentations.

▶ Use of a stimulant medication or atomoxetine is probably the best medication for children with this disorder.

REFERENCES

American Academy of Child and Adolescent Psychiatry. Practice parameter for the assessment and treatment of children and adolescents with attention deficit/hyperactivity disorder. *J Am Acad Child Adolesc Psychiatry*. 2007;46(7):894-921.

Sadock BJ, Sadock VA, Ruiz P. *Kaplan and Sadock's Synopsis of Psychiatry: Behavioral Sciences/Clinical Psychiatry*. 11th ed. Baltimore, MD: Lippincott Williams & Wilkins; 2014.

Stahl SM. Attention deficit hyperactivity disorder and its treatment. *Stahl's Essential Psychopharmacology*. 4th ed. New York, NY: Cambridge University Press; 2013:471-502.

A 7-year-old boy in second grade is brought to a pediatrician by his parents for an evaluation of his eyes. They state that he blinks them repeatedly, and that this behavior seems to be worsening. They first noticed it a year or more ago, but it became very obvious in the past several weeks. They note that their son cannot control the blinking, and that it appears worse at some times of the day compared to others. In the past year, he has also had a twitch of his neck for 2 months and then a shrug of his shoulders for 3 months. The boy's teacher reports that other children tease him because of his rapid eye blinking. The pediatrician observes that in addition to blinking, the child seems to clear his throat frequently, although his nose and throat appear normal on physical examination. The parents report that this behavior occurs several times daily too. The patient is doing well at school, although he sometimes has trouble completing his homework. The patient's father has a history of obsessive-compulsive disorder.

▶ What is the most likely diagnosis?
▶ What is the best therapy for this condition?

ANSWERS TO CASE 4:

Tourette Disorder

Summary: A 7-year-old boy presents to a pediatrician with uncontrollable blinking, which has worsened over the past several weeks. The blinking is worse at some times than at others, and the boy is teased at school because of it. In the past year, he has also had a twitch of his neck for 2 months and then a shrug of his shoulders for 3 months. The child also clears his throat repeatedly, although nothing physically wrong can be found. He is doing well at school although he sometimes has trouble completing his homework. The patient has a paternal history of obsessive-compulsive disorder.

- **Most likely diagnosis:** Tourette disorder.

- **Best treatment:** There is debate as to if the first-line treatment should be an alpha-adrenergic medication such as clonidine or guanfacine as opposed to the atypical antipsychotics. Surveys of actual practice show Risperdal, clonidine, and aripiprazole to be the most commonly utilized medications.

ANALYSIS

Objectives

1. Recognize Tourette disorder in a patient (Table 4–1 for diagnostic criteria).

2. Describe the basic evaluation and treatment of this disorder.

Considerations

A 7-year-old boy currently shows signs of a motor tic in the form of eye blinking. He has had other motor tics as well. These behaviors have been present to some degree for more than a year and have recently worsened. The tics affect how other children at school interact with him. He also exhibits a vocal tic in the form of throat clearing, which has been present for a long period of time. This combination of multiple motor and vocal tics occurring for **at least 1 year** is consistent with Tourette disorder. There is a genetic predisposition to this disease, probably via autosomal dominant inheritance. There are also relationships among Tourette disorder, obsessive-compulsive disorder (OCD), and attention deficit disorder. While haloperidol and pimozide are the only medications with FDA approval to treat Tourette's, today most clinicians treat with alpha-adrenergic agonists or atypical antipsychotics

Table 4–1 • DIAGNOSTIC CRITERIA FOR TOURETTE DISORDER
Presence of both multiple motor and one or more vocal tics during the course of the illness but not necessarily at the same time.
Tics have been occurring for a period of at least a year and may wax and wane in frequency.
Onset must be before 18 years of age.
The disorder must not be due to a substance or a general medical condition.

before utilizing these two agents. This is secondary to up to one-third of patients on haloperidol experiencing extrapyramidal side effects and the need to monitor for cardiovascular side effects with pimozide, which may cause prolongation of the QTc interval and reports of sudden deaths in doses above 10 mg/d. It is important to note that symptoms such as these in a child could also be related to an environmental allergen, and this should be thoroughly worked up before diagnosing Tourette disorder and beginning treatment. In *DSM-5*, Tourette disorder and other tic disorders have been reclassified as a neurodevelopmental disorder.

APPROACH TO:

Tourette Disorders

DEFINITIONS

ATHETOID MOVEMENTS: Slow, irregular, writhing movements.

CHOREIFORM MOVEMENTS: Dancing, random, irregular, nonrepetitive movements.

COPROLALIA: Vocal tic involving the involuntary vocalization of obscenities.

DYSTONIC MOVEMENTS: Slower than choreiform movements, these are twisting motions interspersed with prolonged states of muscular tension.

HEMIBALLISTIC MOVEMENTS: Intermittent, coarse, large-amplitude, unilateral movements of the limbs.

MYOCLONIC MOVEMENTS: Brief, shock-like muscle contractions.

TIC: A sudden, rapid, recurrent, nonrhythmic, stereotyped motor movement or vocalization.

CLINICAL APPROACH

The lifetime prevalence of Tourette disorder is approximately 4 to 5 per 10,000 in the general population, and it tends to be more common in boys. The motor component (eye blinking, shoulder shrugging, neck jerking) usually emerges by 7 years of age, and the vocal component (grunting, sniffing, snorting, using obscene words) by 11 years of age. Epidemiologic studies involving twins indicate a strong genetic etiology, probably via autosomal dominant inheritance. There is a strong relationship between Tourette disorder, OCD, and ADHD, and these disorders run in families. Studies of the causes of tics have centered on the basal ganglia and substantia nigra. Neuropathological studies have suggested imbalances in the input of gamma-aminobutyric acid (GABA) (decreased) and dopamine (increased) in the caudate nucleus.

DIFFERENTIAL DIAGNOSIS

Tic disorders must be differentiated from general medical conditions that can cause abnormal movements. Involuntary movements such as myoclonus, athetosis, dystonias, and hemiballismus can be seen in such diseases as Huntington chorea, Wilson disease, and stroke. The long-term use of a typical antipsychotic such as haloperidol can cause tardive dyskinesia, another involuntary movement disorder. The presence of a family history of these disorders, findings on a physical examination, or a history of long-term use of antipsychotic medication can help rule out these conditions. Children who are treated with or abuse stimulants may develop tics. In such cases stopping the stimulant will often result in a gradual fading of the tics. ADHD in such cases can be treated with atomoxetine or an alpha-adrenergic agonist.

It has long been known that beta-hemolytic streptococci can cause an autoimmune reaction called rheumatic fever that can impact joints, the heart, and even the central nervous system (CNS) (producing Sydenham chorea). Swedo led a group that proposed that some children with a winter-spring seasonal worsening of their tics have a disorder called **pediatric autoimmune neuropsychiatric disorder associated with streptococcal infection (PANDAS).** Studies have shown that OCD, Tourette disorder, and tics are more common in children who have had a streptococcal infection within the last 3 months and much more common in those with multiple streptococcal infections within the last 12 months.

Tics must be differentiated from compulsions seen in OCD. Compulsions are typically fairly complex behaviors performed to ward off the anxiety of an obsession or according to a rigid set of behavioral rules. Certain vocal and motor tics such as barking, coprolalia, or echolalia must be distinguished from the psychotic behavior seen in schizophrenia. However, in the latter case patients have other findings congruent with psychosis, such as hallucinations or delusions. Transient tic disorders last at least 4 weeks but for no longer than 1 year. Patients with a chronic motor or vocal tic disorder can have it for more than 1 year, but there is an absence of multiple motor tics and/or motor and vocal tics occurring simultaneously.

TREATMENT

The treatment of Tourette disorder involves **both somatic therapies and psychotherapies.** In children, tics are often worsened or triggered by anxiety-producing events. Children and families can be taught to reduce the manifested anxiety at home, which in turn can help reduce the triggers for tics. Habit reversal training has the strongest empirical evidence of the psychotherapies. It involves training the child to become aware of the aversive sensation or buildup of tension called a premonitory urge that is relieved by the tics. They are then helped to build a competing response to that urge without engaging in tic behavior along with developing ways of getting social support. Many mild to moderate tics respond to behavioral interventions without the need to add medication. Medication should be reserved for patient with moderate to severe tics where there is significant impairment in the quality of life. Some clinicians believe that alpha-adrenergic agonists such as clonidine and guanfacine should be first-line treatments because of their efficacy and favorable side-effect profile. Some studies have indicated that patients with ADHD and Tourette disorder have a stronger response to these medications than those with pure tic disorder. Clonidine is an alpha-adrenergic agonist that is believed to activate presynaptic autoreceptors in the locus ceruleus to reduce norepinephrine release that may reduce tics. Guanfacine binds to postsynaptic prefrontal alpha-adrenergic cortical receptors to enhance functioning in the prefrontal cortex. Because both drugs can reduce the incidence of tics and can also be used in attention deficit hyperactivity disorder (ADHD) to improve impulsivity, attention, and working memory in children, this makes them possible choices for treating ADHD symptoms in children who have tics. In practice most clinicians utilize the atypical antipsychotics which block dopamine and serotonin receptors, decreasing input from the substantia nigra and ventral tegmentum to the basal ganglia. Risperidone has been the most studied and is effective in doses from 1 to 3.5 mg/d with weight gain, lipid abnormalities, and sedation as the most common side effects. If an atypical antipsychotic is ineffective, consideration can be given to haloperidol or pimozide. These first-generation antipsychotic medications have a greater risk for neurological side effects including dystonias and tardive dyskinesia as well as ECG changes (especially pimozide).

CASE CORRELATION

- See also Case 22 and Case 59. As compared to Tourette disorder, OCD behaviors will more likely include a cognitively-based drive ("I need to avoid contamination with germs") and a particular action that will decrease the anxiety related to the drive ("I need to wash a certain number of times or in a certain order to be clean"). Dystonias are the result of simultaneous contractions of both agonist and antagonist muscles resulting in a distorted posture or movement.

COMPREHENSION QUESTIONS

4.1 When examining a patient with possible Tourette disorder, you should inquire carefully about a family history of which of the following disorders?

A. Obsessive-compulsive disorder

B. Sleep terror disorder

C. Primary insomnia

D. Developmental disability

E. Parkinson disease

4.2 A 9-year-old child presents with a history of motor and vocal tics with obsessive-compulsive symptoms that are worse in the winter and early spring months. Which of the following pathologies would be most important to rule out before starting treatment of Tourette disorder?

A. Streptococcal infection

B. Environmental allergies

C. Autism

D. Marijuana abuse

E. Rett disorder

4.3 A patient's parents have been searching on the Internet for information about Tourette disorder and its treatment. They have a concern about tardive dyskinesia and would like to have the physician prescribe a medication which will minimize that risk. Which of the following medications, given the parents' concern, is the best choice for this patient?

    A. Pimozide

    B. Clonidine

    C. Risperidone (Risperdal)

    D. Haloperidol

    E. Clozapine (Clozaril)

4.4 A patient with ADHD is treated with methylphenidate during the school year. After several months of treatment, his teachers and parents note that he has developed both motor and vocal tics. What should be the first course of action for these symptoms?

    A. Begin treatment with haloperidol.

    B. Discontinue the use of methylphenidate.

    C. Discontinue the use of methylphenidate and switch medication to atomoxetine.

    D. Reduce the dose of methylphenidate.

    E. Administer an anticonvulsant.

ANSWERS

4.1 **A.** Obsessive-compulsive disorder is far more common in families of patients with Tourette disorder than in the general population. Fifty percent of patients with Tourette disorder have significant obsessive-compulsive symptoms.

4.2 **A.** Investigating for a possible case of PANDAS is important in this child, and rapid treatment of streptococcal infections and prevention of reinfection may impact the clinical course of such children.

4.3 **B.** Clonidine is an alpha-2 agonist that does not cause tardive dyskinesia as a side effect. It is moderately effective in the treatment of vocal and motor tics, although not as effective as some antipsychotics. All the other agents are antipsychotic medications, and as such, have a risk of tardive dyskinesia associated with their use. Haloperidol, a typical antipsychotic, has the highest risk of tardive dyskinesia of the group, though tardive dyskinesia is a potential complication seen with all antipsychotic medications.

4.4 **C.** The development of tics as a side effect of stimulant medication is relatively common. While these tics diminish in severity or cease when the dose is reduced, reduction of dose often results in an increase of ADHD symptoms. Because atomoxetine is quite effective for treating ADHD without stimulating tics, a trial on atomoxetine should be considered. If ADHD symptoms and/or tics continue on atomoxetine, then addition of clonidine or guanfacine should be considered.

CLINICAL PEARLS

▶ A diagnosis of Tourette disorder requires both vocal and multiple motor tics and a duration of 1 year.

▶ Vocal tics can consist not only of words but also throat clearing, grunting, and squeaking.

▶ Motor tics can involve complicated movements such as rubbing hair, picking scabs, or other repetitive and intricate hand or arm movements.

REFERENCES

Murphy TK, Lewin AB, Storch EA, Stock S, AACAP Committee on Quality Issues. Practice parameter for the assessment and treatment of children and adolescents with tic disorders. *J Am Acad Child Adolesc Psychiatry*. 2013;52(12);1341-1359.

Sadock BJ, Sadock VA, Ruiz P. *Kaplan and Sadock's Synopsis of Psychiatry: Behavioral Sciences/Clinical Psychiatry*. 11th ed. Baltimore, MD: Lippincott Williams & Wilkins; 2014.

Swain JE, Scahill L, Lombroso PJ, King RA, Leckman JF. Tourette syndrome and tic disorders: a decade of progress. *J Am Acad Child Adolesc Psychiatry*. 2007;46(8):947-968.

A 15-year-old adolescent girl is brought to your office by her family after a recent hospitalization for a suicide attempt. She made this attempt shortly after a party she attended the previous weekend. At this party, she reportedly argued with her best friend and left very angry. Her history at admission shows a several-month history of irritability, worsening performance in school, poor sleep, anhedonia, anergia, and isolation from her family and friends. Her discharge summary has an admitting diagnosis of major depression for which she was started on fluoxetine (Prozac). She sees you 2 weeks after her 3-day hospitalization and is quite cheery, energetic, and happy. She reports no problems and dismisses her earlier suicide attempt as a childish act to get attention. She reports that the staff at the hospital were absolutely wonderful and helped her solve all her problems. She says that she was so impressed with them that she has decided to go into psychiatry herself so she can help others. Later, while meeting with the parents, they report that at home she is sleeping well and appears in a good mood. Nevertheless, they are concerned because they also report that she is worried about whether there were cameras in the doctor's office that were recording her. She also reports that she believes she is being stalked by several of the boys at her school.

▶ What is the most likely diagnosis?
▶ What is the best therapy for this condition?
▶ Should this patient be hospitalized?

ANSWERS TO CASE 5:
Schizoaffective Disorder

Summary: This is a 15-year-old girl who has a diagnosis and evidence of major depression with a suicide attempt. She is treated for this and seems to respond well. The parents, however, note that she has some evidence of paranoia that is still present after the mood symptoms have resolved.

- **Most likely diagnosis:** Schizoaffective disorder (Table 5–1).

- **Best therapy:** An antipsychotic agent (such as haloperidol or risperidone) should be tried initially. If it is ineffective alone, antidepressants (a selective serotonin reuptake inhibitor [SSRI] is generally tried first) should also be administered.

- **Is hospitalization needed:** No. The patient is currently not a danger to herself or others and appears to be able to care for herself. This disorder as presented here should be treated in an outpatient setting unless the suicidal ideation returns and/or worsens.

ANALYSIS
Objectives

1. Recognize schizoaffective disorder in a patient and diagnose it accurately.

2. Know that the disease has two subtypes: depressive and bipolar.

3. Know the recommended pharmacologic treatment for this disorder.

4. Know the indications for hospitalization of a patient with this disorder.

Considerations

This patient has a several-month history of what sounds like mood (depressive) symptoms which seem to have remitted with fluoxetine. However, there is evidence of a paranoid delusion (believing there are cameras in the doctor's office recording her) that persists without mood symptoms. The **psychotic episodes occur during the mood episodes,** but the mood symptoms do not always occur during the psychotic

Table 5–1 • DIAGNOSTIC CRITERIA FOR SCHIZOAFFECTIVE DISORDER
Patients must exhibit psychotic symptoms consonant with the acute phase of schizophrenia.
Psychotic symptoms are accompanied by prominent mood symptoms (mania or depression) during part of the illness.
At other points in the illness, the psychotic symptoms are unopposed; that is, no mood symptoms are present. Periods of illness in which there are only psychotic symptoms, and no mood symptoms, must last for at least 2 wk.
The disorder cannot be caused by a substance or by another medical condition.

episodes, which is the key to the diagnosis. Although the patient was not asked about manic symptoms, the presence of such symptoms is a crucial element in the patient's history because it changes the subtype of schizoaffective disorder from depressive type to bipolar type and in turn affects the pharmacologic treatment choices. Without these symptoms, the patient's disorder would be characterized as depressive type (a mood stabilizer such as valproic acid might be used in a patient with the bipolar type of schizoaffective disorder.). Some studies have demonstrated a more substantial degree of general psychopathology in younger patients with schizoaffective disorder as compared to adults.

Studies have also shown brain matter abnormalities in patients with schizophrenia and schizoaffective disorder. One study confirmed, through MRI, the presence of white matter pathology early in the course of these illnesses. These data support the hypotheses of frontotemporal dysfunction and abnormalities in left-hemisphere lateralization in the pathophysiology of these illnesses.

DSM-5 Considerations: The diagnostic criteria are substantially the same. However, the specifiers used in *DSM-IV* (primary manic type or primary depressive type) have been removed.

APPROACH TO:
Schizoaffective Disorder

DEFINITIONS

ANERGIA: Lack of energy.

ANHEDONIA: Lack of interest in one's usual pleasure-seeking activities, such as hobbies.

TANGENTIAL SPEECH (TANGENTIALITY): A disorder of thought process in which one's thoughts "take off on a tangent" from the initial question or line of thought and do not return to the original line of thinking.

CLINICAL APPROACH

Differential Diagnosis

The key to developing a differential diagnosis for schizoaffective disorder is to carefully examine the longitudinal functioning of patients by reviewing their histories (provided by the patients and ideally by significant others). Periods of psychosis, and psychosis and mood symptoms (mania and/or depression), must be carefully teased out over a time period of years if possible. Conditions causing substance-induced mood disorder (which can be difficult to differentiate from schizoaffective disorder) include cocaine or amphetamine intoxication (manic symptoms), cocaine withdrawal (depressive symptoms), and the effects of a host of prescribed medications including steroids and antiparkinsonian medications. The symptoms of schizophrenia can appear similar, but the mood symptoms sometimes present in that disorder are generally transient and are brief in relation to the total length of the illness. Patients with bipolar disorder, mania, generally have had mood symptoms (euphoria, irritability) predating development of the psychoses, as have patients with major depression with psychotic features (a depressed mood predating the onset of psychosis).

TREATMENT

Patients with schizoaffective disorder generally respond to antipsychotic agents and often require long-term therapy. Although haloperidol (Haldol) and typical antipsychotics were once the treatments of choice (indeed, the only options available), **newer atypical** (second-generation) **antipsychotics** are now used far more frequently because of their more benign side-effect profile. These medications are not known to cause tardive dyskinesia, most extrapyramidal symptoms, or neuroleptic malignant syndrome. They are likely well tolerated because they also produce fewer anticholinergic side effects. However, there is little good evidence that second-generation antipsychotics are better than first generation in terms of efficacy. Both typical and atypical antipsychotic medications have approximately the same duration of action, making once or twice per day dosing feasible in both cases.

Mood stabilizers such as lithium, carbamazepine, and valproic acid should be administered to patients with schizoaffective disorder who exhibit manic symptoms. It is sometimes helpful to combine an antidepressant and an antipsychotic for patients with schizoaffective disorder with a depressed mood. However, such patients should be treated with an antidepressant in addition to their antipsychotic **only** if the antipsychotic alone does not ameliorate the mood symptoms. Other treatment modalities can include hospitalization, particularly when patients are psychotic and unable to care for themselves or suicidal. Psychosocial rehabilitation, such as is used in the treatment of schizophrenia, is often indicated as well because these patients can suffer from the same social isolation, apathy, and disturbed interpersonal relationships that schizophrenics do, although usually not with the same degree of severity.

Transcranial magnetic stimulation (TMS) has more recently shown some utility in the management of psychotic symptoms in both schizophrenic and schizoaffective patients. However, this treatment is still considered experimental and is not yet frequently used.

CASE CORRELATION

- See also Case 6 and Case 8. As opposed to schizophrenia and bipolar disorder with psychotic symptoms, schizoaffective disorder patients must meet criteria for a major mood episode for the majority of the illness, *and* have delusions or hallucinations for 2 or more weeks in the absence of a major mood episode. Essentially, over the lifetime of the illness, the patient must present with just psychotic symptoms (no mood symptoms) for at least some of the disorder, but at other times, have both a mood and psychotic component running concurrently.

COMPREHENSION QUESTIONS

5.1 A 17-year-old adolescent girl is seen in your office after her friends noticed some strange behavior. The patient reports to you that in addition to some long-term depression issues, she has begun to experience some other disturbing events. She reports that over the last 2 months she has been hearing voices—both at work and at home—of people who she does not think are there. She doesn't recognize these voices. Sometimes they just give a dialogue of what she is doing, but more disturbing to her is when they start saying horrible things about her and tell her to do things she does not want to do. You start her on olanzapine and when she returns in 1 week the voices have been gone entirely for 2 or 3 days. However, she continues to experience severe mood symptoms. Her Hamilton Depression rating scale score places her in the moderate to severe range for depression. Which of the following should you do next?

A. Inform the patient that these symptoms are the negative symptoms common to the disorder.

B. Refer the patient for supportive psychotherapy.

C. Treat the patient with fluoxetine (an SSRI).

D. Increase the dose of the antipsychotic.

E. Add a mood stabilizer to the regimen.

5.2 The above patient returns to the office in 1 week and has not improved. In fact, she seems to have worsened. Which of the following might be your best next step?

A. Increase the olanzapine.

B. Add another neuroleptic.

C. Add a mood stabilizer.

D. Add an antidepressant.

E. Consider ordering a urine or serum toxicology for substances of abuse.

5.3 A 28-year-old man is brought to a psychiatrist complaining that he has been hearing voices for the past several weeks. He says that he also heard these voices 3 years ago. He notes that his mood is "depressed" and rates it 3 on a scale of 1 to 10 (with 10 being the best he has ever felt). He does not recall if his mood was depressed the last time he had psychotic symptoms. Which of the following actions should the physician take next?

A. Obtain more detailed information about the time course of the psychotic symptoms and the mood symptoms.

B. Treat the patient with an antipsychotic agent.

C. Treat the patient with an antidepressant medication.

D. Request a urine toxicology screening.

E. Refer the patient to supportive psychotherapy.

5.4 A 40-year-old man with schizoaffective disorder has been hospitalized in an inpatient psychiatry unit for the third time in the last 5 years. During each episode, he becomes noncompliant in taking his medications, develops manic symptoms and auditory hallucinations, and then becomes violent. In the inpatient unit, he physically threatens other patients and staff and is generally agitated. He is put in isolation to help quiet him. The patient is prescribed a mood stabilizer. Which of the following medications might also help relieve this patient's acute agitation?

A. Buspirone

B. Fluoxetine

C. Chloral hydrate

D. Risperidone

E. Benztropine

ANSWERS

5.1 **C.** Although data are not clear as to the efficacy of administering antidepressants to patients with schizoaffective disorder (and depressive symptoms), the continued presence of depressive symptoms makes this treatment worth trying.

5.2 **E.** The possibility of substance use in any psychotic young person is very high. A screening laboratory should always be considered especially in resistant or worsening cases. A number of illicit drugs could cause hallucinations and they will not clear up until the substance use has been addressed.

5.3 **A.** The time course of the mood symptoms and psychotic symptoms determines the treatment of the patient because the diagnosis is likely schizoaffective disorder versus major depression (with psychosis). Although the patient should undergo a urine toxicology screening, this should not be done until a complete history is obtained so that further targeting of laboratory testing can be accomplished.

5.4 **D.** Atypical neuroleptics such as risperidone or quetiapine are shown to be effective in managing manic symptoms especially in the acute state while mood stabilizers reach therapeutic levels.

CLINICAL PEARLS

► Unlike patients with schizophrenia, patients with schizoaffective disorder have mood symptoms that occur during significant portions of their illness.

► Once a very clear longitudinal history of symptoms and functioning is obtained, it is often possible to diagnose either a bipolar illness or schizophrenia in a patient with schizoaffective disorder.

► Patients with schizoaffective disorder and manic mood symptoms should be treated with a mood stabilizer and an antipsychotic. Patients with schizoaffective disorder and depressive mood symptoms should be treated with an antipsychotic alone; if this is not effective, an antidepressant should also be used.

► Younger patients with schizoaffective disorder may exhibit more severe symptomatology than adult patients.

REFERENCES

American Psychiatric Association. *Diagnostic and Statistical Manual of Mental Disorders.* 5th ed. Washington, DC: American Psychiatric Publishing; 2013.

Black BW, Andreasen NC. *Introductory Textbook of Psychiatry.* 6th ed. Washington, DC: American Psychiatric Publishing; 2014:164-170, 551-570.

Kindler J, Homan P, Flury R, Strik W, Dierks T, Hubl D. Theta burst transcranial magnetic stimulation for the treatment of auditory verbal hallucinations: results of a randomized controlled study. *Psychiatry Res.* August 30, 2013;209(1):114-117. doi: 10.1016/j.psychres.2013.03.029. Epub May 4, 2013.

Sadock BJ, Sadock VA, Ruiz P. *Kaplan and Sadock's Synopsis of Psychiatry: Behavioral Sciences/Clinical Psychiatry.* 11th ed. Baltimore, MD: Lippincott Williams & Wilkins; 2014.

A 26 year-old man presents to the emergency department (ED) in handcuffs, escorted by two policemen for an evaluation "for causing a ruckus outside the grocery store and threatening store customers." The patient refuses to engage in much of the interview. He yells, "Let me go or they are going to get me! They have been after me for years! You can't let them get me!" He denies depressed mood, suicidal ideation (SI), homicidal ideation (HI), auditory or visual hallucinations, and prior psychiatric or medical problems. He denies taking prescription medications or illicit drugs. In response to marijuana use, he retorts, "it's legal now." He prematurely ends the interview, refusing to answer any further questions because "they can hear us." The patient refuses to provide any contacts from which to gather collateral information.

On mental status examination, the patient appears disheveled and dirty. He acts suspicious and guarded, avoiding eye contact. His speech is difficult to follow, and he often turns his head away and mumbles to himself. The patient's affect appears blunted. He looks around abruptly several times and appears to be responding to internal stimuli.

▶ What conditions need to be ruled out before a psychiatric diagnosis can be made?
▶ Does this patient require psychiatric hospitalization?

ANSWERS TO CASE 6:

Schizophrenia

Summary: A 26-year-old man with no known psychiatric or medical history is brought to the emergency department by the police after exhibiting bizarre and threatening behavior. He does not endorse SI or HI. His substance abuse history is positive only for marijuana. The patient's mental status examination reveals poor hygiene, paranoid behavior, and a disorganized thought process. His statements demonstrate persecutory delusions, and he appears distracted by internal stimuli.

- **What conditions are important to rule out before a psychiatric diagnosis can be made?** Substance intoxication or withdrawal, substance or medication-induced psychotic disorder, and psychotic disorder due to another medical condition must be ruled out before idiopathic (ie, primary psychiatric) diagnoses can be considered.

- **Should this patient be hospitalized?** Yes. The patient poses a potential danger to himself and others. He exhibits paranoid behavior and objectively appears to be experiencing hallucinations. His ability to care for himself seems compromised. This may be an episode of first break psychosis, thus necessitating a thorough workup, psychoeducation, and stabilization on appropriate medication.

ANALYSIS

Objectives

1. Understand the diagnostic criteria for schizophrenia.

2. Understand which conditions should be excluded prior to making a diagnosis of schizophrenia.

3. Understand the criteria for involuntary psychiatric admission and recognize when a patient warrants admission.

Considerations

This case captures the presentation of a young man suffering from first break psychosis. He exhibits the two main diagnostic criteria for schizophrenia: **delusions** (persecutory) and **hallucinations (Table 6–1).** Although he does not explicitly endorse either of these symptoms, they are evident from his behavior. It appears that his symptoms have been present for at least 6 months. ("They have been after me for years.") He ~~de~~nies history of psychiatric and medical problems, although these would need to be ~~furth~~er investigated by physical examination, laboratory workup, and more history ~~of th~~e patient and collateral sources. Like many patients with psychotic symptoms, ~~he is guard~~ed and not forthcoming with information. As rapport builds, he may feel ~~comfortable r~~evealing more. In the ED setting, the clinician should focus on assessing ~~the safety of the~~ patient and those around him. If the patient is **at risk of harming him-** ~~self or others~~ **or unable to care for himself, a psychiatric admission is warranted.**

Table 6–1 • DIAGNOSTIC CRITERIA FOR SCHIZOPHRENIA
At least two of the following symptoms of psychosis have been present for 1 mo: • Delusions • Hallucinations • Disorganized speech • Disorganized or catatonic behavior • Negative symptoms
There has to be significant social and/or occupational dysfunction.
Some symptoms are required to be present for at least 6 mo; they can include only negative symptoms or less intense positive symptoms.
Both schizoaffective disorder and mood disorder with psychotic features need to be ruled out.
A substance (either of abuse or medication) or another medical condition cannot cause the symptoms.

APPROACH TO:
Schizophrenia

DEFINITIONS

ACTIVE-PHASE OF SCHIZOPHRENIA: Phase of schizophrenia characterized by the presence of positive and negative symptoms.

CATATONIA: A neuropsychiatric syndrome occurring in psychiatric or medical disorders that presents with three or more psychomotor symptoms, including stupor, catalepsy, waxy flexibility, mutism, negativism, posturing, grimacing, mannerism, stereotypy, agitation, echopraxia, or echolalia.

DELUSIONS: Fixed, false beliefs which lack cultural sanctioning.

DISORGANIZED SPEECH: The expression of thoughts lacking logical connections between the ideas (*loose associations*) or between the individual words (*word salad*).

HALLUCINATIONS: False perceptions in any sensory modality without an external stimulus. Auditory hallucinations (AHs) are most common in schizophrenia spectrum disorders, often in the form of voices.

IDEAS OF REFERENCE: Misinterpretation of aspects of the external environment as having particular significance for the individual. For example, a patient may think that the television or radio station has a special message specifically directed at him.

NEGATIVE SYMPTOMS OF SCHIZOPHRENIA: Symptoms that are characterized by the lack of emotional responses and thought processes present in the general population, that is, decreased expression of emotions, flattening of affect, alogia (decreased spontaneous speech), and avolition (decreased motivation).

POSITIVE SYMPTOMS OF SCHIZOPHRENIA: Symptoms experienced b those with psychotic disorders that are not experienced by most people in the ge eral population. These include hallucinations, delusions, ideas of reference, grossly disorganized speech or behavior.

CLINICAL APPROACH

Schizophrenia encompasses a heterogeneous constellation of symptoms with core features of impaired reality testing, perceptual disturbances, disorganized thought process, and deterioration in social relatedness. The time course for schizophrenia lasts at least **6 months** and includes at least **1 month of active-phase symptoms** with two or more of the following present: **delusions, hallucinations, or disorganized speech.** The disorder is typically chronic with significant functional impairment and socioeconomic sequelae. The lifetime prevalence of schizophrenia is approximately 1% in the general population. The average age of onset for men is early to mid twenties, whereas women typically first experience symptoms in their late twenties.

Safety Assessment

Although some schizophrenic patients can be aggressive, the majority of them are not. More frequently, they suffer from victimization. Risk factors for aggression include a history of violence and impulsivity, substance abuse, younger age, male gender, and lack of treatment.

Twenty percent of individuals with schizophrenia attempt suicide; 5% complete it. Specific risk factors include command AHs to harm oneself or others, depressive symptoms, substance abuse, unemployment, recent psychotic episode or hospital discharge, younger age, and male gender.

CHANGES FROM *DSM-IV* TO *DSM-5*

- The *DSM-IV* subtypes (paranoid, disorganized, catatonic, undifferentiated) have been replaced in *DSM-5* with dimensions to rate core symptoms on a severity scale.

- The *DSM-5* eliminates the importance of Schneiderian first-rank symptoms (two or more voices conversing or voices commenting on one's behavior) and bizarre delusions.

DIFFERENTIAL DIAGNOSIS

Psychotic symptoms are not pathognomonic for schizophrenia or any other psychiatric disorder. Prior to diagnosing a primary psychotic disorder, the following must be ruled out: substance intoxication/withdrawal, substance/medication-induced psychotic disorder, and psychotic disorder due to another medical condition. A thorough history, vital signs, physical examination, blood alcohol level, urine toxicology screen, and serum drug levels can reveal a medical etiology or substance use as a causal factor. A meticulous review of the patient's medications may indicate a potential cause of psychosis, particularly if these include steroids and anticholiner-͏. Specifically inquire about over-the-counter (OTC) drugs and herbal supple-͏ as many patients do not consider these to be medications or feel reluctant to ͏heir use to a physician.

͏hotic disorders represent a spectrum of psychopathology. From the ͏t information, a clinician needs to delineate if the signs and symp-͏ or multiple domains of dysfunction. For example, a patient expe-͏ with no other psychotic symptoms present for at least 1 month would be diagnosed with delusional disorder. Note that patients with schizophrenia suffer from extreme social dysfunction and isolation due to **negative symptoms** that sets them apart from those with other psychotic disorders.

Assess the timeline of symptoms: **brief psychotic disorder (1 day to 1 month), schizophreniform disorder (1-6 months), and schizophrenia ($\geq$ 6 months).**

Distinguishing schizophrenia from both schizoaffective disorder and mood disorders with psychotic features can be challenging. The temporal pattern of the mood and psychotic symptoms determines the diagnosis. In mood disorders with psychotic features, **psychosis occurs only in the context of mood symptoms** (depression, mania, or mixed state). By contrast, **psychotic symptoms occur for at least 2 weeks** even in the **absence of mood symptoms** in **schizoaffective disorder.** Clarification of the diagnosis aids in determining treatment and prognosis.

Prognosis from best to worst:

Mood disorder with psychotic features $\rightarrow$ Schizoaffective disorders $\rightarrow$ Schizophrenia

TREATMENT

Utilize a holistic approach process in determining the treatment plan. Along with medication, take into account the patient's home situation and support system. Provide psychoeducation for the patient, family, and caregiver(s). Consider linking the patient with a case manager and local community resources. Evaluate whether or not the patient is willing to take a medication. Only prescribe a medication if the patient can adhere to the dosing regimen and necessary laboratory follow-up. Increase adherence by prescribing once daily dosing, disintegrating tablets, and long-acting injectables.

Review a patient's history of response to prior psychotropic trials, including allergies or side effects, medical problems that could be exacerbated, potential interactions with current medications, family history of medication response, and side-effect profile of the current treatment options. Often clinicians begin with the **atypical or second-generation antipsychotics** (SGAs) because of their reduced risk of side effects and increased efficacy in treating negative symptoms. More recent data on atypicals suggest that they have less effect on negative symptoms than previously thought. SGAs have their own set of problems, such as increased risk of **metabolic syndrome**, which consists of abdominal obesity, dyslipidemia, hyperglycemia, and hypertension. Clozapine and olanzapine tend to have the most metabolic side effects, whereas ziprasidone and aripiprazole have the least. Studies have shown that **Clozapine** is the most effective antipsychotic medication in treating schizophrenia. Despite this, the risk of **agranulocytosis** prevents Clozapine from being used as a first-line drug.

Typical antipsychotics have a higher likelihood of causing **extrapyramidal symptoms** (akathisia, dystonias, parkinsonism), **hyperprolactinemia**, and **tardive dyskinesia. Acute dystonias** are involuntary muscle contractions, which can be disconcerting but are rarely life threatening. Dystonias can be treated with **anticholinergics, such as benztropine or diphenhydramine.** Depending on the severity of the dystonia, the offending agent may be decreased or switched. **Akathisia**, the sensation of inner restlessness, may respond to benzodiazepines or a beta-blocker, such as propranolol. **Parkinsonian** symptoms, typically **bradykinesia** and **muscle rigidity (eg, cogwheeling),** can be managed by adding benztropine. **Tardive dyskinesia** manifests as characteristic involuntary movements with long-term antipsychotic use. **Neuroleptic malignant syndrome (NMS)** is the most severe, potentially life-threatening complication with altered mental status, fever, dysautonomia, and muscle rigidity. Immediate discontinuation of the offending agent and intensive supportive measures are a necessity. In severe cases, the patient may require treatment with dantrolene and/or bromocriptine.

> ## CASE CORRELATION
>
> - See also Case 7 and Case 54. The diagnosis of schizophrenia is only made when the cause of the psychotic symptoms has been determined to be unrelated to either an underlying medical or substance cause. Schizotypal personality disorder patients will only appear psychotic for short periods of time under stress, and will have subthreshold symptoms that are more associated with persistent personality features.

COMPREHENSION QUESTIONS

6.1 A 29-year-old woman with no medical or psychiatric history is brought to the ED by her husband because of her bizarre behavior. She has been ranting about being a victim of gang stalking ever since she lost her job at the postal service. "I know they are after me," she states repeatedly. Her husband states that since being laid off, the patient has been spending much of her time "with the neighborhood druggies." Which of the following would the initial workup include?

    A. CT of the head

    B. Brain MRI

    C. Urine drug screen

    D. Spinal tap

    E. Ceruloplasmin level

6.2 A 45-year-old man with a history of schizophrenia and alcohol use disorder was brought in by an ambulance after he was found sleeping on the floor of a local homeless shelter. He appears drowsy, but arousable, and mumbles, "the voices are killing me." He admits to taking a bottle of lorazepam because "I just couldn't take it anymore." Which of the following antipsychotics has been associated with decreased suicide attempts?

    A. Haldol

    B. Clozapine

    C. Quetiapine

    D. Lurasidone

    E. Paliperidone

6.3 A 50-year-old man with a past history of chronic, treatment-resistant schizo-phrenia was admitted last night after reemergence of command auditory hal-lucinations telling him to "do bad things." He had been recently hospitalized and stabilized on clozapine. He denies missing any doses. What addiction is the most common form of substance abuse in patients with schizophrenia and likely contributed to the patient's recent psychotic episode?

A. Alcohol

B. LSD

C. Marijuana

D. Nicotine

E. PCP

ANSWERS

6.1 **C.** Although the complete workup may ultimately include all the given options depending on the clinical findings, the urine drug screen (UDS) needs to be one of the initial laboratory tests ordered. A UDS should be checked for all psychiatric patients. In this case, the suspicion is fairly high for positive find-ings. If there is a history of recent head trauma or focal neurologic findings, obtain head imaging and consider performing a lumbar puncture. Ceruloplas-min is only necessary if Wilson disease is suspected. The standard psychiatric laboratory tests include, at minimum, complete blood count with leukocyte differential, comprehensive metabolic panel (electrolytes, BUN, creatinine, and hepatic markers), urinalysis, thyroid stimulating hormone, UDS, medica-tion levels, and a pregnancy test. The APA guidelines recommend addition-ally checking cholesterol, triglycerides, and RPR/FTA-ABS. HIV, Hepatitis C, heavy metal toxins, EEG, and brain MRI or CT of the head may also be indicated. Further workup may include ammonia, vitamin B12, folate, ESR, ANA, prolactin, and karyotype.

6.2 **B.** Clinical trials have demonstrated that clozapine reduces suicide attempts in patients suffering from schizophrenia and schizoaffective disorder.

6.3 **D.** Nicotine is the most frequently used substance by schizophrenics. Patients with schizophrenia are three times more likely to be addicted to nicotine com-pared to the general population (75%-90% vs 25%-30%). Smoking induces cytochrome P450 1A2 (CYP1A2) enzyme activity, which results in signifi-cantly lower clozapine serum concentrations. This patient likely returned to smoking upon discharge, which led to lower clozapine concentrations, and resulted in reemergence of psychotic symptoms. Try to obtain an accurate smoking history, encourage smoking cessation, but take into account that the patient may return to old habits after discharge.

CLINICAL PEARLS

▶ Before diagnosing any psychiatric disorder, remember to rule out substance use, medications, or medical conditions that could be causing, contributing to, or exacerbating the symptoms.

▶ Algorithm for approaching psychiatric disorders:

  ▶ Step 1. Rule out substance or medication induced:

    ▶ Adverse effect, toxicity, or withdrawal

    ▶ Look for common offenders, including Rx and OTC medications, herbals/supplements, illicit substances

    ▶ Workup: UDS, BAL, serum drug levels

  ▶ Step 2. Rule out identifiable medical disorders:

    ▶ Screen for endocrinopathies, neurologic diseases, etc

    ▶ Workup: blood glucose, UA, CBC, CMP, TSH, pregnancy test

  ▶ Step 3. Characterize the psychiatric disorder

▶ Although **catatonia** has been historically associated with schizophrenia, there are many other etiologies, including **medical conditions** and **mood disorders.**

▶ **Positive symptoms** of schizophrenia include **hallucinations, delusions, paranoia, and grossly disorganized speech or behavior**.

  ▶ When asking about AH, differentiate if the sound comes from "inside" versus "outside" the patient's head to help distinguish between their own thoughts versus true AH.

  ▶ In schizophrenia spectrum disorders, patients often misinterpret their own thoughts or vocalizations as an external experience.

  ▶ Determine the patient's level of insight into the perceptual experiences to help delineate **actual hallucinations (lack of insight)** from **hallucinosis (insight intact).**

▶ **Negative symptoms** of schizophrenia remain the most **challenging symptoms** to target and often continue after the positive symptoms have resolved. Severe **impairment in social functioning** characterizes schizophrenia, unlike the other psychotic disorders.

▶ **Clozapine** stands out as **the most efficacious antipsychotic** medication for schizophrenic patients, but is often reserved for treatment-resistant cases due to the risk of **agranulocytosis**.

▶ **Clozapine** is the only antipsychotic with **antisuicidal properties** for patients with schizophrenia.

REFERENCES

American Psychiatric Association. *Diagnostic and Statistical Manual of Mental Disorders*. 5th ed. Washington, DC: American Psychiatric Association; 2013.

Sadock BJ, Sadock VA, Ruiz, P. *Kaplan & Sadock's Synopsis of Psychiatry*. 11th ed. Baltimore, MD: Lippincott Williams & Wilkins; 2014.

Tandon R, Gaebel W, Barch DM, et al. Definition and description of schizophrenia in the DSM-5. *Schizophr Res*. 2013;150(1):3-10. http://dx.doi.org/10.1016/j.schres.2013.05.028. Accessed July 8, 2014.

A 36-year-old woman with a history of epilepsy is brought to the emergency department by her husband for evaluation after she insists that she can see "our future children." The patient describes seeing three young boys playing silently in the backyard since yesterday. She feels "a sense of longing" but denies any depressive symptoms. She does not have any personal or family history of psychiatric illness. The husband denies anything else unusual in his wife's behavior but relays that last week she suffered from a cluster of seizures. She had recovered uneventfully. The husband discloses that the couple has not been able to conceive despite multiple attempts. He thought that his wife had given up on the idea years ago. The patient's seizures have been relatively well controlled on Depakote for the last 10 years. She has no history of substance use. Family history is negative for psychiatric illness. No abnormalities are apparent on physical and mental status examination.

▶ What is the likely diagnosis for this patient?
▶ What further diagnostic workup should be completed?

ANSWERS TO CASE 7:

Psychosis Due to Another Medical Condition

Summary: A 36-year-old woman with a known history of epilepsy and no past psychiatric history has new-onset visual hallucinations after experiencing a cluster of seizures. The patient's psychotic symptoms lasted over the course of a day following a week-long **"lucid" interval.** Her epilepsy had been fairly well controlled prior to this, and she denies any changes in her antiepileptic drug (AED) regimen. She has no other psychiatric symptoms and no family history of psychiatric disorder.

- **Most likely diagnosis:** Psychosis due to another medical condition.

- **Diagnostic tests:** The standard psychiatric laboratory workup for first break psychosis includes complete blood count with leukocyte differential, comprehensive metabolic panel (electrolytes, BUN, creatinine, and hepatic markers), urinalysis, thyroid stimulating hormone, urine drug screen, medication levels, and a pregnancy test. Given the patient's known history of epilepsy, electroencephalogram (EEG) monitoring is needed to determine if the nature of the patient's seizures has changed. Other tests that may be considered include RPR/FTA-ABS, HIV, hepatitis C, ceruloplasmin, heavy metal toxins, ammonia, vitamin B12, ESR, ANA, prolactin, karyotype, brain MRI, or CT of the head.

ANALYSIS

Objectives

1. Understand the diagnostic criteria for psychosis due to another medical condition.

2. Know the common medical conditions that cause psychosis.

Considerations

Investigate potential underlying medical etiologies when patients present with new-onset psychotic symptoms, particularly when there is an unusual aspect to the presentation such as late age of onset. As demonstrated in this case, the strongest diagnostic indicator is a temporal relationship between the onset or exacerbation of a medical disease and the psychotic symptoms. Primary psychotic disorders may elicit hallucinations in any sensory modality, but most commonly present with auditory hallucinations and less typically manifest with **visual, olfactory, and gustatory** perceptions.

In this case, the patient's visual hallucinations are a **direct pathophysiologic result of her known medical condition.** The psychotic symptoms, involving **visual hallucinations** and possibly delusions, manifest a week after a cluster of seizures. Afterward, there was a period of minimal symptoms and clear sensorium, known as a lucid interval.

The relationship between epilepsy, particularly temporal lobe epilepsy, and psychosis has been well established. Psychosis can occur in the ictal (during the seizure), **postictal** (after the seizure), or **interictal** (between seizures) period. Of these, postictal psychosis is most common, occurring in up to 8% of patients with epilepsy.

Postictal psychosis may manifest as hallucinations, delusions, and agitation lasting for hours to weeks. Interictal psychosis often occurs after long-term inadequately treated or treatment resistant childhood-onset epilepsy. The highest risk occurs in a chronically epileptic patient who experiences a flurry of seizures (partial complex, clonic-tonic, or both). Other risk factors include bilateral seizure focus and a family history of psychiatric illness.

APPROACH TO:

Psychotic Disorder Due to Another Medical Condition

DEFINITIONS

FORMICATION: Tactile hallucination of insects crawling on or under the skin. Heavy use of cocaine and amphetamines can result in formication.

PSYCHOSIS: A condition characterized by deterioration of mental functioning, impaired reality testing, perceptual disturbances, and disorganized thought process.

CLINICAL APPROACH

The diagnostic criteria for psychosis due to another medical condition are summarized in Table 7–1. Remember that psychiatric disorders are essentially diagnoses of exclusion. **No pathognomonic symptoms differentiate** primary from secondary psychiatric disorders. **Any brain disturbance can manifest in the same manner as a psychiatric disorder.** Patients with a psychiatric history who present with somatic symptoms are often written off as having a "psych" issue without an appropriate workup. One should complete a thorough medical evaluation before determining that a presentation is primarily psychiatric in nature. The extensive differential diagnosis includes neurologic, infectious, immune, endocrine, metabolic, nutritional, and toxin-related etiologies. Psychotic symptoms that are determined to be part of a psychologic response to a severe illness, contrastingly, do not fall into the category of psychosis due to another medical condition.

Table 7–1 • DIAGNOSTIC CRITERIA FOR PSYCHOSIS DUE TO ANOTHER MEDICAL CONDITION
Prominent hallucinations or delusions
Evidence that the disturbance is the direct pathophysiologic consequence of a medical condition based on the history, physical examination, and/or laboratory studies
Symptoms are not accounted for by another mental illness
Symptoms do not only occur during delirium

DIFFERENTIAL DIAGNOSIS

The differential diagnosis for psychotic symptoms includes delirium, primary psychotic disorders, and substance/medication-induced psychosis. Psychosis occurring as part of delirium (ie, with acutely fluctuating levels of attention and awareness) does not fit into the category of psychotic disorders. Moreover, primary psychotic disorders cannot be diagnosed if the symptoms are thought to be due to another medical condition or a medication/substance. A primary mood disorder with psychotic features should be considered when mood symptoms and psychosis coexist. The temporal relationship of symptoms to medication, toxin, or substance exposure is important to elicit. If symptoms occur during intoxication/withdrawal or within 4 weeks of exposure, a diagnosis of substance/medication-induced psychosis should be considered. This diagnosis is not applicable, however, if an individual retains intact reality testing and accurately attributes the perceptual disturbance to intoxication or withdrawal. If this is the case, a more appropriate diagnosis would be substance intoxication (or withdrawal) with perceptual disturbances. In some cases, both diagnoses, psychotic disorder due to another medical condition and substance/medication-induced psychotic disorder, may be appropriate.

CAUSES OF PSYCHOSIS

Alcohol/Illicit Drugs

- *Intoxication:* alcohol, cannabis, hallucinogens, phencyclidine (PCP); inhalants; sedatives/hypnotics/anxiolytics; stimulants (eg, cocaine, amphetamines)

- *Withdrawal:* alcohol; sedatives/hypnotics/anxiolytics

Medications

- *Intoxication:* anesthetics/analgesics, anticholinergics, anticonvulsants, antihistamines, antihypertensives, antimicrobials, antineoplastics, corticosteroids, muscle relaxants, antidepressants, disulfiram

- *Withdrawal:* sedatives/hypnotics/anxiolytics (eg, benzodiazepine)

Toxins

- *Intoxication:* organophosphate insecticides, nerve gases, carbon monoxide, carbon dioxide, fuel, paint

Medical Conditions

- *Neurologic:* epilepsy, TBI, neoplasms, Huntington disease, multiple sclerosis, migraine, CNS infection, HIV encephalitis, neurosarcoidosis

- *Endocrine:* thyroid dysfunction, parathyroid dysfunction, Cushing syndrome

- *Metabolic:* hypoglycemia, electrolyte imbalances

- *Autoimmune disorders:* systemic lupus erythematosus (SLE), N-methyl-D-aspartate (NMDA) receptor autoimmune encephalitis

TREATMENT

The treatment of psychosis due to another medical condition is accomplished by correction of the underlying medical problem. For example, psychosis due to a vitamin deficiency will resolve with repletion. Antipsychotics may be useful in the short term while waiting for resolution of the underlying problem or in situations in which the medical condition cannot be effectively treated. Patients with psychosis due to epilepsy need to continue treatment with an AED, but may also benefit from the addition of benzodiazepines and antipsychotics.

CASE CORRELATION

- See also Case 12 and Case 46. Delusions or hallucinations in the presence of a major or minor neurocognitive disorder would be diagnosed as a delirium, not a psychosis due to another medical condition. A major depression with psychotic features might display hallucinations and/or delusions, but no medical cause would be found for the psychosis, and prominent mood symptoms would be present.

COMPREHENSION QUESTIONS

7.1 A 25-year-old man with a history of traumatic brain injury (TBI) and autoimmune hypoparathyroidism was brought to the ED by his wife because of his increasingly irritable and aggressive behavior. His wife reports that the patient's irritability and aggression increased after the TBI, but his symptoms also worsen with hypocalcemia and improve with calcium correction. On examination, the patient exhibits agitation, paranoia, and tangential thought process. He admits to occasionally hearing an unfamiliar man's voice making derogatory comments about him. Laboratory work is remarkable for hypocalcemia. Serum phosphate is within normal limits. Which of the following should be administered first?

A. Calcium

B. Haloperidol

C. Topiramate

D. Lorazepam

E. Donepezil

7.2 A 33-year-old woman with no known medical or psychiatric history presents to her physician complaining of "smelling fire." She has called the fire department several times but they have not been able to locate a source of the fumes. No abnormalities are noted on mental status examination. Which of the following symptoms are most indicative of a psychosis due to a temporal lobe seizure?

A. Command auditory hallucinations

B. Olfactory hallucinations

C. Disorganized thought content

D. Persecutory delusions

E. Pressured speech

7.3 A 41-year-old man with a longstanding history of epilepsy presents to the ED complaining of a growing concern about his neighbors. He claims that his neighbors used to watch him through the ceiling vents on occasion, but they have now become more intrusive. The patient states that he has tried to get the police to intervene but they ignored his concerns and told him to "go to a shrink." He admits that he and his wife divorced 10 years ago because "She kept cheating on me with them. It all started when they installed those cameras in our house." Since the divorce, he keeps to himself but maintains his job as a janitor at the local high school. He has been to the ED several times in the past because of uncontrolled seizures and has difficulty adhering to his AED regimen. He has no personal or family history of psychiatric illness. What is the most likely diagnosis?

A. Postictal psychosis

B. Brief psychotic disorder

C. Interictal psychosis

D. Schizophrenia

E. Delusional disorder

ANSWERS

7.1 **A.** Correction of the calcium level (as well as vitamin D and magnesium) should be the first step in treatment. In psychotic disorders due to another medical condition, always attempt to address the underlying etiology. If the patient's psychotic symptoms remain after treating his hypoparathyroidism, consider adding an antipsychotic such as haloperidol. Given the patient's history of TBI, a benzodiazepine such as lorazepam may be disinhibiting. Topiramate and donepezil are not indicated.

7.2 **B.** Olfactory hallucinations have a higher association with temporal lobe seizures. The other symptoms are not specific for temporal lobe tumors. Have a high level of suspicion for an underlying medical etiology when a patient presents with perceptual disturbances of olfaction, gustation, and/or vision.

7.3 **C.** This man most likely suffers from interictal psychosis, which may develop in patients with poorly controlled epilepsy since childhood. He has had ongoing symptoms of paranoia and increasing social isolation, consistent with the chronic, progressive course of interictal psychosis. Risk factors for interictal psychosis include frequent seizures, multiple seizure types, low intelligence, and other neurologic abnormalities. Brain imaging often reveals focal damage, periventricular gliosis, and enlarged cerebral ventricles. In contrast to interictal psychosis, postictal psychosis occurs episodically. In patients with uncontrolled epilepsy, psychotic symptoms may initially present in a postictal pattern before progressing to an interictal pattern. Whereas schizophrenia typically interferes with one's socioeconomic functioning, this patient has maintained gainful employment.

CLINICAL PEARLS

▶ A psychiatric disorder due to another medical condition should be listed separately from the contributing medical condition in a patient's problem list. The contributing medical condition should immediately precede the psychosis listing.

▶ A positive finding on workup of psychosis does not establish causality. Some abnormal findings may simply be coincidental. Response of the patient's symptoms to correction of an abnormality may provide insight into the cause.

▶ **Symptoms occurring during delirium** do not fall within the category of psychotic disorders.

REFERENCES

American Psychiatric Association. *Diagnostic and Statistical Manual of Mental Disorders*. 5th ed. Washington, DC: American Psychiatric Association; 2013.

Kaufman D, Milstein, M. *Clinical Neurology for Psychiatrists*. 7th ed. London, England: Elsevier; 2013.

Sadock BJ, Sadock VA, Ruiz P. *Kaplan & Sadock's Synopsis of Psychiatry*. 11th ed. Baltimore, MD: Lippincott Williams & Wilkins; 2014.

A 14-year-old boy is brought to the emergency department after being found in the basement of his home by his parents during the middle of a school day. The parents came home after receiving a call from the school reporting that their son had not attended school for 4 days. The boy was furiously working on a project he claimed would solve the fuel crisis. He had started returning home from school after his parents left for work because his science teacher would no longer let him use the school laboratory other than during regular class time. The patient was involved in an altercation with the school janitor after being asked to leave the school because it was so late. The boy claimed that the janitor was a foreign spy trying to stop his progress.

The parents are very proud of their son's interest in science but admit that he has been more difficult to manage lately. He can't stop talking about his project, and others cannot get a word in edgewise. His enthusiasm is now palpable. For the past few weeks, he reads late into the night and gets minimal sleep. Despite this, he seems to have plenty of energy and amazes his parents' friends with detailed plans of how he is going to save the world. His friends have not been able to tolerate his increased interest in his project. His train of thought is difficult to follow. He paces around the examination room, saying "[I am] anxious to get back to my project before it is too late." Although he has no suspects in mind, he is concerned that his life may be in danger because of the importance of his work.

▶ What is the most likely diagnosis?
▶ What is the best treatment?

ANSWERS TO CASE 8:
Bipolar Disorder (Child)

Summary: A 14-year-old boy is brought to the emergency department by his parents because he has been skipping school to work feverishly on a project he says will save the world. The problem appears to have escalated over the past few weeks. He does not sleep, yet he has plenty of energy. His thoughts are disordered, and he has no insight into his intrusiveness or how much he annoys people with his excessive, incessant talking. He is irritable and labile. He has paranoid and grandiose thoughts.

- **Most likely diagnosis:** Bipolar I disorder, single manic episode, with mood-congruent psychotic features.

- **Best treatment:** Mood stabilizer (such as valproic acid or lithium) and atypical antipsychotic agent. According to American Academy of Child and Adolescent Psychiatry (AACAP) guidelines, monotherapy with the traditional mood stabilizers lithium, divalproex, and carbamazepine or the atypical antipsychotics olanzapine, quetiapine, and risperidone is the first-line treatment if no psychosis is present. **The majority of the guideline panel recommended lithium or divalproex as the first medication of choice for nonpsychotic mania.** Lithium is the only mood stabilizer with FDA approval for treatment of bipolar disorder in children aged 12 years or older. Divalproex has been used for seizure disorder treatment for years in younger children and has a well-established safety and risk profile, so it may be a better choice in children aged less than 12 years. Given that this patient has signs of significant thought disorder and paranoia, he should be started on both a mood stabilizer and an atypical antipsychotic medication.

ANALYSIS

Objectives

1. Understand the diagnostic criteria for bipolar disorder.

2. Understand the criteria for inpatient psychiatric treatment for this disorder.

3. Understand the initial plan for the treatment of bipolar disorder.

Considerations

The patient presents with grandiosity, inflated self-esteem, paranoia, a decreased need for sleep, an increased energy level, pressured speech, and an increased motor activity level. It seems as if the symptoms have been building for several weeks. The boy does not appear distressed and neither were his parents until his behavior became more troublesome, and his school performance was affected. It is unclear whether this is the first such episode for this patient. Although this patient presents with classical euphoric mania, it is important to remember that children with bipolar disorder often present with a mixed or dysphoric picture characterized by short periods of intense mood lability and irritability. Is there a need for hospitalization? Yes. The patient does not appear to be an acute danger to himself or to others, although he has clearly become increasingly difficult to manage. His parents were unaware that he had been leaving school early and are unsure what other activities he engaged in or where he might have been. The patient is at high risk for engaging in impulsive actions that have the potential for painful consequences (sexual indiscretions, buying sprees, or other pleasurable but risky behaviors). An inpatient setting would be ideal for starting treatment with medications rapidly and titrating to efficacy. Because the patient is a minor, his parents can sign him into a hospital voluntarily. After starting a mood stabilizer and atypical antipsychotic medication, the patient should be monitored closely. If there is only a partial response to therapeutic doses of the medications, then addition of another mood stabilizer would be indicated. If no response is seen, a switch to a new mood stabilizer would be the best course of action.

APPROACH TO:
Bipolar Disorder (Child)

DEFINITIONS

BIPOLAR TYPE I DISORDER: A syndrome with complete manic symptoms occurring during the course of the disorder.

BIPOLAR TYPE II DISORDER: Characterized by depression and episodes of hypomania (elevated, expansive, or irritable mood and increased activity or energy that do not meet the full criteria for manic syndrome).

HYPOMANIA: Symptoms are similar to those of mania, although they do not reach the same level of severity or cause the same degree of social impairment. Although hypomania is often associated with an elated mood and very little insight into it, patients do not usually exhibit psychotic symptoms, racing thoughts, or marked psychomotor agitation.

RAPID-CYCLING BIPOLAR DISORDER: Occurrence of at least four mood episodes—both retarded depression or hypomania/mania—in a year. These episodes have to be separated by either a full or partial remission of at least 2-month duration or a full switch from one pole to the other (from full mania to major depression).

LABILE: A mood and/or affect that switches rapidly from one extreme to another. For example, a patient can be laughing and euphoric 1 minute, followed by a display of intense anger and then extreme sadness in the following minutes of an interview.

CLINICAL APPROACH

The *Diagnostic and Statistical Manual of Mental Disorders, 5th edition (DSM-5)*, criteria for a diagnosis of bipolar disorder in children (Table 8–1) are the same as those for adults. The proper diagnosis of bipolar disorder in children and adolescents is one of the most controversial areas in psychiatry. Some authors suggest that many juveniles with bipolar disorder have a presentation of severe mood dysregulation with multiple, intense, prolonged mood swings or temper outbursts every day consisting of short periods of euphoria followed by longer periods of irritability. These children can average between three and four cycles per day. As a result, these authors hold that the clinician should diagnose bipolar disorder in youth who do not meet the *DSM-5* criteria but have this mood dysregulation. Others hold that many youth who are episodically explosive and emotionally labile really have temperament problems as part of an early personality disorder and these individuals are improperly being called bipolar. In *DSM-5* many of these individuals with recurrent temper outbursts will be diagnosed with disruptive mood dysregulation disorder.

In adults the overall prevalence of mood disorders is about 1% and increases with increasing age. The prevalence of adolescent bipolar disorder in the general population is also about 1%. The fact that these two rates are the same is of concern because bipolar disorder is a lifelong condition and the overall prevalence rates in youth should be lower than in adults. This also implies that some children diagnosed with bipolar really have problems that are being misattributed to bipolar disorder. Bipolar disorder is rare in preschool-age children. The rate of occurrence of bipolar I disorder is 0.2% to 0.4% in prepubertal children.

Studies indicate that youth who are diagnosed as having bipolar disorder that does not meet the previous *DSM-IV* criteria for mania (bipolar disorder NOS)

Table 8–1 • DIAGNOSTIC CRITERIA FOR BIPOLAR DISORDER (MANIC EPISODE) IN CHILDREN[a]
A distinct period of abnormally and persistently elevated, expansive, or irritable mood *and* persistent increased energy lasting at least 1 wk (or any duration if hospitalization is required).
Three or more of the following symptoms during the period of mood disturbance and increased energy: • Inflated self-esteem or grandiosity   • Decreased need for sleep   • Greater talkativeness than usual or pressure to keep talking   • Flight of ideas or subjective experience that thoughts are racing   • Distractibility   • Increase in goal-directed activity or psychomotor agitation   • Excessive involvement in pleasurable activities with a high potential for painful consequences (buying sprees, sexual activity, foolish investments)
Criteria for a mixed episode are not met.
The impairment must be severe enough to cause impairment in functioning, hospitalization is necessary, OR there are psychotic features.
Disturbance is severe enough to cause impairment in normal functioning.
Symptoms are not caused by the effect of a substance or a medical condition.

[a]*The current* Diagnostic and Statistical Manual of Mental Disorders *diagnosis for bipolar disorder does not have any modifications for the disorder in children.*

have an increased incidence of having various types of psychopathology as adults, but not an increased incidence of bipolar disorder.

The bottom line is that clinicians must be extremely cautious about making a diagnosis of bipolar disorder in youth and must constantly question the accuracy of the diagnosis if made by others, especially if the patient does not meet full *DSM-5* criteria for bipolar disorder. The AACAP practice parameters hold that all criteria for bipolar, including the duration criterion of 1 week for mania and 2 weeks for major depression, should be followed when making a diagnosis of mania or hypomania in children or adolescents.

Mood disorders tend to cluster in families. The rate of mood disorders in the children of adults with these disorders is at least three times the rate seen in the general population with a lifetime risk of 15% to 45%. The finding that identical twins have a concordance rate of 69% for bipolar disorder compared to a 19% rate for dizygotic twins indicates a strong genetic component but also suggests an effect of psychosocial issues on the development of mood disorders.

Bipolar I disorder is rarely diagnosed before puberty because of the absence of episodes of mania. Usually, an episode of major depression precedes an episode of mania in an adolescent with bipolar I. Mania is recognized by a definite change from a preexisting state and is usually accompanied by grandiose and paranoid delusions and hallucinatory phenomena. **In adolescence, episodes of mania are often accompanied by psychotic features** and hospitalization is frequently necessary. Hypomania must be differentiated from attention deficit hyperactivity disorder (ADHD), which is characterized by distractibility, impulsivity, and hyperactivity that are present on a daily basis consistently since before the patient is 7 years old. Children with ADHD will frequently develop oppositional defiant disorder (ODD), where the patient defiantly opposes the wishes of others and breaks minor rules, or conduct disorder (CD), where the youth defiantly breaks major social rules. **A youth who has both ADHD and ODD or CD can present with a pattern of distractibility, motor agitation, and impulsive angry outbursts that can be mistaken for bipolar disorder. The history of the behavior in the preschool age then becomes a key piece of information, as bipolar disorder is extremely rare in this age range whereas ADHD and ODD are very common. With the release of** *DSM-5*, **some children who were previously diagnosed with bipolar disorder will be diagnosed with disruptive mood dysregulation disorder.**

DIFFERENTIAL DIAGNOSIS

The psychomotor agitation or increase in activity level often associated with bipolar disorder must be carefully differentiated from the symptoms of ADHD, especially if the child also has ODD or CD. If the episode occurring is a depressive one, other mood disorders must be ruled out, including major depression or an adjustment disorder with depressed mood. Mood disorders related to substance intoxication, anxiety disorders, the side effects of a medication, or a general medical condition must also be excluded.

WORKING WITH CHILDREN AND THEIR FAMILIES

Treatment guidelines of the AACAP note that the family is essential in providing the detailed past history and current observations needed to make an accurate diagnosis. In the process of taking a history, it is critical to consider if the parents or other family members have been diagnosed as having bipolar disorder or if the family members have undiagnosed or untreated bipolar disorder. In such cases, assuring that the family members are receiving adequate treatment for their illnesses can have major beneficial effects on the child's environment. Finally, it is critical to make sure that the families fully understand what bipolar disorder is, its clinical course, how it can be effectively treated, and the availability of bipolar disorder support groups.

TREATMENT

Medications play a significant role in the treatment of bipolar disorder, and AACAP treatment algorithms should be consulted when providing care to juveniles with bipolar disorder. Often **mood-stabilizing agents such as lithium carbonate, carbamazepine, and divalproex** can be helpful in preventing and treating manic phases. Lithium is the only mood-stabilizing agent approved by the FDA for treatment of bipolar disorder in youth aged 12 years and older. All must have blood levels monitored to assure dosing in a therapeutic range. Treatment guidelines developed by the AACAP note the lack of good research data in treating depressed bipolar youth but do note that lithium can be recommended as a treatment option in youth with bipolar depression. Meta-analysis of traditional mood stabilizers suggest antimanic efficacy with a need for more double-blinded studies. Other anticonvulsants have a lack of evidence for efficacy.

Patients on lithium need to have thyroid and kidney function monitored on a regular basis, whereas those on carbamazepine need close monitoring for rare aplastic anemia or agranulocytosis. In addition to monitoring for liver function and platelet levels if the patient is on divalproex, a number of studies have suggested a high rate of polycystic ovarian syndrome in women with epilepsy who are treated with divalproex, raising concerns about its long-term use in young women with bipolar disorder. Many mood stabilizers have shown evidence of **teratogenic effects.** For this reason, pregnancy tests should be performed on all females of childbearing age before prescribing these drugs.

Atypical antipsychotics such as olanzapine, risperidone, and quetiapine have also been used as monotherapy to control episodes of mania. They do not have the teratogenic effects noted with lithium, divalproex, and carbamazepine. Patients placed on atypical antipsychotics should be carefully monitored for development of a metabolic syndrome consisting of weight gain, diabetes mellitus, and hypercholesterolemia. **Tardive dyskinesia** is a possible side effect of the atypical antipsychotics, and an assessment of abnormal movements should be done at baseline and regular intervals using the Abnormal Involuntary Movement Scale (AIMS). Interestingly, double-blind placebo-controlled studies of atypical antipsychotics show greater efficacy than open-label studies.

Off-label utilization of selective serotonin reuptake inhibitors (SSRIs) and bupropion can also be considered during bipolar-depressed phases based on the AACAP guidelines, and lamotrigine and divalproex are other treatment options noted. **Many antidepressants are believed to be able to trigger or "unmask" mania,** and so they should be used carefully, and patients should be observed closely for emergent manic symptoms.

The treatment of bipolar disorder in childhood can be very difficult. There are numerous comorbid psychiatric diseases, particularly ADHD. If treatment of the bipolar disorder is adequate, but comorbid psychiatric disorders are not addressed, the child will continue to have academic and functional impairment. The lack of recognition of the high degree of comorbidity could lead to false assumptions about treatment success and repeated unnecessary medication trials.

The **treatment of bipolar disorder in children involves both psychotherapy and psychopharmacotherapy.** The school and the family should be included in the treatment, as the ramifications of bipolar disorder in an individual can have far-reaching effects. **Cognitive therapy** is often an important component of treatment and focuses on **reducing negative thoughts and building self-esteem. Family therapy** can be indicated in situations where family dynamics might be a factor contributing to the symptoms.

CASE CORRELATION

- See also Case 3 and Case 20. ADHD can look like bipolar disorder and be confused for it, especially in children and adolescents, because rapid speech, distractibility, and racing thoughts may be common to both. However, these symptoms appearing in a discrete episode mark the diagnosis as bipolar rather than ADHD. Patients with GAD have anxious ruminations which may look like racing thoughts, and attempts to minimize the anxiety may appear as impulsive behavior. However, a careful history should discriminate between the two.

COMPREHENSION QUESTIONS

8.1 Which of the following medications would be the best choice for mood-stabilization of nonpsychotic mania in a 10-year-old boy?

A. Isotretinoin (Accutane)

B. Beclomethasone

C. Lithium

D. Divalproex

E. Risperidone

8.2 A 16-year-old girl has been admitted with a 3-week history of sudden irritability, impulsive buying, and disappearing at night with older men. Her need for sleep is decreased; she has flight of ideas and grandiose thoughts about being an advisor to a presidential candidate. Test results indicate she is pregnant. Which of the following is a statement that should be made to her parents?

A. Treatment with an SSRI antidepressant is a reasonable alternative to mood stabilizers in a pregnant girl.

B. Given the fact that she is pregnant, she should be kept secluded on an inpatient unit during the first trimester of pregnancy with no medications.

C. An atypical antipsychotic may be the best choice for managing both psychotic features and mood disturbance associated with her bipolar disorder, especially during the first trimester.

D. Psychotherapy will have little role in the treatment of her bipolar disorder.

E. Lithium, divalproex, and carbamazepine are all reasonable first-choice mood stabilizers for this patient.

8.3 Parents of a 10-year-old boy note that their son does well with his family until he is not allowed to do something he wants to do. When this occurs, he will get irritable, impulsively aggressive, and agitated for several hours. Once he calms, or gets his way, he is happy and pleasant again. At school he has no trouble focusing but if he does not want to do something he becomes argumentative. Which of the following is the most likely diagnosis?

A. Oppositional defiant disorder

B. Bipolar disorder-mania

C. Attention deficit hyperactivity disorder combined type

D. Major depression

E. Disruptive mood dysregulation disorder

ANSWERS

8.1 **D.** Mood stabilizers are used to treat bipolar disorder. Lithium is the only mood-stabilizing medication that has received FDA approval for the treatment of bipolar disorder in youth older than 12 years, but divalproex has a longer safety profile in young individuals given its long history of use for seizures even though this is an off-label use.

8.2 **C.** Atypical antipsychotics are good choices for controlling mania in pregnancy given the strong teratogenic effects of most mood stabilizers. SSRIs will only make the mania worse. The patient may need psychotherapy focused on helping her sort out her feelings about the pregnancy.

8.3 **A.** The pattern described best fits oppositional defiant disorder, because the patient can be seen to calm down and be pleasant after he gets his way. A child with bipolar disorder might be seen to have these kinds of outbursts, but the mood dysregulation continues, even after the child "gets his way." Children in the midst of a bipolar disorder never "calm down and become pleasant." Depressed children would also have a persistent mood shift. The symptoms of inattention and distractibility are not present so the patient does not have ADHD. Disruptive mood dysregulation disorder is a persistent angry and irritable mood with episodic temper outbursts and is the best fit here.

CLINICAL PEARLS

▶ The AACAP practice parameters hold that all the DSM criteria, including the duration criterion of 1 week for mania and 2 weeks for depression, should be followed when making a diagnosis of mania or hypomania in children or adolescents.

▶ The majority of the AACAP treatment guideline panel recommended lithium or divalproex as the first medication choice for nonpsychotic mania.

▶ There is a high degree of psychiatric comorbidity in bipolar disorder in childhood.

▶ Mood-stabilizing agents have a significant risk for teratogenicity.

REFERENCES

American Academy of Child and Adolescent Psychiatry. Practice parameter for the assessment and treatment of children and adolescents with bipolar disorder. *J Am Acad Child Adolesc Psychiatry.* 2007;46(1):107-125.

Liu HA, Potter MP, Woodworth KY, et al. Pharmacologic treatments for pediatric bipolar disorder: a review and meta-analysis. *J Am Acad Child Adolesc Psychiatry.* 2011;50(8):749-762.

Sadock BJ, Sadock VA, Ruiz P. *Kaplan and Sadock's Synopsis of Psychiatry: Behavioral Sciences/Clinical Psychiatry.* 11th ed. Baltimore, MD: Lippincott Williams & Wilkins; 2014.

A 19-year-old college freshman is brought to the emergency department by his dorm roommate. The roommate states that his fellow freshman has been up until 4 AM for the last two nights, painting for an art final. The roommate complains the patient's behavior precludes him from being able to sleep or work in their shared space. He states that his colleague continuously paces between the easel and the window. He describes his roommate's mood as "obnoxiously happy" especially in the context of finals week. The patient describes a history of good moods during which he has bursts of energy and creativity while requiring less sleep. These episodes are typically followed by feeling down and depleted, even with sufficient sleep. The patient denies any associated suicidality or psychotic symptoms. He denies substance use, medications, or medical problems.

▶ What is the next step?
▶ What is the most likely diagnosis?

ANSWERS TO CASE 9:
Cyclothymic Disorder

Summary: The patient's behavior has been disruptive enough that his roommate brought him in for evaluation. The severity and duration of the patient's symptoms do not meet the full criteria for a hypomanic episode. He exhibits an elevated mood and increased energy and goal-directed activity (painting) for 2 to 3 days. The patient needs less sleep than usual and displays psychomotor agitation with his continuous pacing. He reports a history of chronic fluctuations between episodes of elevated and depressive mood states. The patient denies substance use or significant medical history.

- **Next diagnostic step:** Order the typical laboratory tests for a psychiatric workup, including urine toxicology, blood alcohol level, and medical screens. Substance use and medical conditions must be ruled out before a diagnosis of cyclothymic disorder can be established.

- **Most likely diagnosis:** Cyclothymic disorder.

ANALYSIS

Objectives

1. Understand the criteria for cyclothymic disorder (Table 9–1).

2. Learn how to differentiate cyclothymic disorder from other psychiatric disorders, particularly bipolar II disorder.

3. Become familiar with the treatment strategy.

Considerations

This clinical vignette describes a patient with cyclothymic disorder. The patient exhibits hypomanic symptoms but does not meet the full criteria for a hypomanic episode. From the history gathered, the patient has experienced years of fluctuating, subclinical mood symptoms. His reported good health and alcohol/drug abstinence make a primary psychiatric diagnosis more likely, but a complete workup will help confirm the history.

Patients typically seek help for depression, while patients are brought in by others for evaluation during (hypo)manic episodes. Often the damage done during

Table 9–1 • DIAGNOSTIC CRITERIA FOR CYCLOTHYMIC DISORDER
At least **2 y** of **fluctuating hypomanic** and **depressive symptoms without ever meeting full criteria for hypomanic, manic, or major depressive** episodes. These symptoms have been present for **at least half the time** and have not been **absent for > 2 mo**.
Not better explained by another psychiatric disorder.
Not induced by substances or a medical condition.
Symptoms lead to significant distress and/or impaired functioning.

(hypo)mania leads to problems which can worsen overall well-being. Irritability and disruptive behaviors often lead to relationship conflict.

APPROACH TO:
Cyclothymic Disorder

DEFINITIONS

BIPOLAR I DISORDER: At **least one manic episode required.** Hypomanic and major depressive episodes are common but not required for diagnosis.

BIPOLAR II DISORDER: Hypomanic episode + major depressive episode.

HYPOMANIC EPISODE: Essentially the same criteria as a manic episode, except **shorter duration** and **less intense. Elevated, expansive, or irritable mood** with **increased energy/activity** for **4 days or more** with **three or less associated symptoms:** grandiosity, impulsivity, distractibility, risky behaviors, pressured speech, flight of ideas/racing thoughts, decreased need for sleep, and increased goal-directed activity/psychomotor agitation.

MANIC EPISODE: Elevated, expansive, or irritable mood with **increased energy/ activity** for at **least 7 days** with **three or more associated symptoms:** grandiosity, impulsivity, distractibility, risky behaviors, pressured speech, flight of ideas/racing thoughts, decreased need for sleep, and increased goal-directed activity/psychomotor agitation. Considered a manic episode if **psychotic features** are present or **hospitalization** is required.

MAJOR DEPRESSIVE EPISODE: Depressed mood or anhedonia for **2 weeks** with **four or more other associated symptoms:** suicidal ideation, fatigue, impaired concentration, excessive guilt, psychomotor retardation/agitation, hypersomnia/insomnia, and unintentional change in appetite/weight.

MIXED SYMPTOMS: Mood episodes encompassing simultaneous symptoms from the opposite poles of the mood spectrum, such as depressed symptoms during a manic episode or manic symptoms during a major depressive episode.

CLINICAL APPROACH

Cyclothymic disorder is a chronic, fluctuating mood disorder with less severe hypomanic and depressive episodes compared to bipolar II disorder. Symptoms can occasionally be equally intense as bipolar II disorder but for a shorter duration. Most individuals with cyclothymia experience mixed symptoms with prominent irritability. Patients may be described as temperamental or unreliable due to their unpredictable mood changes. Cyclothymia has an insidious onset but typically begins in adolescence or early adulthood. Some patients diagnosed with cyclothymic disorder go on to develop bipolar I or II disorder. In order to be classified as a disorder, there needs to be significant distress or functional impairment as a consequence of the mood disturbance.

Changes from *DSM-IV-TR* to *DSM-5*: *DSM-5* specifies that cyclothymia can only be diagnosed if full criteria are **not** met for a hypomanic episode and a major depressive episode.

DIFFERENTIAL DIAGNOSIS

The differential for cyclothymic disorder is broad. Mood fluctuations due to **substance-induced** or **another medical condition must be ruled out first.** Medications and illicit drugs—particularly stimulants and steroids—can induce mood swings. Gather a thorough history with collateral information, perform a physical examination, and order a urine drug screen. If the patient's mood stabilizes after cessation of a substance, this likely indicates the substance as culprit. Evaluate for chronic medical conditions such as hyperthyroidism or epilepsy. Carefully assess for a medical etiology particularly when onset occurs later in life.

Bipolar disorders I and II with rapid cycling may appear similar to cyclothymic disorder because of the frequent changes in mood. Rapid cycling involves at least **four episodes within a 12-month period.** Bipolar II disorder is characterized by episodes of depression and episodes of hypomania. Bipolar I disorder by definition encapsulates a manic episode and often also involves a major depression. Patients with bipolar disorder can present with a "mixed state," exhibiting elements of both depression and (hypo)mania. Psychotic disorders with mood symptoms could be considered, but the presence of psychotic features would rule out cyclothymia. Borderline personality disorder also presents with mood lability and relationship difficulties and may co-occur with cyclothymic disorder.

TREATMENT

The treatment for cyclothymic disorder mirrors bipolar disorder regarding medication regimen. Mood stabilizers such as lithium and valproate are first-line agents. Atypical antipsychotics can also be used in both the acute and maintenance phases. Lamotrigine can be used to address depressive symptoms. Avoid antidepressants in cyclothymic disorder as patients have increased sensitivity to antidepressant-induced (hypo)mania. Educate the patient and family about the illness and treatment options. Supportive or insight-oriented psychotherapy can help patients increase their awareness of the symptoms and develop healthy coping mechanisms.

CASE CORRELATION

- See also Case 8 and Case 57. Note that in cyclothymic disorder, the criteria for a major depressive, manic, or hypomanic episode have never been met. By contrast, these criteria must have been met for the patient to receive a diagnosis of bipolar disorder with rapid cycling. Borderline personality disorder patients have frequent and marked shifts of mood. If the criteria for borderline personality disorder and cyclothymic disorder are both met, then both diagnoses must be given.

COMPREHENSION QUESTIONS

9.1 A 65-year-old retired engineer presents to his primary care physician at the insistence of his wife. The patient reports not needing as much sleep as he used to—only a few hours for the last few nights. He is considering going back to work because he wants to share his knowledge with "all the young fledgling engineers—they need my guidance." His wife notes that he has been very irritable and overly talkative lately. The patient has no previous psychiatric or medical history. He denies use of drugs or alcohol. Which of the following is the best next step?

    A. Admit to the inpatient psychiatric unit.

    B. Order a urinalysis.

    C. Perform a physical examination.

    D. Start a mood-stabilizing drug.

    E. Start an antipsychotic drug.

9.2 A 20-year-old musician comes to his primary care physician's office because he has been feeling depressed, fatigued, and unmotivated for the last few weeks. He wants help getting his "muse" back. Physical examination and laboratory studies are unremarkable. He is prescribed fluoxetine with plan to follow-up in a month. The patient's girlfriend brings him back to clinic 2 weeks later, concerned that he is "acting different." She reports that the patient plays guitar all day and late into the night. She complains that he has spent all their money on new guitars and keyboards. She does not want to "crush his dreams, but he's reaching a bit high trying to book tours with the Rolling Stones." The patient reports feeling, "Better than ever!" He talks quickly and informs the physician that he has to get going so he can keep practicing for "the big gig." What is the most likely diagnosis?

    A. Antidepressant-induced bipolar disorder

    B. Bipolar disorder due to another medical condition

    C. Major depressive disorder

    D. Narcissistic personality disorder

    E. Schizoaffective disorder

9.3 A 32-year-old woman with cyclothymia presents to the obstetrician at 22 weeks pregnant for a routine prenatal visit. She has continued her prescription of valproate during pregnancy. Which of the following is the most likely abnormality that might be found on an ultrasound examination due to the effects of the mood stabilizer?

    A. Fetal abdominal wall defect

    B. Fetal microcephaly

    C. Fetal renal dysplasia

    D. Fetal spina bifida

    E. Fetal tetralogy of Fallot

ANSWERS

9.1 **C.** Late-onset mood and behavioral changes without any past psychiatric history should lead to high suspicion of a medical etiology. All patients deserve a proper medical workup, including physical examination and laboratory studies. This would include a urinalysis as well as a urine drug screen, but the next best step is the physical examination. While hospital admission may be necessary if the patient's behavior escalates, he does not currently warrant inpatient admission. Prior to admission, a physical examination should be performed. Both a mood stabilizer and/or an antipsychotic may also be helpful, but first try to determine if there is an underlying, resolvable etiology.

9.2 **A.** This case demonstrates the point that patients with major depression can cycle into (hypo)manic state due to antidepressants. Many patients with bipolar spectrum disorders initially present with depression. Screen carefully for past history of (hypo)manic symptoms and proceed cautiously when initiating treatment in antidepressant-naïve patients. The patient in this vignette has recently completed a medical workup without any positive findings, thus an underlying medical etiology is less likely. Given the emergence of hypomanic symptoms, major depressive disorder would be incorrect. The patient appears grandiose but it is unclear if he has demonstrated truly delusional thinking. Otherwise, he does not appear thought-disordered or disorganized, thus schizoaffective disorder would not be the most likely diagnosis. The patient's display of grandiosity is a new-onset phenomenology, not a pervasive pattern as would be the case in narcissistic personality disorder.

9.3 **D.** Maternal use of valproate is associated with an increased risk of fetal neural tube defects such as spina bifida. Increasing folic acid supplements (1-4 mg daily) can help reduce the risk of birth defects. For women in the reproductive age, ensure appropriate contraception if prescribing a medication associated with teratogenicity.

CLINICAL PEARLS

▶ Patients often seek help for depression but are typically brought in by others during (hypo)manic episodes.

▶ Carefully assess for a medical etiology especially when the onset occurs later in life.

▶ Avoid antidepressants as cyclothymic patients are particularly susceptible to antidepressant-induced (hypo)mania.

▶ Patients diagnosed with cyclothymic disorder may later develop bipolar I or II disorder.

▶ Provide thorough psychoeducation to patients about the medications and possible side effects.

▶ For women in the reproductive age, ensure appropriate contraception if prescribing a medication with potential teratogenicity. Increase daily folic acid to decrease risk of birth defects.

REFERENCES

American Psychiatric Association. *Diagnostic and Statistical Manual of Mental Disorders*. 5th ed. Washington, DC: American Psychiatric Association; 2013.

Sadock BJ, Sadock VA, Ruiz, P. *Kaplan & Sadock's Synopsis of Psychiatry*. 11th ed. Baltimore, MD: Lippincott Williams & Wilkins; 2014.

A 55-year-old woman presents to a psychiatrist with complaints of a depressed mood for the past 3 months. She notes that her mood has been consistently low, and she describes her recent state as "just not me." She has also noticed a decrease in energy and a weight gain of 6 to 7 lb occurring over the same period of time, although her appetite has not increased. She denies any past psychiatric history and does not remember ever feeling this depressed for this long a period of time. She denies any medical problems and takes no medications, except for multivitamins. She drinks one to two times per week, one glass of wine per time. She smokes five cigarettes per day and denies illicit drug use. Her family history is positive for schizophrenia in one maternal aunt.

On mental status examination, the patient appears well dressed and groomed. She acts tired but is cooperative, with good eye contact. She has some psychomotor retardation but no tremors. Her speech is somewhat slowed but otherwise unremarkable. Her mood is "depressed," with a congruent affect, although she has a full range. Her thought processes are linear and logical. She is not suicidal or homicidal and does not report hallucinations or delusions. Her cognition is grossly intact. Her insight is good. Her judgment and impulse control are not impaired.

Her physical examination reveals a blood pressure of 110/70 mm Hg and a temperature of 98°F (36.7°C). Her thyroid gland is diffusely enlarged but not painful. Her heart has a regular rate and rhythm. She has coarse, brittle hair but no rashes.

▶ What is the most likely diagnosis?
▶ What is the next most appropriate diagnostic step?

ANSWERS TO CASE 10:

Depressive Disorder Due to Hypothyroidism

Summary: A 55-year-old woman presents to a psychiatrist with a depressed mood, decreased energy, and weight gain with a normal appetite. She has never had these symptoms before and denies past psychiatric history. Her mental status examination is significant for a depressed-appearing female but is otherwise unremarkable. Her physical examination is notable for a diffusely enlarged thyroid gland and coarse, brittle hair.

- **Most likely diagnosis:** Depressive disorder due to another medical condition (hypothyroidism).

- **Next diagnostic step:** Obtain thyroid studies for this patient, including determinations of thyroid stimulating hormone (TSH), triiodothyronine, and thyroxine levels.

ANALYSIS

Objectives

1. Recognize a mood disorder occurring due to another medical condition.

2. Use the most likely diagnosis of hypothyroidism in this patient to guide the laboratory examination(s) required.

Considerations

Although this patient's history is consistent with that of a major depressive episode, two elements are atypical. While weight gain is observed in patients in a major depression with atypical features, this condition is usually accompanied by an increase in appetite. Weight gain in the absence of an increased appetite is a clue to the metabolic changes caused by this patient's hypothyroidism. An enlarged thyroid is not seen in patients with major depression, but it is a sign that guides the specific laboratory examinations chosen in this case.

APPROACH TO:

Depressive Disorder Due to Another Medical Condition

CLINICAL APPROACH

Diagnosis of this disorder requires a prominent and persistent period of depressed mood or markedly diminished interest or pleasure in activities, thought to be related to the direct pathophysiological effects of another medical condition. The depressive episode must cause significant distress or impairment in functioning. Note that a similar diagnosis is bipolar and related disorder due to another medical condition.

This is characterized by a persistent period of abnormally elevated or irritable mood and increased activity or energy, due to the direct physiological consequences of another medical disorder. In either case, the patient's history, physical examination, or laboratory findings must demonstrate a causal relationship between the medical illness and the change in mood; in other words, the depression or mania cannot result only from the *stress* of having a medical condition. In addition to the above criteria, the mood episode cannot occur only during the course of a delirium.

DIFFERENTIAL DIAGNOSIS

The differential diagnosis for a depressive or bipolar disorder due to another medical condition is extensive given the numerous medical and neurologic conditions that can cause depression or mania. Table 10–1 lists many of them. Also important in this differential diagnosis are substance/medication-induced depressive and bipolar disorders caused not only by alcohol and illicit drugs (both in intoxication and withdrawal) but also by a large number of medications. See Table 10–2 for a partial list of medications that can cause depressive symptoms. Making a distinction

Table 10–1 • MEDICAL CONDITIONS CAUSING MOOD DISORDERS	
Medical Condition	**Mood Disorder**
Parkinson disease	Depression
Huntington disease	Depression or mania
Wilson disease	Mania
Cerebrovascular accident	Depression or mania
Cerebral neoplasm	Depression or mania
Cerebral trauma	Depression or mania
Encephalitis	Depression or mania
Multiple sclerosis	Depression or mania
Temporal lobe epilepsy	Mania
Hyperthyroidism	Depression or mania
Hypothyroidism	Depression
Hyperparathyroidism	Depression
Hypoparathyroidism	Depression
Uremia	Depression or mania
Cushing syndrome	Depression
Addison disease	Depression
Systemic lupus erythematosus	Depression
Rheumatoid arthritis	Depression
Folate deficiency	Depression
Vitamin B_{12} deficiency	Depression or mania
Human immunodeficiency virus disease	Depression

Table 10–2 • MEDICATIONS CAUSING DEPRESSIVE SYMPTOMS	
Antihypertensive agents with catecholamine effects	**Analgesics**
• Clonidine	• Indomethacin
• Propranolol	• Opiates
• Reserpine	**Antibiotics and anti-infectives**
• Lidocaine	• Ampicillin
• Methyldopa	• Clotrimazole
GI motility drugs	• Griseofulvin
• Metoclopramide	• Metronidazole
Sedatives and hypnotics	• Sulfonamides
• Barbiturates	• Tetracycline
• Chloral hydrate	• Interferon
• Benzodiazepines	**Insecticides**
Steroids and hormones	• Organophosphates
• Corticosteroids	**Antineoplastic agents**
• Oral contraceptives	• Azathioprine
• Prednisone	• Vincristine
• Triamcinolone	• Bleomycin
Neurologic agents	• Trimethoprim
• Amantadine	• Cycloserine
• Carbamazepine	• Vinblastine
• Levodopa	• Amphotericin B
• Phenytoin	• Procarbazine
Heavy metals	**Histamine 2 receptor antagonists**
• Mercury	• Cimetidine
• Lead	• Ranitidine

between primary (psychiatric) and secondary (induced) mood disorders can sometimes be difficult, especially because stressors such as medical illnesses themselves may trigger episodes of both major depression and mania.

TREATMENT

The treatment of a depressive (or bipolar) disorder due to another medical condition entails attending to and treating the underlying medical condition first, if possible, and subsequently achieving improvement or resolution of the mood symptoms. For example, in the previously described case, if the woman is diagnosed with clinical hypothyroidism and treated with thyroid supplementation, she will likely experience a diminishing of her depressive symptomatology. Depressive symptoms caused by medical or neurologic conditions that are recurrent, chronic, or otherwise untreatable (eg, dementias, strokes, malignancies) often respond to typical psychopharmacologic treatments such as selective serotonin reuptake inhibitors, serotonin-norepinephrine reuptake inhibitors, tricyclic antidepressants, mood stabilizers, and electroconvulsive therapy.

CASE CORRELATION

- See also Case 11 and Case 13. It may be difficult to differentiate whether a major depressive episode is being caused by a medical condition itself, or by the medication used to treat that medical condition. Clinical judgment and a careful history regarding the timing of the appearance of symptoms will be helpful in these cases. Likewise, patients with other medical conditions do become depressed, and the clinician will be left with deciding if the disorder presented is a major depression, or one due to a medical condition. Helpful clues to this will be the presence/absence of depressive symptoms in history before the presentation of the medical condition, and whether or not the particular medical condition is known for a propensity to cause major depressive symptoms.

COMPREHENSION QUESTIONS

For the following clinical vignettes (Questions 10.1-10.5), choose the one most likely diagnosis (A-E):

  A. Adjustment disorder with depressed mood

  B. Bipolar I disorder, manic

  C. Major depressive disorder

  D. Mood (depressive or bipolar) disorder due to another medical condition

  E. Substance/medication-induced mood (depressive or bipolar) disorder

10.1 An 18-year-old single man presents with 3 days of an irritable mood, decreased desire for sleep, talkativeness, increased energy, and distractibility. He has no past or family psychiatric history and no current medical problems. His mental status examination is remarkable for psychomotor agitation and an irritable affect. He is paranoid but denies delusions or hallucinations. His physical examination is notable for a slightly elevated pulse rate and blood pressure, as well as markedly dilated pupils bilaterally. The result of his urine toxicology screen is positive for cocaine.

10.2 A 39-year-old married woman presents with 1 month of a gradually worsening depressed mood, with increased sleep, low energy, and difficulty concentrating, but no appetite or weight changes. Her medical history is significant for multiple sclerosis, but she is currently not taking any medications. Her mental status examination is notable for psychomotor slowing and a depressed and blunted affect. Her physical examination demonstrates several different sensory and motor deficits.

10.3 A 52-year-old divorced man executive presents with the new onset of depression, early-morning awakening, decreased energy, distractibility, anhedonia, poor appetite, and weight loss for the past 3 months. His symptoms began shortly after he suffered a myocardial infarction. Although he did not experience significant sequelae, he has felt less motivated and fulfilled in his life and work, believing that he is now "vulnerable." As a result, he does not push himself as he used to, and his work output is beginning to decline. He feels "empty" but denies suicidal ideation.

10.4 An 80-year-old widowed woman without past psychiatric history is seen for a follow-up appointment after suffering from a left-sided cerebral vascular accident that has left her paralyzed on her right side. Since her stroke, she complains of an absence of pleasure in anything that she formerly enjoyed. She describes frequent crying spells, sleeping more than usual, a decreased appetite with weight loss, and feelings of hopelessness and helplessness. She admits to passive thoughts of suicide, without plan or intent.

10.5 A 36-year-old married man with a past history of a major depressive episode is brought into the emergency room by the police after stopping traffic on the highway proclaiming that he is "the Messiah." His wife is contacted who states that he has been walking throughout the house all night for the last 4 nights, talking "nonstop," and starting many home repair projects that remain unfinished. She confirms that he is taking sertraline for his depression and propranolol for high blood pressure. His blood alcohol level is less than 10, and his urine toxicology screen is negative.

ANSWERS

10.1 **E.** The most likely diagnosis for this man is cocaine-induced bipolar disorder. Although he presents with classic symptoms of a manic episode (irritable mood, decreased sleep, etc), he has no psychiatric or family history of mood disorder. His physical examination reveals several findings not necessarily consistent with mania, namely, elevated vital signs (pulse rate and blood pressure) and dilated pupils. The important factor in this case is his cocaine use, which can produce symptoms mimicking those of acute mania.

10.2 **D.** The most likely diagnosis is depressive disorder due to multiple sclerosis. Although this woman displays the characteristic symptoms of an episode of major depression (depressed mood, increased sleeping, low energy), she does not exhibit the appetite or weight changes commonly seen in this illness. Steroids can often cause mood symptoms such as depression or mania, but she is currently not taking any medication. The results of her physical examination are also consistent with a flare-up of her multiple sclerosis and demonstrate a temporal relationship to her depression. There has been found to be some association between depression in patients with multiple sclerosis and neuropathology in the left anterior temporal/parietal regions.

10.3 **C.** The most likely diagnosis for this man is major depressive disorder. He has symptoms which are typical of the disorder, both a depressed mood and neurovegetative symptoms (changes in sleep, appetite, and energy) lasting for more than 2 weeks. Although his condition was preceded by a heart attack, it is not likely a physiologic cause of his depression. Rather, his medical illness (and subsequent feeling of vulnerability) was the stressor that brought on his episode of depression.

10.4 **D.** The most likely diagnosis in this case is depressive disorder due to a cerebral vascular accident. The patient has obvious symptoms of a depressive illness, including anhedonia and neurovegetative symptoms. These symptoms also have a clear temporal relationship to her stroke, which has left her with significant motor deficits. Cerebral vascular events have been shown to not infrequently result in depression.

10.5 **E.** The most likely diagnosis for this patient would be antidepressant-induced bipolar disorder, in other words mania brought on by antidepressant treatment. He has classic symptoms and signs of mania, such as decreased need for sleep, talkativeness, increased activity, risky behavior, and delusions of grandeur. He also has a history of a major depressive episode and has been taking an antidepressant which likely has caused a switch into his current manic episode. According to the *DSM-5*, manic episodes caused by antidepressant treatment are considered substance induced, unless his manic symptoms persist beyond the physiological effects of the antidepressant. Although he is taking a beta-blocker for hypertension, it would be more likely to cause depression than mania, and there is not strong evidence that beta-blockers actually cause depressive symptoms.

CLINICAL PEARLS

▶ A complete medical history, physical examination, and routine laboratory tests, including thyroid studies, are essential in the workup for an individual presenting with the first episode of a mood (depressive or bipolar) disorder.

▶ Atypical symptoms, for example, weight gain without an increase in appetite, suggest a depressive disorder due to another medical condition.

▶ For a mood (depressive or bipolar) disorder due to another medical condition to be diagnosed, the medical condition is required to have a causal, physiologic relationship to the mood episode.

▶ The incidence of depressive episodes after a stroke is significant.

REFERENCES

Ayerbe L, Ayis S, Wolfe CD, Rudd AG. Natural history, predictors and outcomes of depression after stroke: systematic review and meta-analysis. *Br J Psychiatry*. 2013;202:14.

Hage MP, Azar ST. The Link between Thyroid Function and Depression. *J Thyroid Res*. 2012;2012: 590648. http://dx.doi.org/10.1155/2012/590648. Last accessed September 1, 2014.

Ko DT, Hebert PR, Coffey CS, Sedrakyan A, Curtis JP, Krumholz HM. Beta-blocker therapy and symptoms of depression, fatigue, and sexual dysfunction. *JAMA*. 2002;288(3):351.

Sadock BJ, Sadock VA. *Kaplan & Sadock's Synopsis of Psychiatry*. 9th ed. Baltimore, MD: Lippincott Williams & Wilkins; 2007:738-739.

Siegert RJ, Abernethy DA. Depression in multiple sclerosis: a review. *J Neurol Neurosurg Psychiatry*. 2005;76:469-475.

A 16-year-old girl comes to the emergency department at the insistence of her parents with a chief complaint of suicidal ideation. She states that for the past week she has felt that life is no longer worth living and that she has been planning to kill herself by getting drunk and taking her mother's alprazolam (Xanax). She says that her mood is depressed, she has no energy, and she is not interested in doing things she normally enjoys. Prior to 1 week ago, she had none of these symptoms. The patient states that she has been sleeping 12 to 14 hours a day for the past week and eating "everything in sight." She says she has never been diagnosed with major depression or been seen by a psychiatrist. She is not aware of any medical problems. The patient states that up until 9 days ago she used cocaine on a daily basis for a month, but then stopped it when school started.

On mental status examination, the patient appears alert and oriented to person, place, and time. Her speech is normal, but her mood is "depressed," and her affect is constricted and dysphoric. She denies having hallucinations or delusions but has suicidal ideation with a specific intent and plan. She denies having homicidal ideation.

▶ What is the most likely diagnosis for this patient?
▶ What is the next step in the treatment?

ANSWERS TO CASE 11:

Substance/Medication-Induced Depressive Disorder (Cocaine)

Summary: A 16-year-old patient presents to the emergency department with suicidal ideation 9 days after she stopped using cocaine. For the past 1 week, she has noted a depressed mood, hypersomnia, decreased energy, anhedonia, and an increased appetite. She has no medical problems and has never been diagnosed with major depression. On a mental status examination, her mood is seen to be depressed, and her affect is dysphoric and constricted. She has suicidal ideation with a specific intent and a plan.

- **Most likely diagnosis:** Substance/medication-induced mood disorder (cocaine).

- **Next step:** Discontinuing use of the offending drug is usually enough to cause the mood disorder symptoms to abate. An antidepressant is generally not needed initially; however, if the depressive symptoms continue, treatment with an antidepressant can be indicated. This patient certainly needs substance abuse treatment to deal with her substance abuse problems. A more detailed substance abuse history should be taken. Because she is suicidal with specific intent and a plan, she should be hospitalized on a psychiatric inpatient unit.

ANALYSIS

Objectives

1. Recognize substance/medication-induced depressive disorder (Table 11–1 for diagnostic criteria).

2. Know the treatment recommendations for a patient with this disorder.

Considerations

The primary consideration in this case is that the patient did not start having mood symptoms until *after* she stopped taking cocaine. On withdrawing from the drug, the patient noted a severely depressed mood with suicidal ideation. In addition, she noted many of the signs/symptoms of cocaine withdrawal, including fatigue, decreased energy, hypersomnia, and an increased appetite. The patient has no history of major depression.

Table 11–1 • DIAGNOSTIC CRITERIA FOR SUBSTANCE/MEDICATION-INDUCED DEPRESSIVE DISORDER
A. A persistent, prominent disturbance in mood that is characterized by depressed mood or markedly diminished interest or pleasure.
B. There is evidence from the history, physical examination, or laboratory findings of both:
1. The symptoms developed during or soon after substance intoxication or withdrawal or after exposure to a medication.
2. The involved substance/medication is capable of producing the symptoms.
C. The disturbance is not better explained by a depressive disorder that is not substance/medication induced.
D. The disturbance does not occur exclusively during the course of a delirium.
E. The disturbance causes clinically significant distress or impairment in functioning.

APPROACH TO:

Substance/Medication-Induced Depressive Disorder

DEFINITIONS

ANHEDONIA: Loss of interest or pleasure in normally enjoyable activities.

HYPERACTIVITY: Excessive level of activity significantly above that expected for the developmental stage and setting.

HYPERSOMNIA: An increase in the amount of sleep (and a subjective feeling of a need for sleep) above what is normal for a particular person.

IMPULSIVITY: Taking action without appropriate thought and consideration that can often lead to a dangerous situation.

CLINICAL APPROACH

Cocaine has been used at least once by 25 million people in the United Sates with 2.7% of the population having had cocaine dependence at one time. (The lifetime prevalence of bipolar disorder is only 1.6%.) Cocaine-induced mood disturbance can occur during use, intoxication, or withdrawal from the drug. During use and intoxication, cocaine is more likely to produce a manic state; depressed states are more common during withdrawal.

Substances, including medications used to treat nonpsychiatric disorders, neuroactive chemicals, or recreational agents, can induce mood changes. Antihypertensive agents (especially beta-blockers), interferon, and cytotoxic agents may destabilize mood. Depression, mania with or without psychotic symptoms, or mixed depression and mania can result. Both intoxication with and withdrawal from a substance can lead to a mood disturbance.

DIFFERENTIAL DIAGNOSIS

Care must be taken to determine if substance intoxication or substance withdrawal is currently present. Realize that patients will often lie to health care providers regarding their substance use. A toxicology screen and ancillary history from family and friends can be extremely helpful in determining actual substance use patterns. If no substance use is identified, a primary mood disorder should be considered. Depressive disorder due to another medical condition should be considered if a medical condition is thought to account for the depressive symptoms. Finally, a careful review of the patient's history should indicate whether episodes of mania or depression have occurred, and if so, a diagnosis of bipolar disorder should be considered.

TREATMENT

The main treatment for a substance/medication-induced depressive disorder is cessation of use of the causative substance. This is particularly true of alcohol and opioids. On the other hand, cessation of the use of some substances can initially result in a worsening of mood; for instance, discontinuing cocaine use often leads to a "crash," which quite commonly includes a severely dysphoric mood. However, even in such cases, the vast majority of mood symptoms resolve on their own without psychopharmacologic intervention, usually within several weeks. If the symptoms of a substance/medication-induced depressive disorder do not resolve with removal of the offending substance after several weeks, the use of psychotropic medications may be indicated. For example, a patient whose substance/medication-induced mood disorder takes the form of a manic presentation should be treated like a patient with bipolar disease and given a mood stabilizer. After a sufficient washout period, a patient with this disorder who remains depressed should be treated like a patient with major depression and given antidepressant medication. There is some suggestion that individuals with co-occurring depression and cocaine use may respond to tricyclic antidepressants (TCAs) over selective serotonin reuptake inhibitors (SSRIs).

Referral for substance abuse treatment is always indicated. Many patients need more than 10 attempts at substance abuse treatment in order to finally achieve sobriety.

CASE CORRELATION

- See also Case 10 or Case 13. Individuals with medical conditions often take medications for those conditions, and it may sometimes be difficult to discern which (the medical condition or the medication used to treat it) may be causing the depressive disorder. The history often provides a basis for judgment, or a medication change may be needed to sort out the diagnosis. A depressive disorder should be diagnosed when it is judged that the substance/medication in question is *not* etiologically related to the symptoms of depression.

COMPREHENSION QUESTIONS

11.1 A 35-year-old man is brought to a psychiatrist's office by his wife. He had previously suffered a major depressive episode 2 years prior and ceased medications 6 months ago. More recently, the patient had been working many overtime hours for several weeks to complete a project at work, and had slept much less than normal without apparent ill effect. When the project was completed, the patient continued to sleep little, and shifted his activities to socializing and drinking with his work colleagues. The patient admits he has not drunk this heavily since college. For the past few days, the patient has "crashed" back into depression. Which of the following is the most likely explanation for this patient's condition?

A. Exacerbation of major depression

B. Substance/medication-induced depressive disorder (alcohol)

C. Bipolar disorder

D. Adjustment disorder

E. Circadian rhythm sleep disorder

11.2 A 22-year-old woman presents to the emergency department with complaints of depression and suicidal ideation. She admits that up until 24 hours ago, she was heavily abusing cocaine. Which of the following findings would be most common with this presentation?

A. Miosis, slurred speech, drowsiness

B. Nystagmus, hypertension, muscle rigidity

C. Conjunctival injection, increased appetite, dry mouth

D. Fatigue, increased appetite, vivid and unpleasant dreams

E. Mydriasis, gooseflesh, rhinorrhea, muscle aches

11.3 A 23-year-old man is referred from an outpatient drug rehabilitation program to a psychiatrist for significant depression. The patient endorses having used "everything I can get my hands on, as often as I can get it." A drug screen is positive for an illicit substance. The psychiatrist, however, doubts that the drug identified is responsible for the patient's symptoms of depression. Which of the following drugs is most likely to be present on the drug screen?

A. Cannabis

B. Cocaine

C. Alcohol

D. Methamphetamine

E. Inhaling spray paint or "huffing"

11.4 Which of the following scenarios is most clearly consistent with a diagnosis of a substance/medication-induced depressive disorder?

A. A 23-year-old woman who has newly been diagnosed with lupus, experiences profound depression after her first course of steroids.

B. A 40-year-old man who has had problems with depression and drinking since adolescence, and has a strong family history of depression and suicide attempts.

C. A 23-year-old graduate student who has had issues with depression for 5 years and smokes marijuana once a month.

D. A 35-year-old military combat veteran, who begins drinking more heavily to drown out nightmares of when his truck was hit by an Improvised explosive device (IED), killing and wounding several members of his unit.

E. A newly widowed 89-year-old woman begins drinking a small glass of wine every night so she can go to sleep.

ANSWERS

11.1 **C.** The patient describes a pattern of decreased need for sleep, yet with no decrease in energy level, which is highly suggestive of a diagnosis of bipolar disorder. He may have had similar episodes in the past, but such patients generally seek help when they are depressed, as opposed to hypomanic or manic. Increased goal-directed activity and excessive pleasure-seeking activities such as drug use are hallmarks of a manic episode. However, it is often very difficult to distinguish between a primary mood disorder and a substance/medication-induced one, without an extended period of abstinence accompanied by continuing mood complaints. Adjustment disorder or circadian rhythm disorder does not explain this patient's array of symptoms.

11.2 **D.** A is consistent with opioid intoxication. B describes phencyclidine intoxication. C is cannabis intoxication. E is consistent with opioid withdrawal.

11.3 **A.** *Diagnostic and Statistical Manual of Mental Disorders, 5th edition (DSM-5)* does not specifically recognize cannabis-induced mood disorders. Mood disorders would be much more common with the other substances listed.

11.4 **A.** In A, the timing and the likely offending agent are most consistent with a substance/medication-induced depressive disorder. In B, there is likely a strong genetic component to his depression, and there is no mention of his depression's relationship to any periods of sobriety. In C, cannabis is not clearly likely to induce depression, especially at low doses. D is more consistent with posttraumatic stress disorder (PTSD). E is most consistent with bereavement.

CLINICAL PEARLS

▶ The symptoms can occur during the period of time the substance is being used or up to a month after use of the substance has ceased.

▶ In order for the mood symptoms to be accurately assessed, the patient should not be acutely intoxicated or undergoing the withdrawal process.

REFERENCES

DSM-5 Task Force *Diagnostic and Statistical Manual of Mental Disorders*. 5th ed. Washington, DC: American Psychiatric Publishing; 2013.

Ketter TA, Chang KD. Bipolar and Related Disorders. *Textbook of Psychiatry*. 6th ed. Washington, DC: American Psychiatric Publishing; 2014:379-382.

A 16-year-old student is brought to the emergency department by her parents. She says that for the past 6 weeks, she feels as if she "just can't cope with all the pressure at school." She broke up with her boyfriend 6 weeks ago. Since that time, she cannot sleep more than 3 or 4 hours a night. She has lost 15 lb without trying to, and her appetite is decreased. She says that nothing interests her and that she cannot even concentrate long enough to read a magazine, much less her text-books. Her energy level is very low. She is not doing things with her friends like she was in the past and says that when she is with them "things just aren't fun like they used to be." She tends to be irritable and gets angry with slight provocation.

On a mental status examination, she is observed to be a well-dressed teenager with good hygiene. She notes that her mood is very depressed, 2 on a scale of 1 to 10. Her affect is dysphoric and constricted. She admits to hearing a voice telling her that she is "no good." She has heard this voice at least daily for the past week. She admits to having had thoughts of suicide frequently over the past several days but denies that she would act on these thoughts because it would be a "sin." She does not have a suicide plan. No delusions are present, and she is alert and oriented to person, place, and time.

▶ What is the most likely diagnosis?
▶ What is the next step?

ANSWERS TO CASE 12:

Major Depression with Psychotic Features

Summary: A 16-year-old girl experienced a depressed mood with anhedonia, anergia, insomnia, and a decreased appetite with weight loss because her boyfriend broke up with her 6 weeks previously. She also has decreased energy, suicidal ideation, and **mood-congruent auditory hallucinations.** Even with all these symptoms, she is well dressed and has good hygiene. Her mood and affect are dysphoric, and she has noted an increase in her irritability. She is suicidal but does not have a specific intent or plan.

- **Most likely diagnosis:** Major depressive disorder, severe, single episode with mood-congruent psychotic features (auditory hallucinations).

- **Best treatment:** She should be **offered a psychiatric admission** because her major depression is severe. Although she is not committable, she could still be hospitalized by her parents because she is a minor. She should be started on a selective serotonin reuptake inhibitor (SSRI) and an atypical antipsychotic medication. When stabilized, the patient should be seen weekly for at least 4 weeks by the physician or qualified mental health professional to assess for any increase in suicidal thinking in compliance with current Food and Drug Administration (FDA) warnings for antidepressant use in children.

ANALYSIS

Objectives

1. Recognize major depression in a patient.

2. Understand admission criteria for a patient with major depression with psychotic features.

Considerations

This patient has clear-cut major depression with psychotic features. Although the depression seems to have been precipitated by her break-up with her boyfriend, the combination of **vegetative symptoms, suicidal ideation,** and auditory hallucinations points to major depression. An adjustment disorder would not have all these features. Children and adolescents with major depression often report their mood as angry or mad as opposed to sad or depressed. This patient is obviously quite depressed, reporting suicidal ideation and auditory hallucinations; thus hospital admission is a reasonable decision choice. However, she does not appear to be in imminent danger to herself or to others, nor is there evidence that she cannot take care of herself; therefore she is not committable. However, a minor can be hospitalized with a parent's permission, and this certainly should be sought.

In this patient's case, the description of the disorder is major depression, *severe with mood-congruent psychotic features* (Table 12–1).

Table 12–1 • DIAGNOSTIC CRITERIA FOR MAJOR DEPRESSION WITH PSYCHOTIC FEATURES
The patient must have five or more of the following symptoms, which should be present during a 2-wk period; this symptom picture must be significantly different from the patient's usual functioning. At least one of the symptoms must be depressed mood or anhedonia. <ul><li>Depressed mood</li><li>Significantly decreased pleasure or interest in usual activities</li><li>A significant decrease or increase in appetite, weight loss (without dieting), or weight gain (> 5% of body weight)</li><li>Daily insomnia or excessive sleeping</li><li>Psychomotor slowing (retardation) or agitation</li><li>Decreased or absent energy</li><li>A sense of worthlessness or unusual feelings of guilt</li><li>Decreased ability to concentrate or slowed thinking</li><li>Thoughts of death (not just fear of death) or suicide</li></ul>
The symptoms are not those of an episode of bipolar disorder, mixed.
The symptoms must cause the patient considerable distress or a decrease in functioning (social life, job, activities of daily living).
The symptoms are not the effects of a medical illness or a substance (prescription or street drug).
The symptoms are not part of normal bereavement following a loss.

APPROACH TO:

Major Depression with Psychotic Features

DEFINITIONS

ANHEDONIA: Loss of a subjective sense of pleasure.

MOOD-CONGRUENT DELUSIONS OR HALLUCINATIONS: The content of the delusions or hallucinations reflects the nature of the illness. For example, in major depression, delusions and hallucinations are often about being defective, deficient, diseased, or guilty and deserving of punishment.

PSYCHOSIS: A syndrome characterized by hallucinations and/or delusions (fixed, false beliefs). The individual's ability to assess reality is impaired.

SOMATIC DELUSIONS: False beliefs about one's body; in depression, these are beliefs regarding illness, for example, that one has cancer and is about to die.

VEGETATIVE SYMPTOMS: Symptoms of depression that are physiologic or are related to body functions, such as sleep, appetite, energy, and sexual interest. Other symptom categories for depression are cognitive (poor concentration, low self-esteem) and emotional (crying spells).

CLINICAL APPROACH

Differential Diagnosis

Studies suggest the prevalence of major depression is 0.3% in preschoolers, 3% in elementary school children, and 6% to 7% in adolescents. Genetic factors, loss of a parent at an early age (before the age of 11), and adverse early life experiences are significant predictors for major depression in childhood and adulthood. **Depressed youths often present first to their pediatricians with complaints of sudden onset of anger and irritability, lack of interest in fun activities, decreased energy, sudden poor grades** (caused by decreased ability to concentrate), **staying up late** (under the claim of wanting to watch TV but really because the patient has trouble falling asleep), and **withdrawal from friends and family.** It is then important to inquire about psychotic symptoms and suicidal thoughts. Suicide is the third leading cause of death in adolescents. The rate is 18.25/100,000 in males and 3.48/100,000 in females. Females attempt more often, but males use more lethal means. Suicide rates in children and adolescents aged 5 to 19 years have shown a steady decrease from 1988 until 2003, in large part because of the increased recognition of depression in youth and the subsequent provision of treatment. Interestingly, while most depressed persons who commit suicide seek professional help in 1 month prior to committing suicide, most are not on an antidepressant at the time of suicide. This suggests that a lack of implementing effective treatment is a major problem. Diagnosis is often complex because there are many comorbid disorders such as anxiety disorders, disruptive behavior disorders, or substance abuse that can confuse the picture. Similarly, many personality disorders can begin to be seen in adolescence and need to be considered as well. Many medical conditions and substances can also cause mood disorders. (See Tables 10–1 and 10–2 for a listing of the general medical illnesses and substances that can cause mood symptoms.)

Other mood disorders such as bipolar illness and dysthymia can be difficult to differentiate from major depression. **Sometimes a patient with bipolar disorder has several episodes of depression before the first episode of mania,** and examining a carefully recorded family history and clinical history can raise the clinician's suspicion of bipolar disorder. Sometimes a patient has an episode of major depression superimposed on lifelong dysthymia, making the diagnosis difficult. Schizoaffective disorder includes both depressive and psychotic symptoms; knowledge of the history and course of the illness is often necessary to make a diagnosis. Patients with schizophrenia can experience episodes of depression, but these usually develop later in the course of the illness, and the predominant picture is one of psychosis and negative symptoms. An active substance dependence makes the diagnosis of depression difficult because depressive and psychotic symptoms accompany the use of many substances (such as alcohol or cocaine); these can be indistinguishable from major depression. Often a patient must abstain from the substance for several weeks before a diagnosis can be confirmed.

In normal bereavement, especially during the first 2 months after the loss of a significant other, an individual can have symptoms of major depression. However, these gradually diminish with time. Indications that a bereaved person can be developing major depression include a preoccupation with guilt, feeling that one has caused the death of the loved one, and suicidal thoughts. It is important to remember that in children and adolescents with normal bereavement, they will often have hallucinatory phenomena where they will see or hear the deceased loved one, often with messages that are reassuring and comforting. These are not usually signs of a psychotic depression. Hostile accusatory hallucinations are more typical of major depression with psychotic features.

TREATMENT

In October 2004, the Federal Food and Drug Administration issued a black box warning regarding the possible increase in risk in suicidality as evidenced by a two-fold increase of suicidal behavior in pediatric populations who were not actively suicidal at the time antidepressants were prescribed. Debate about this finding continues with opinions ranging from this finding being the result of inadequate dosing with antidepressants that allowed the depression to progress, the result of an adverse effect of akathisia, or a medication-produced switch from depression to a bipolar mixed state. The effect of the warning on many physicians and the general public was marked. Gibbons et al found that from 2003 to 2005, the use of antidepressants decreased in all patient populations with a 20% decrease in children up to the age of 14 years. At the same time, the suicide rates for youth aged 5 to 19 years increased 14% from 2003 until 2004. Today most psychiatrists would hold that youth with major depression should receive antidepressant treatment with close monitoring. A study in 2013 indicated that 3.9% of US adolescents were on antidepressants, usually for depression or anxiety disorders.

The American Academy of Child and Adolescent Psychiatry (AACAP) has developed practice parameters for the treatment of major depression. According to AACAP, this patient should initially be started on an SSRI and an atypical neuroleptic along with supportive psychotherapy to help stabilize her. The doses of either medication should be increased gradually until a therapeutic response is achieved, a maximum dose for body size is reached with no response, or the patient is experiencing side effects. If the patient's depression has no response or only a partial response to an adequate trial of the first SSRI, an alternative SSRI should be tried. If that fails to produce a response, consideration should be given to switching to a different class of antidepressant. Similarly, if one atypical antipsychotic does not control the psychotic symptoms with adequate dosing, a switch to another should be considered.

If the child suffering from major depression with psychotic features responds to the combination of antidepressant and atypical antipsychotic, the atypical antipsychotic should be continued for 3 months and then tapered off. The antidepressant should be continued for 6 to 12 months and then tapered over 2 to 3 months.

Once the patient is stable, a course of cognitive behavioral psychotherapy along with medication should be utilized. This psychotherapy focuses on automatic negative thinking on the part of the child that occurs when stressful events happen. This adds to the stress of the event and can predispose patients to depressive episodes.

CASE CORRELATION

- See also Case 5 and Case 13. Major depressive disorder with psychotic features is a subcategory of major depressive disorder. The qualifier of 'with psychotic features' is added when patients fulfill criteria for a major depressive disorder and in addition, have evidence of delusions and/or hallucinations appearing *after* the onset of the depressive symptoms. Schizoaffective disorder patients must meet criteria for a major mood episode for the majority of the illness, *and* have delusions or hallucinations for 2 or more weeks in the *absence* of a major mood episode. Essentially, over the lifetime of the illness, the schizoaffective patient must present with just psychotic symptoms (no mood symptoms) for at least some of the disorder, but at other times, have both a mood and psychotic component running concurrently.

COMPREHENSION QUESTIONS

12.1 A 10-year-old girl is brought in for treatment by her father following the unexpected death of her mother due to a heart attack 6 weeks previously. The father is worried because the child is not sleeping well, has lost 7 lb because of a decreased appetite, seems to be tired much of the time, and is preoccupied with memories of her mother. He notes that she cannot concentrate on her usual favorite television shows and has lost interest in many of her previous social activities. The patient reports that she deeply misses her mother, and she smiles in recalling many pleasant memories of their life together. Which of the following is the most likely diagnosis?

A. Adjustment disorder with depressed mood

B. Major depression

C. Normal bereavement

D. Sleep disorder

E. Dysthymic disorder

12.2 A 17-year-old honors student is brought to the emergency department by his parents. In the last academic quarter, his grades have suddenly dropped, he is irritable with friends and family, has no energy, does not go to bed until 1 am, and has a poor appetite. He also has auditory hallucinations in which a man's voice tells him that he is a "lazy bastard" and that his family "would be better off with him dead." Which of the following would be the most appropriate initial pharmacologic treatment plan?

A. Benzodiazepine

B. Antidepressant and antipsychotic medications

C. Antidepressant medication

D. Antipsychotic medication and a benzodiazepine

E. Antidepressant medication and lithium

12.3 Psychotic depression is diagnosed in a 14-year-old boy, and he is treated with an antipsychotic agent (risperidone), and an antidepressant. Three months later, his mood symptoms have resolved, and he is no longer psychotic. Which of the following best describes the next step?

A. Both medications should be discontinued via a taper.

B. The antipsychotic medication should be discontinued via a taper.

C. The antidepressant medication should be discontinued via a taper.

D. Both agents should be continued for 6 to 9 months.

E. The antipsychotic medication should be stopped immediately.

ANSWERS

12.1 **C.** Normal bereavement. This patient's symptoms fulfill the criteria for major depression, but she is in the very early stages of bereavement when such behavior is considered normal. Her sleep problems are part of bereavement. If her symptoms do not diminish in the subsequent 4 months, the clinician should make a reassessment for major depression. Reassessment should be sooner if suicidal or homicidal ideation occurs or if the patient becomes psychotic.

12.2 **B.** An antidepressant combined with an antipsychotic agent is needed for this patient who has major depression with psychotic symptoms. A benzodiazepine can address neither the depressive nor the psychotic symptoms. Lithium is an augmenting agent that can be considered later if necessary.

12.3 **B.** The antipsychotic agent should be discontinued via a gradual taper because the psychotic symptoms have abated. The antidepressant should be continued for approximately 6 to 12 months in a patient with the first onset of major depression, and for longer (perhaps indefinitely) for a patient with recurrent depression.

CLINICAL PEARLS

▶ Psychotic symptoms indicate severe depression and should prompt a serious consideration of hospitalization.

▶ Children and adolescents with major depression often report their mood as angry or mad as opposed to sad or depressed.

▶ Patients with depression are relieved when the clinician inquires about suicidality; asking about suicidal thoughts does not increase the risk that patient will kill him- or herself. Suicide rates in 15 to 19 year olds have quadrupled over the last four decades and are usually in the top three or four causes of death in adolescents. Always ask about suicide in depressed children and adolescents. (Have you ever wanted to die? Have you ever thought about or tried to kill yourself?)

▶ According to AACAP practice parameters, youth suffering from major depression with psychosis should initially be started on an SSRI and an atypical neuroleptic with doses of both increased gradually until a therapeutic response is achieved, a maximum dose for body size is reached with no response, or the patient is experiencing side effects.

▶ If the child suffering from major depression with psychotic features responds to the combination of antidepressant and atypical antipsychotic, the atypical antipsychotic should be continued for 3 months and then tapered off. The antidepressant should be continued for 6 to 12 months and then tapered over 2 to 3 months.

REFERENCES

AACAP. Practice parameter for the assessment and treatment of children and adolescents with depressive disorders. *J Am Acad Child Adolesc Psychiatry*. 2007;46(11):1503-1526.

Gibbons RD, Hendricks B, Hur K, et al. Early evidence on the effects of regulators' suicidality warnings on SSRI prescriptions and suicide in children and adolescents. *Am J Psychiatry*. 2007;164(9): 1356-1363.

Olfson M, He JP, Merikangas KR. Psychotropic medication treatment of adolescents: results from the National Comorbidity Survey-Adolescent Supplement. *J Am Acad Child Adolesc Psychiatry*. 2013;52(4):378-388.

A 42-year-old man comes to his outpatient psychiatrist with complaints of a depressed mood, which he states is identical to depressions he has experienced previously. He was diagnosed with major depression for the first time 20 years ago. At that time, he was treated with imipramine, up to 150 mg/d, with good results. During a second episode, which occurred 15 years ago, he was treated with imipramine, and once again his symptoms remitted after 4 to 6 weeks. He denies illicit drug use or any recent traumatic events. The man states that although he is sure he is experiencing another major depression, he would like to avoid imipramine this time because it produced unacceptable side effects such as dry mouth, dry eyes, and constipation.

▶ What is the best therapy?
▶ What are the side effects of the proposed therapy?

ANSWERS TO CASE 13:

Major Depressive Disorder

Summary: A 42-year-old man complains of symptoms of major depression identical to two prior episodes he experienced in the past. Previously, he was successfully treated with a tricyclic antidepressant (TCA), although this class of medication often produces anticholinergic side effects such as dry mouth, dry eyes, and constipation, of which this patient complains. The question becomes what medication should be used to treat recurrent major depression when tricyclics are not an option.

- **Best therapy:** A selective serotonin reuptake inhibitor (SSRI), such as sertraline, paroxetine, citalopram, fluoxetine, or fluvoxamine, is one of the first-line choices of medication for this patient. Selective serotonin-norepinephrine reuptake inhibitors (SNRIs) such as venlafaxine, desvenlafaxine, duloxetine and levomilnacipran are also first-line treatment options. Other antidepressant options are bupropion and mirtazapine.

- **Common side effects: Gastrointestinal symptoms**—stomach pain, nausea, and diarrhea—occur in early stages of the treatment. Minor sleep disturbances—either sedation or insomnia—can occur. Other common side effects include tremor, dizziness, increased perspiration, and **male and female sexual dysfunction** (most commonly delayed ejaculation in men and decreased libido in women). **Bupropion** is one of the few antidepressants that does not cause sexual side effects.

ANALYSIS

Objectives

1. Understand the treatment of uncomplicated major depressive disorder without psychotic features.

2. Be able to counsel a patient regarding the common side effects of SSRIs, SNRIs, bupropion, and mirtazapine.

Considerations

Although the patient has been successfully treated with a **TCA** (imipramine) two times in the past, these medications are no longer considered first-line treatments because of their **side effect profiles and their potential lethality in overdose** (cardiac arrhythmias). For a patient such as this one, one might consider using imipramine again. However, the patient specifically requests another type of medication because of his previous discomfort with the side effects. Current first-line treatments for patients with major depression, SSRIs, SNRIs, bupropion, and mirtazapine, are thus logical choices; they have fewer side effects and are safer.

Table 13–1 lists the criteria for major depressive disorder.

Table 13–1 • DIAGNOSTIC CRITERIA FOR MAJOR DEPRESSIVE DISORDER

Five or more of the following symptoms have been present during the same 2-wk period (at least one of the symptoms must be depressed mood or anhedonia):
  • Depressed mood
  • Anhedonia
  • Significant weight change or change in appetite
  • Insomnia or hypersomnia
  • Psychomotor agitation or retardation
  • Fatigue or loss of energy
  • Feelings of worthlessness or excessive guilt
  • Decreased ability to concentrate or indecisiveness
  • Thoughts of death or suicidal ideation

There has never been a manic, hypomanic, or mixed episode.
Symptoms cause significant distress or impairment in functioning.
Symptoms are not caused by substance abuse, medication, or a medical condition.
Symptoms are not better accounted for by schizophrenia, schizoaffective disorder, delusional disorder, or a psychotic disorder not otherwise specified.
Symptoms are not better accounted for by bereavement (ie, symptoms last longer than 2 mo; marked functional impairment, suicidal ideation, and/or psychotic symptoms are noted).

APPROACH TO:
Major Depressive Disorder

DEFINITIONS

ANHEDONIA: Loss of interest or pleasure in activities that were previously pleasurable.

SELECTIVE SEROTONIN REUPTAKE INHIBITOR: An agent that blocks the reuptake of serotonin from presynaptic neurons without affecting norepinephrine or dopamine reuptake. These agents are used as antidepressants and in treating eating disorders, panic, obsessive-compulsive disorder, and borderline personality disorder (for symptom-targeted pharmacotherapy).

SELECTIVE SEROTONIN-NOREPINEPHRINE REUPTAKE INHIBITOR: An agent that blocks reuptake of norepinephrine. These agents are used as antidepressants and for generalized anxiety disorder. Duloxetine may also be used for painful diabetic neuropathy.

OTHER ANTIDEPRESSANTS

Bupropion: An agent that blocks norepinephrine and dopamine reuptake. Bupropion is primarily used for depression, anxiety associated with depression, and smoking cessation.

Mirtazapine: A tetracyclic antidepressant agent believed to work through noradrenergic and serotonergic mechanisms. It is not a reuptake inhibitor. Mirtazapine is used to treat depression, anxiety disorders, and to induce sleep.

CLINICAL APPROACH

Major depression is a common problem. **In the United States, approximately one in seven individuals will suffer from this disorder at some time in their lives.** Women are affected twice as often as men, with a mean age of occurrence at 40 years. A common hypothesis concerning the etiology of major depressive disorder involves the alteration of biogenic amines, particularly norepinephrine and serotonin. Genetics plays a role, as evidenced by family studies.

Given the frequency with which depression is a presenting complaint in the primary care setting, a mnemonic is helpful in remembering the criteria for an episode of major depression. This simple mnemonic can help you evaluate patients smoothly and effectively: "Depression **Is** Worth Studiously Memorizing Extremely Grueling Criteria. Sorry." The initials (DIWSMEGCS) stand for the nine symptoms of depression, at least five of which must be present for at least 2 weeks to meet the criteria of a major depressive episode.

Depressed Mood

Interest (lack of)

Weight (loss or gain)

Sleep (most usually decreased, may be increased)

Motor activity (usually decreased though may be agitated)

Energy (decreased)

Guilt (excessive)

Concentration (decreased)

Suicide (thoughts of, plans for, intent to perform)

DIFFERENTIAL DIAGNOSIS

It is important to rule out other disorders that could be causing a depressed state, including medical diseases (eg, hypothyroidism or multiple sclerosis), medications (eg, antihypertensives), or substances (eg, alcohol use or cocaine withdrawal). Obtaining a thorough history, performing a physical examination, and ordering appropriate laboratory studies are crucial in the assessment of any new onset of depression.

Many psychiatric illnesses are characterized by depressive symptoms, including psychotic disorders, anxiety disorders, and personality disorders. A critical distinction to make, especially in recurrent episodes of depression, is between major depressive disorder and bipolar disorders. This distinction is essential not only for making the correct diagnosis but also for proper treatment. **Standard therapies for major depression can be less effective and actually worsen bipolar** illnesses. It is necessary to obtain any current or past history of episodes of mania, as well as any family history of bipolar disorder.

ASSESSMENT OF SUICIDE RISK

One of the most important determinations a clinician must make in the case of a depressed individual is the risk of suicide. The best approach is to ask the patient directly using questions such as, "Are you or have you ever been suicidal?" "Do you want to die?" A patient with a specific suicide plan is of special concern. The psychiatrist should also be alert to warning signs such as an individual becoming uncustomarily quiet and less agitated after a previous expression of suicidal intent or making a will and giving away personal property. Risk factors for suicide include older age, alcohol or drug dependence, prior suicide attempts, male gender, and a family history of suicide.

Adults with major depressive disorder being treated with antidepressants should be observed for worsening depressed mood and suicidality, especially during the initial few months of a course of drug therapy, or at times of dose changes (either increases or decreases).

The results of a careful mental status examination, risk factors, prior suicidal attempts, and suicidal thoughts and intent must be all considered when assessing suicidal risk.

DEPRESSIVE DISORDER WITH PERIPARTUM ONSET

As many as 20% to 40% of US women report some emotional disturbance or problem with cognitive functioning during the peripartum and postpartum period. Fifty percent of "postpartum" major depressive episodes begin prior to delivery. These episodes are collectively referred to as peripartum episodes. Many experience what is known as the "baby blues," in which there **is sadness, strong feelings of dependency, frequent crying spells, and dysphoria.** These feelings, which do not constitute a major depressive episode and therefore should not be treated as such, seem to be attributable to a combination of the rapid hormonal shifts occurring during the postpartum period, the stress of childbearing, and the sudden responsibility of caring for another human being. The "baby blues" **usually last for several days to a week.** In rare cases, peripartum and/or postpartum episodes exceed in both severity and length that which is observed in the "baby blues" and are **characterized by suicidality and severely depressed feelings.** Women with a major depressive episode with peripartum onset need to be treated as one would treat a patient with major depression, taking care to educate them as to the risks of breastfeeding an infant because the antidepressant appears in the milk. Left untreated, a major depressive episode with peripartum onset can worsen to the point that the patient becomes **psychotic,** in which case antipsychotic medication and hospitalization can become necessary.

TREATMENT

In individuals who suffer from major depression, there is an **85% lifetime recurrence rate and a 1-year recurrence rate of about 40%.** The risk of recurrence increases not only with each subsequent episode but also with the occurrence of residual symptoms of depression between episodes, comorbid psychiatric disorders, and chronic medical conditions. Therefore, adequate treatment resulting in full remission is the goal. The treatment options for recurrent episodes of major depression are not significantly different from those for a first episode: pharmacotherapy, psychotherapy (for mild or moderate symptomatology), a combination of the two, or **electroconvulsive** therapy (ECT) in **major depression with psychotic features or where a rapid response is required. For patients who tolerate medication poorly, repetitive transcranial magnetic stimulation (rTMS) can be offered in an outpatient setting as an alternative.**

Common first-line pharmacotherapy for episodes of major depression includes SSRIs (such as fluoxetine, fluvoxamine, sertraline, paroxetine, and citalopram), SNRIs (such as venlafaxine and desvenlafaxine), bupropion, and mirtazapine. Side effects vary among the specific medications and include sedation or activation, weight gain, headache, gastrointestinal symptoms, tremor, elevated blood pressure (for venlafaxine at higher doses), and **sexual dysfunction,** particularly with **SSRIs and venlafaxine.** Although efficacy is essentially equivalent among all classes of antidepressants, **TCAs** such as desipramine and nortriptyline are usually **not considered first-line agents** because their **side effects are less well tolerated.** These side effects include **anticholinergic effects, orthostasis, and cardiac effects** leading to lethality in overdose. **Monoamine oxidase inhibitors (MAOIs)** are used less frequently because of their significant **drug–drug interactions** and because **dietary restrictions** are necessary.

A rule of thumb in managing recurrent episodes of major depression is that the particular medication that achieved remission in past episodes is likely to achieve remission in subsequent episodes, often at the same dose. Additional factors to consider when choosing a medication are prior side effects, drug–drug interactions, cost, and patient preference.

CASE CORRELATION

- See also Case 14. The man in the present case reports a depressed mood that he states is identical to previous episodes occurring 20 years ago and 15 years ago. The fact that this man has episodes of major depression (with the assumption of normal euthymic functioning *between* episodes) differentiates him from Case 14, in which the patient has had a depressed mood that occurs almost all the time, and has done so for at least 2 years.

COMPREHENSION QUESTIONS

13.1 A 30-year-old man presents to your office complaining of being "down" the last month. He has been suffering from difficulty falling and staying asleep, severe fatigue, guilt, poor appetite, and thoughts of wanting to take his life. He does not ever recall feeling this bad. He has stopped talking with his friend and has no interest in doing anything. You believe he is suffering from a major depressive disorder. In order to diagnose this, which symptom must be present?

 A. Decreased appetite

 B. Fatigue

 C. Insomnia

 D. Loss of interest (anhedonia)

 E. Suicidal ideation

13.2 A 44-year-old woman comes to your office for a follow-up visit. She recently received a diagnosis of major depressive disorder and began treatment with citalopram (an SSRI) 6 weeks ago. She claims to feel "happy again," without further depression, crying spells, or insomnia. Her appetite has improved, and she has been able to focus at work and enjoys time with her family. Although she experienced occasional headaches and loose stools at the beginning of her treatment, she no longer complains of any side effects. Which of the following is the most appropriate next step in her treatment?

A. Consider a different class of antidepressants.

B. Discontinue the citalopram.

C. Increase the dose of citalopram.

D. Lower the dose of citalopram.

E. Maintain the current dose of citalopram.

13.3 Which of the following side effects common to SSRIs is the woman in Question 13.2 most likely to complain of in the future?

A. Anorgasmia

B. Headaches

C. Insomnia

D. Nausea

E. Tremor

13.4 The woman in Questions 13.2 and 13.3 is seen 1 year later for a return visit. She has remained on the citalopram at the same dose, and she is tolerating it well, but she worries about "always having to take medication," and requests it to be discontinued. What is her lifetime risk of reoccurrence if not maintained on medication?

A. 10%

B. 25%

C. 50%

D. 85%

E. 100%

ANSWERS

13.1 **D.** Although a change in appetite, insomnia, fatigue, and suicidal ideation are all criteria used in diagnosing major depressive disorder, one of the symptoms *must* be either a depressed mood or anhedonia.

13.2 **E.** The proper strategy in the management of an episode of major depression that has recently remitted is to continue treatment at the same dose if it can be tolerated. Early discontinuation of medication can lead to an early relapse. A general rule of thumb is, "The dose that got you better will keep you well." A reasonable duration for continuing the medication is 6 to 12 months.

13.3 **A.** Although activation (causing insomnia), gastrointestinal symptoms (including nausea), and tremor are common side effects of SSRIs, only sexual dysfunction generally occurs later in the treatment course (after weeks to months).

13.4 **D.** The recommendations for maintenance therapy in major depressive disorder should be made on a case-by-case basis. However, the illness tends to run a chronic course, especially if treatment is discontinued. Indeed, 85% of individuals will suffer from at least one further episode in their lifetime.

CLINICAL PEARLS

▶ It is important to rule out an underlying substance (eg, alcohol and cocaine withdrawal), medication (eg, antihypertensives, steroids), or medical condition causing depression (eg, hypothyroidism, multiple sclerosis), especially if the patient does not have a prior history of depression.

▶ More than 50% of patients who have had one episode of major depression will have recurrent episodes.

▶ The risk of further episodes of major depression increases with the number of prior episodes, the occurrence of residual symptoms of depression between episodes, and any comorbid psychiatric or chronic medical illnesses.

▶ The treatment that was successful for prior episodes of major depression has a higher likelihood of achieving remission in future episodes.

▶ Selective serotonin reuptake inhibitors, selective serotonin-norepinephrine reuptake inhibitors as well as bupropion, and mirtazapine, are all first-line treatment options for major depressive disorder.

REFERENCES

American Psychiatric Association. *Diagnostic and Statistical Manual of Mental Disorders.* 5th ed. Arlington, VA: American Psychiatric Publishing; 2013:160-168.

Black BW, Andreasen NC. *Introductory Textbook of Psychiatry.* 6th ed. Washington, DC: American Psychiatric Publishing; 2014:164-170, 551-570.

Hales RE, Yudofsky SC, Roberts LW. *The American Psychiatric Publishing Textbook of Psychiatry.* 6th ed. Washington, DC: American Psychiatric Publishing; 2014:363-372.

A 34-year-old man comes to the psychiatrist with a chief complaint of a depressed mood lasting "for as long as [he] can remember." The patient states that he never feels as if his mood is good. He describes it as being 4 on a scale of 1 to 10 (10 being the best the patient has ever felt). He states he does not sleep well but has a "decent" energy level. His appetite has fluctuated for the past several years, although he has not lost any weight. He feels distracted much of the time and has trouble making decisions at his job as a computer operator. He feels his self-esteem is low, although he denies thoughts of suicide. He notes he was hospitalized once 5 years ago for major depression and was treated successfully with an antidepressant, although he does not remember which one. He also notes he has felt depressed for at least the last 10 years and that the feeling is constant and unwavering. He denies manic symptoms, psychotic symptoms, or drug or alcohol abuse. He has no medical problems.

▶ What is the most likely diagnosis for this patient?
▶ Should this patient be given any medication?

ANSWERS TO CASE 14:

Persistent Depressive Disorder

Summary: A 34-year-old man suffered from major depression in the past and, according to his history, at least a 10-year-period of depressed mood with insomnia, a fluctuating appetite, and a decreased ability to concentrate. He also notes that his self-esteem is low. He is experiencing no suicidal ideation, psychotic symptoms, or weight loss and is able to continue working. He denies any other psychiatric symptoms or medical problems.

- **Most likely diagnosis:** Persistent depressive disorder

- **Best medical therapy:** Selective serotonin reuptake inhibitors (SSRIs), selective-norepinephrine reuptake inhibitors (SNRIs), and other antidepressants such as bupropion or mirtazapine can be helpful in many patients with this disorder. Although other antidepressants such as tricyclic antidepressants (TCAs) and monoamine oxidase inhibitors (MAOIs) can be effective, SSRIs and SNRIs have better side effect profiles and are usually the first choice.

ANALYSIS

Objectives

1. Understand the diagnostic criteria for persistent depressive disorder (Table 14–1).

2. Be aware of the pharmacologic treatment options available for this disorder.

Considerations

This patient has at least a 10-year history of a depressed mood; this duration fulfils the **2-year requirement** for a diagnosis of persistent depressive disorder to be made.

Table 14–1 • DIAGNOSTIC CRITERIA FOR PERSISTENT DEPRESSIVE DISORDER
A subjective or objective depressed mood most of the day for more days than not for at least 2 y; can be only 1 y for children and adolescents.
The presence of two or more depressive symptoms such as appetite changes, sleep changes, a low energy level, low self-esteem, poor concentration or indecisiveness, or feelings of hopelessness.
During the 2-y time period the person has never been without the depressive symptoms for more than 2 mo.
The criteria for major depression may be continuously present for 2 y.
No manic, hypomanic, or mixed episodes or cyclothymic disorder have ever been present. Not related to a psychotic disorder exclusively.
Symptoms are not caused by substances or due to another medical condition and must cause clinically significant impairment.
The symptoms cause clinically significant distress or impairment in social, occupational, or other important areas of functioning.

Although he experiences a fluctuating appetite and insomnia, neither appears to be severe. (The patient is able to continue to work and has not lost any weight.) He complains of other symptoms consistent with persistent depressive disorder, such as poor concentration, difficulty making decisions, and low self-esteem. He **does not have psychotic symptoms or suicidal ideation,** either of which suggests a more severe disorder. He experienced a major depression in the past, but does not currently meet criteria. The patient denies alcohol, drug abuse, or medical problems, all of which can mimic persistent depressive disorder; however, a complete history, physical examination, and laboratory studies should still be performed.

APPROACH TO:
Persistent Depressive Disorder

CLINICAL APPROACH

Persistent depressive disorder affects approximately 1.5% to 3% of the population. It is more common in women. Whereas major depression is typically characterized by discrete episodes, persistent depressive disorder is usually chronic and nonepisodic. Other mental disorders frequently coexist with persistent depressive disorder, such as major depressive disorder, anxiety disorders (particularly panic disorder), substance abuse, and borderline personality disorder.

DIFFERENTIAL DIAGNOSIS

As in all affective disorders, substances of abuse (such as alcohol), medications (such as beta-blockers), and medical conditions (such as hypothyroidism) must be ruled out as potential causes of the depressive symptoms. Often, it can be difficult to make the distinction between persistent depressive disorder and major depressive disorder (Table 14–2). Although there is a **significant overlap between the two,** there are important differences. **Persistent depressive disorder tends to have an earlier onset** (in the teenage years and in early adulthood) and a **more chronic course** than major depressive disorder, which tends to be more episodic. In other words, **persistent depressive disorder can be viewed as a less-intense, longer-lasting depressive illness** compared to major depressive disorder. When an individual with persistent depressive disorder develops an episode of major depression, the condition is often referred to as "double depression," which has a poorer prognosis than either illness alone.

TREATMENT

Although psychotropic medications were previously viewed as being ineffective in individuals with persistent depressive disorder, more recent research demonstrates a significant benefit from antidepressants. As in major depressive disorder, **SSRIs, SNRIs, bupropion, mirtazapine TCAs, and MAOIs can all be useful in treating persistent depressive disorder.** Because of its chronic nature, a significant therapeutic effect can require up to 8 weeks, and treatment is often continued for many years or for life in some cases. Other modalities useful in treating persistent depressive

Table 14–2 • CHARACTERISTICS OF VARIOUS AFFECTIVE DISORDERS	
Disorder	Criteria
Major depression	Five or more *"Depression Is Worth Studiously Memorizing Extremely Grueling Criteria. Sorry"* criteria for at least 2 wk
Bipolar I disorder (manic)	Meets criteria for **mania** (three or more criteria for at least 1 wk causing **marked impairment or psychosis**) with or without depression (if present, major)
Bipolar II disorder (hypomania)	Meets criteria for **hypomania** (three or more criteria for at least 4 d **not** causing marked impairment or psychosis) with or without depression (if present, major)
Persistent depressive disorder	Depressed mood for most of the day on more days than not, for 2 y (1 y for adolescents and children), no mania or hypomania
Cyclothymia	Numerous episodes of hypomania and persistent depressive disorder for 2 y (1 y for adolescents and children)

Depression Is Worth Studiously Memorizing Extremely Grueling Criteria. Sorry: Depressed Mood, Interest, Weight, Sleep, Motor Activity, Energy, Guilt, Concentration, Suicide

disorder include various psychotherapies. Whereas **cognitive behavioral therapy** is the best studied, insight-oriented therapy and interpersonal therapy are also likely to be of benefit. Because of the pervasive nature of this illness, it is not unusual for patients to be treated with both pharmacotherapy and psychotherapy. This combination can be more efficacious than either treatment alone.

> ### CASE CORRELATION
>
> - See also Case 13. Differentiating these two disorders is done by paying attention to the duration of the illness. Those with persistent depressive disorder must show evidence of a depressive mood plus two or more symptoms meeting criteria for persistent depressive disorder for 2 years or more, while the diagnosis of a major depressive disorder may be made after the presence of symptoms for 2 weeks.

COMPREHENSION QUESTIONS

14.1 A 22-year-old woman is referred to your office by her family physician for evaluation of depression. Her primary care doctor is unsure whether she is suffering from persistent depressive disorder or a major depressive disorder. Which of the following characteristics is more consistent with persistent depressive disorder than major depression?

A. Episodic course.

B. Numerous neurovegetative symptoms.

C. Presence of psychotic symptoms.

D. Severe impairment in functioning.

E. Symptoms are of a low intensity.

14.2 The patient in Question 14.1 is evaluated fully and is determined to have persistent depressive disorder. Which of the following medications is the most appropriate first-line treatment for her?

A. Desipramine

B. Lithium

C. Lorazepam

D. Phenelzine

E. Sertraline

14.3 The patient in Questions 14.1 and 14.2 returns to your office for a medication check. Sertraline was started 4 months ago. The dose has been increased twice, and the patient has been taking 200 mg for 2 months. She feels the medication has provided some, but not total, relief from her symptoms, and she has tolerated the medication well. You augment with 40 mg of duloxetine. The next morning the patient calls to report she is not feeling well. She has a headache, chills, her heart is racing, and her temperature is 102°F (38.9°C). What instructions should you give your patient?

A. Have her call her primary care physician.

B. Have her come to your office this afternoon when you have an opening.

C. Nothing. It is probably a virus.

D. Tell the patient to go directly to the emergency department.

E. Tell her to take ibuprofen to control the temperature and headache and report back in the morning.

ANSWERS

14.1 **E.** Although the distinction between persistent depressive disorder and major depressive disorder can sometimes be challenging (especially if the major depressive illness is chronic and/or recurrent), patients with persistent depressive disorder tend to have an earlier onset of lower-intensity symptoms, a more chronic course, fewer neurovegetative symptoms, lack of psychosis, and less severe psychosocial or occupational impairment when compared to individuals with major depression.

14.2 **E.** SSRIs (such as sertraline), SNRIs, bupropion, and mirtazapine have demonstrated efficacy in treating persistent depressive disorder. Although TCAs and MAOIs are also beneficial, newer antidepressants such as SSRIs or SNRIs are better tolerated and safer in overdose. Neither lithium nor lorazepam is indicated for persistent depressive disorder.

14.3 **D.** The symptoms the patient reports occurred directly after a medication change which should always be a red flag. Headache, rapid heartbeat, fever, and chills are all symptoms of serotonin syndrome, which can be life threatening. She needs to seek immediate medical care.

CLINICAL PEARLS

▶ Patients with persistent depressive disorder can function relatively well in their lives but experience subjective symptoms of a depressed mood and mild vegetative symptoms.

▶ Persistent depressive disorder can be diagnosed in children if they are symptomatic over a 1-year time period (instead of the 2 years required for adults).

▶ Persistent depressive disorder can be successfully treated with antidepressant medication, psychotherapy, or a combination of the two.

REFERENCES

American Psychiatric Association. *Diagnostic and Statistical Manual of Mental Disorders*. 5th ed. Arlington, VA: American Psychiatric Publishing; 2013:168-171.

Black BW, Andreasen NC. *Introductory Textbook of Psychiatry*. 6th ed. Washington, DC: American Psychiatric Publishing; 2014:171-173.

Hales RE, Yudofsky SC, Roberts LW. *The American Psychiatric Publishing Textbook of Psychiatry*. 6th ed. Washington, DC: American Psychiatric Publishing; 2014:372-376.

A 33-year-old female artist presents to the clinic requesting a referral for marriage counseling. She reports that she and her husband have been fighting since they got married last year. She tearfully discloses that her husband has threatened to divorce her. She describes a longstanding history of periodic irritability "when I just can't stand anyone." During these episodes, she readily angers and berates her loved ones. Her husband now takes the brunt of her verbal abuse. After inquiry, the patient acknowledges that these symptoms typically occur prior to her menses. She experiences "a sense of release" and alleviation of the irritability after the onset of her menses. She denies any changes in sleep regimen or energy level. She denies suicidal ideation, homicidal ideation, or psychotic symptoms.

▶ What is the most likely diagnosis?
▶ How should the patient's symptoms be managed?

ANSWERS TO CASE 15:

Premenstrual Dysphoric Disorder

Summary: A 33-year-old woman presents to clinic describing cyclical episodes of irritability, anger, and increased interpersonal conflicts. These episodes occur prior to her menses and resolve after its onset. The symptoms are leading to relationships issues, particularly marital discord. The patient denies any other symptoms, including those of mania and/or psychosis.

- **Most likely diagnosis:** Premenstrual dysphoric disorder (PMDD).

- **Management:** Selective serotonin reuptake inhibitors (SSRIs) are first-line treatment.

ANALYSIS

Objectives

1. Become familiar with the diagnostic criteria for PMDD (Table 15–1).

2. Learn the treatment strategies for PMDD.

Considerations

This case captures a classic presentation of PMDD, namely irritability and associated symptomatology reoccurring in a premenstrual pattern. PMDD manifests with a

---

Table 15–1 • DIAGNOSTIC CRITERIA FOR PREMENSTRUAL DYSPHORIC DISORDER

During the **majority of menstrual cycles** over the last year, multiple **symptoms begin the week before menses, improve within days after the onset of menses,** and are **minimal/absent during the postmenses** week.

At least **five** symptoms total from both mood and associated symptom categories:

Mood Symptoms
- Depression, hopelessness, self-deprecation
- Affective instability, mood swings, rejection sensitivity
- Increased irritability, anger, or interpersonal conflicts
- Significant anxiety and tension

Associated Symptoms
- Decreased interest
- Concentration difficulty
- Insomnia or hypersomnia
- Fatigue or decreased energy
- Easily overwhelmed
- Change in appetite or specific cravings
- Weight gain, bloating, muscle/joint pain, breast tenderness, or swelling

Symptoms cause significant distress or impairment in functioning.

Symptoms are not caused by substance abuse, medication, or a medical condition.

perimenstrual surge and subsequent recession of mood, behavior, and physical symptoms. Although exacerbation of psychiatric and medical conditions can occur premenstrually, PMDD better accounts for the clinical picture. This patient's mood is predominately irritable, rather than depressed, but she does not exhibit any other signs of mania. The first-line treatment for PMDD is SSRIs. The patient would also likely benefit from individual therapy to learn better coping strategies for her anger. Couples therapy may help develop healthier ways of conflict resolution, but both parties must be willing partners to engage meaningfully in the treatment.

APPROACH TO:
PMDD

DEFINITIONS

AFFECTIVE LABILITY: Rapid changes in affect, for example, mood swings.

FOLLICULAR PHASE OF MENSTRUATION: Begins with onset of menses through the day before the luteinizing hormone (LH) surge. Phase length is approximately 14 to 21 days.

LUTEAL PHASE OF MENSTRUATION: Begins on the day of the LH surge through onset of menses. Ovulation occurs about 36 hours after the LH surge. Phase length is 14 days.

CLINICAL APPROACH

Patients with PMDD present with a premenstrual pattern of symptoms in at least half of their cycles over the course of the year. These luteal phase symptoms most frequently manifest as irritability and mood swings, as well as associated behavioral and somatic symptoms. The typical physical complaints tend to be bloating and breast tenderness. Symptom resolution begins with the onset of menses and reaches quiescence during the follicular phase prior to ovulation. PMDD disrupts patients' education, career, and/or relationships.

The premenstruum, along with postpartum and perimenopause, are all periods of hormonal fluctuation and thus windows of vulnerability for mood disorders. These physiologic hormonal changes trigger mood symptoms for some women. PMS/PMDD can be considered a significant risk factor for postpartum depression. Many women suffer from mild nonpathologic premenstrual issues; 2% to 5% of premenopausal women experience clinical symptoms that cause impairment in functioning. PMDD may begin at anytime after menarche and symptoms remit after menopause. Cyclical hormone replacement can potentially retrigger PMDD symptoms.

Changes from *DSM-IV-TR* to *DSM-5*: PMDD was moved from the appendix in DMS-IV to the main body of the text in *DSM-5*.

DIFFERENTIAL DIAGNOSIS

As always, rule out a substance or another medical condition as the underlying cause. Thyroid dysfunction, fibromyalgia, and irritable bowel syndrome may manifest similarly. Exogenous hormones prescribed to alleviate premenstrual symptoms may sometimes cause or exacerbate the problem. Evaluate if the symptoms occur after initiation of hormonal therapy and if they resolve with medication discontinuation.

Premenstrual syndrome (PMS) is generally less severe than PMDD with fewer symptoms and without significant mood changes. There is a higher prevalence of PMS compared to PMDD. Dysmenorrhea describes pain associated with menses, but lacks mood changes. The pain begins with the onset of menses versus in PMDD in which the symptoms improve during menses. Perimenopause presents similarly as PMS but without the cyclicity.

Mood disorders including major depressive disorder (MDD), persistent depressive disorder, and bipolar disorder may be on the differential. The key aspect in delineating a diagnosis involves examining the timing of symptom onset in relation to the premenstrual phase. Clinical trials have revealed that mood swings and irritability are the most severe of the affective symptoms while depressed mood was least, which further distinguishes PMDD from MDD. Although bipolar disorder commonly presents with irritability and mood lability, the predictable perimenstrual pattern is specific to PMDD.

Symptoms of psychiatric and medical conditions can worsen during the premenstrual phase, but the symptoms do not resolve postmenstruation. In addition to gathering a thorough history and collateral information, ask the patient to use daily prospective ratings for at least two consecutive cycles to obtain more objective data.

TREATMENT

SSRIs have emerged as first-line therapy for PMDD, targeting irritability, depression, and associated physical symptoms within days. Notably, SSRIs work faster in PMS/PMDD compared to any other psychiatric disorder. SSRIs can be administered continuously throughout the menstrual cycle or limited to the luteal phase. Continuous therapy may be more effective for patients with erratic menstrual cycles or in those who cannot follow the dosing regimen. Continuous dosing is ideal in the case of comorbid mood/anxiety disorders or SSRI discontinuation syndrome. Some studies indicate that PMDD symptoms respond better to SSRIs compared to Serotoninnorepinephrine reuptake inhibitors (SNRIs). Previous studies indicate that tricyclic antidepressants are generally not efficacious, with the exception of clomipramine. Combination oral contraceptives suppress ovulation, thus eliminating the luteal phase and predominately address the associated physical discomfort. Oral contraceptive pills (OCPs) should be used with caution, as some studies have shown exogenous hormones to negatively impact mood. Cognitive behavioral therapy may be useful in helping patients better manage their symptoms.

CASE CORRELATION

- See also Case 13 and Case 14. Many women with MDD or persistent depressive disorder believe they have PMDD. However, when asked to provide daily ratings of their mood and compared to the timing of their menstrual cycles, it is clear that there is no correlation between the two. This method is invaluable in distinguishing between these diagnoses.

COMPREHENSION QUESTIONS

15.1 A 40-year-old G3P2 banker at 33-week gestational age is referred to psychiatry by her obstetrician after the patient did not make appropriate weight gains during the pregnancy. The patient admits that she has had depressive symptoms, irritability, and suicidal thoughts "on and off" since the birth of her first child. She reports that the symptoms worsened again after the delivery of her second child. Her husband recently left her, claiming she was "always PMSing." For the last few months, she has struggled to raise the children as a single parent. She denies any plan to hurt herself, her other children, or the fetus. She voices her concern about caring for her children and the newborn after delivery. What is the most likely diagnosis?

    A. Borderline personality disorder

    B. Bipolar disorder

    C. Major depressive disorder, with peripartum onset

    D. Posttraumatic stress disorder

    E. Premenstrual dysphoric disorder

15.2 A 33-year-old writer is brought to the ER by her sister who voices concern that her sibling is acting "out of control." The patient laughs at her sister's accusation and rapidly retorts, "I feel great! She's the one with something wrong." The patient paces around the room, speaking rapidly. The ER physician attempts to redirect the interview several times, but the patient keeps talking. Her sister reports that the patient was like this several months ago, but otherwise has been normal. She remembers that both episodes seemed to occur around the time of her sister's period. The patient responds by chanting, "Yes! Yes! I've got the PMS!" The patient has no known medical problems, substance use, or family history of psychiatric illness. What is the most likely diagnosis?

    A. Bipolar disorder

    B. Premenstrual dysphoric disorder

    C. Premenstrual syndrome

    D. Schizophrenia

    E. Substance-induced bipolar disorder

15.3 A 23-year-old graduate student presents to her primary care physician complaining of severe abdominal cramps, bloating, and difficulty concentrating. She reports concern about her studies suffering over the last few days due to these symptoms. The patient recalls that these same troublesome symptoms occurred last month around the same time, but resolved on their own after her period started. Her boyfriend accompanies the patient. When she steps out to use the restroom, the boyfriend confides in the physician, "She has been so mean over the last few days. It's like anything I do or say sets her off." He does not recall any other changes in her behavior. Which of the following is the first-line treatment for these symptoms?

A. Fluoxetine

B. Lithium

C. Maprotiline

D. Methylphenidate

E. Spironolactone

ANSWERS

15.1 **C.** Based on the information given, the leading diagnosis is major depressive disorder with peripartum onset, commonly referred to as postpartum depression. The patient notes that during this pregnancy and after previous pregnancies, she felt depressed. Further exploration of mood symptoms correlating with her menstrual cycle would be helpful, but this is not a clear diagnosis from the history gathered. Her husband's accusation of premenstrual syndrome (PMS) may have been unfounded, especially given that he made this statement while she was pregnant and not menstruating. Although she may have some degree of mood-related estrogen sensitivity, her symptoms are not reported to correlation with her menstrual cycle. Premenstrual syndrome patients do not necessarily have a change in mood or a minimum of five depressive symptoms. In all patients with postpartum depression, maintain a high clinical suspicion for bipolar disorder which often initially presents as depression after delivery. From the current clinical data, there is no report of manic symptoms. Borderline personality disorder may be considered given the patient's history of chronic suicidality, but more information needs to be gathered. The patient has had a recent rupture in her relationship and she should be screened carefully for abuse. Pregnancy is a particularly vulnerable time for women. From the information gathered by the Centers for Disease Control (CDC), each year 324,000 pregnant women suffer from intimate partner violence. Given that many never report their abuse, this statistic is likely underestimated. A trauma-informed history should be taken. From the history gathered, she does not meet criteria for PTSD.

15.2 **A.** The most likely diagnosis is bipolar disorder. The patient presents in a manic state with elevated mood, irritability, psychomotor agitation, and rapid, pressured speech. Substance-induced bipolar disorder would need to be ruled out with the aid of a urine drug screen. As per collateral information, the patient does not use drugs. These symptoms appear episodically, with otherwise normal functioning. Although the patient's behavior seems strange, there are no overt signs or symptoms of psychosis. Thus schizophrenia is unlikely, but schizoaffective disorder should be kept on the differential. Although the patient reports having PMS, neither PMS or PMDD would account for the patient's manic symptoms. Patients with other psychiatric and medical disorders sometimes experience an exacerbation of symptoms during the premenstrual phase; this does not imply PMDD as the etiology.

15.3 **A.** SSRIs are the first-line therapy for PMDD and can reduce symptoms within days. Some studies have shown that spironolactone may help with the physical symptoms of PMDD, but would not be selected as the initial treatment. Studies have not shown maprotiline or other tricyclic antidepressants to be efficacious, with the exception of clomipramine. Lithium does not have any known benefits in PMDD, but would be the gold standard maintenance treatment for bipolar disorder. Besides irritability, the patient and her boyfriend do not describe previous or current manic symptoms. Concentration impairment does not indicate use of a stimulant, such as methylphenidate, unless ADHD is specifically diagnosed.

CLINICAL PEARLS

▶ Carefully screen for perimenstrual exacerbation of other psychiatric or medical problems.

▶ Take into account all comorbid diseases when choosing a treatment regimen. Utilize medications that may concurrently treat multiple disorders and avoid agents that may worsen other conditions.

▶ SSRIs are first-line treatment for PMDD.

▶ Use OCPs with caution because they may negatively impact mood.

▶ PMS/PMDD is a significant risk factor for PPD in the year after delivery, thus carefully monitor pregnant patients with a history of PMS/PMDD.

REFERENCES

American Psychiatric Association. *Diagnostic and Statistical Manual of Mental Disorders.* 5th ed. Washington, DC: American Psychiatric Association; 2013.

Centers for Disease Control and Prevention. Intimate Partner Violence. 2013. http://www.cdc.gov/reproductivehealth/violence/IntimatePartnerViolence/Sept 3, 2014.

Epperson CN, Steiner M, Hartlage SA, et al. Premenstrual dysphoric disorder: evidence for a new category for DSM-5. *Am J Psychiatry*. May 2012;169(5):465-475.

Hartlage SA, Freels S, Gotman N, Yonkers K. Criteria for premenstrual dysphoric disorder secondary analyses of relevant data sets. *Arch Gen Psychiatry*. 2012;69(3):300-305.

International Society for Premenstrual Disorders. ISPMD consensus on the management of premenstrual disorders. *Arch Womens Ment Health*. Aug 2013;16(4):279-291.

A 36-year-old woman presents to the emergency department with a chief complaint of "I think I'm going crazy." She states that for the past 3 months, she has been experiencing abrupt episodes of intense fear, along with palpitations, sweating, trembling, shortness of breath, chest pain, dizziness, and feeling as if she is going to die. The first instance occurred when she was walking down the street, "not thinking about anything in particular." The episode lasted approximately 15 minutes, although she felt as if it lasted much longer. Since that time she has had similar episodes at least once per day that have occurred unexpectedly in different situations. As a result she finds herself worrying nearly continuously regarding when she will have another attack. She denies other psychiatric symptoms. However, she has been to the emergency department twice in the past 2 weeks, convinced that she is having a heart attack, although the results of her physical and laboratory examinations have been unremarkable. She denies drug use and drinks alcohol only "occasionally," in fact decreasing since the episodes began. She has a medical history of hypothyroidism for 1 year, for which she takes levothyroxine (Synthroid).

▶ What is the differential diagnosis?
▶ What is the next diagnostic step?

ANSWERS TO CASE 16:

Panic Disorder versus Medication-Induced Anxiety Disorder

Summary: A 36-year-old woman presents to the emergency department with a chief complaint and symptoms consistent with panic disorder (intense fear/anxiety, associated with panic attacks: feeling as if she is going crazy or going to die, chest pain, shortness of breath, palpitations, sweating, trembling, and dizziness). The episodes last approximately 15 minutes. The episodes have occurred at least once a day for several months, and there are no clear precipitating factors. The patient spends a great deal of time between attacks worrying about having another attack. She has been to the emergency department several times with the same symptoms, and no physical problems were found. She denies alcohol or drug abuse, and her only medical problem is hypothyroidism.

- **Top two diagnoses in the differential:** Panic disorder versus medication (Synthroid)-induced anxiety disorder.

- **Next diagnostic step:** Obtain a thyroid profile and look for elevated levels of thyroid hormone, which, if present, could explain her symptoms.

ANALYSIS

Objectives

1. Correctly diagnose panic disorder in a patient.

2. Be aware that medical illnesses (as well as some substances and medications) can cause panic attacks.

3. Be able to rule out a medical condition, medication, or substance use as a cause of anxiety or panic with appropriate studies.

Considerations

This woman presents with classic symptoms of a panic attack. The **attacks first appeared "out of the blue"** and have occurred at least **once a day, every day, for the past several months.** They are short-lived in duration, lasting about 15 minutes per episode. The patient spends a lot of time in between the attacks worrying about having another attack, which is a classic feature of the disease. She does not have any symptoms of any other psychiatric disorder. She denies drug or alcohol use other than the occasional use of alcohol (which should be carefully quantified). She has hypothyroidism that is being treated with levothyroxine (Synthroid), which may cause panic attacks if the dose is too high; thyroid studies should be used to rule out this possibility. If the thyroxine level were elevated, the patient's diagnosis would be medication-induced anxiety disorder and not anxiety disorder due to hyperthyroidism, as might be considered. If the patient has panic disorder, she should be treated with a combination of a selective serotonin reuptake inhibitor (SSRI) and a course of cognitive-behavioral therapy. A short-acting benzodiazepine (alprazolam) can be added for immediate control of her symptoms, but should be discontinued after the first several weeks. If the patient is determined to have medication (Synthroid)-induced anxiety disorder, the dose should be decreased, and the panic symptoms ought to remit.

APPROACH TO:
Panic Disorder

DEFINITIONS

AGORAPHOBIA: Marked or intense fear or anxiety triggered by the real or anticipated exposure to a wide range (at least two) of situations. These situations include using public transportation, being in open spaces, being in enclosed spaces, standing in line or being in a crowd, or being outside the home alone.

PANIC ATTACK: An abrupt surge of intense fear that reaches a peak within minutes, associated with at least four of the symptoms listed in Table 16–1. The criteria for panic disorder are given in Table 16–2.

CLINICAL APPROACH

The *Diagnostic and Statistical Manual of Mental Disorders, 5th edition* (DSM-5) requires that at least one panic attack be followed by 1 month of **concern about having additional attacks, worry about the consequences of the attacks, or a maladaptive change in behavior related to the attacks.**

The DSM-5 has established separate diagnostic criteria for **agoraphobia** (anxiety triggered by real or anticipated exposure to a wide range of situations) irrespective of the presence of panic disorder.

Table 16–1 • DEFINITION OF PANIC ATTACK
Panic attack consists of discrete episodes of intense fear or discomfort associated with at least four of the following: • Palpitations • Sweating • Trembling • Shortness of breath • Feelings of choking • Chest pain • Nausea • Dizziness • Derealization or depersonalization • Fear of losing control or "going crazy" • Fear of dying • Numbness or tingling (paresthesias) • Chills or hot flashes

Table 16–2 • CRITERIA FOR PANIC DISORDER
Recurrent, unexpected panic attacks.
Attacks followed by 1 mo of one of the following: concerns about having additional attacks or worry about the consequences of attacks, and/or a maladaptive change in behavior related to the attacks.
Attacks are not caused by the physiological effects of a substance, a medication, or a medical condition.
Attacks are not better accounted for by another mental disorder.

Often, the first panic attack an individual experiences is spontaneous; however, it can also follow an emotional or fearful event. The attacks begin within a 10-minute period of rapidly intensifying symptoms (extreme fear or a sense of impending doom) and last up to 20 to 30 minutes. Patients with an additional diagnosis of agoraphobia avoid being in situations where obtaining help from friends or loved ones would be difficult. These individuals may need to be accompanied when traveling or when in enclosed areas (eg, tunnels, elevators). Some severely affected individuals are unable to leave their own homes.

In the general population, the lifetime prevalence rate of panic disorder is approximately 6%. The median age of onset is 20 to 24 years of age, with women being two times more likely to be affected than men. Approximately one-third of patients with panic disorder also have agoraphobia.

DIFFERENTIAL DIAGNOSIS

At the top of the differential diagnosis list for panic disorder are the numerous medical conditions that can cause panic attacks. Table 16–3 lists some of them. Intoxication caused by amphetamines, cocaine, or hallucinogens, and withdrawal from alcohol or other sedative-hypnotic agents can mimic panic disorder. Medications such as steroids, anticholinergics, and theophylline are also well known to produce anxiety. Underlying endocrine disorders should also be considered. In cases of difficult-to-manage hypertension accompanied by physical symptoms such as racing heart, sweating, nervousness, headache, muscle tension, chest pain, and abdominal distress, pheochromocytoma should be suspected. Tachycardia, heat intolerance, weight loss, and anxiety are features of hyperthyroidism which may mimic an anxiety disorder. Obtaining a thorough history (including details of alcohol and substance use), performing a physical examination, and ordering appropriate laboratory studies (eg, TSH, plasma metanephrine) can usually clarify the diagnosis. With the exception of the elevated blood pressure and pulse rate found in most anxious states, no abnormalities are seen on examination in individuals with panic disorder. Any additional abnormal findings discovered should prompt a further workup for a nonpsychiatric cause. Treating the underlying conditions, adjusting medications, and/or initiating a detoxification process should likely resolve the anxiety symptoms.

Distinguishing panic disorder from other anxiety disorders can often be confusing. Panic attacks can be seen in many other anxiety states, such as posttraumatic stress disorder, obsessive-compulsive disorder, as well as in depression. In fact, a

Table 16-3 • MEDICAL CONDITIONS CAUSING PANIC ATTACKS
Cardiac
• Angina
• Arrhythmias
• Congestive heart failure
• Infarction
Endocrine
• Cushing disease
• Addison disease
• Hyperthyroidism
• Hypoglycemia
• Hypoparathyroidism
• Premenstrual dysphoric disorder
Neoplastic
• Carcinoid
• Insulinoma
• Pheochromocytoma
Neurologic
• Seizure disorder
• Vertigo
• Huntington disease
• Migraine
• Multiple sclerosis
• Transient ischemic attacks
• Wilson disease
Pulmonary diseases
• Asthma
• Chronic obstructive pulmonary disease
• Hyperventilation
• Pulmonary embolus
Other diseases
• Anaphylaxis
• Porphyria

significant percentage of patients with panic disorder also have major depressive disorder. The **hallmark of panic disorder is *unexpected* panic attacks not provoked by any particular stimulus;** this is in contrast to other anxiety disorders, where panic attacks are because of exposure to a certain cue. For example, a car backfiring might provoke a panic attack in a patient with posttraumatic stress disorder, or being near a dog might provoke a panic attack in someone with a specific phobia to dogs. The other important characteristic to remember is that in panic disorder the fear is of *having an attack*, not of a specific situation (contamination in the case of obsessive-compulsive disorder or public speaking in the case of social phobia) or of a number of events (as in generalized anxiety disorder).

TREATMENT

Antidepressants such as SSRIs, SNRIs (such as venlafaxine), and tricyclic antidepressants are highly effective in treating panic disorder. Another efficacious option is cognitive behavioral therapy (CBT). Cognitive behavioral therapy teaches the patient about the disorder, helps reduce or eliminate core fears, and specifically addresses the restrictions on lifestyle present in individuals with this condition. **There may be a slight benefit in combining both medication and CBT, particularly in treatment refractory patients.** As in depression, a significant therapeutic effect from medications may not be seen for several weeks. Treatment with a **benzodiazepine may be needed on a short-term basis to provide more immediate relief.** In fact, alprazolam and clonazepam are not only effective but FDA approved for the treatment of panic disorder. Given the addictive potential of benzodiazepines, as well as the significant comorbidity of alcohol abuse in panic disorder, the goal should be to use as small a dose for as short a period of time as possible, with the intention of discontinuing this medication once the antidepressant reaches full effect.

> ## CASE CORRELATION
>
> - See also Case 21 for another presentation of anxiety/panic. These three disorders (panic disorder, substance/medication-induced anxiety disorder, and anxiety due to another medical condition) must be teased apart by a careful history into the patient's medical condition, medications or substances used/abused, and a time course of the anxiety symptoms.

COMPREHENSION QUESTIONS

16.1 A 28-year-old businessman describes a persistent fear of speaking in public. Although he does not have difficulty with one-on-one situations, when giving a lecture to a group he becomes extremely anxious, worrying that he will be humiliated. He relates one episode in which he was forced to speak at the last minute, which resulted in his experiencing panic, shaking, abdominal cramps, and a fear that he would defecate on himself. Because of this problem, he has been held back from promotion at his place of employment. Which of the following is the most likely diagnosis?

A. Agoraphobia

B. Generalized anxiety disorder

C. Panic disorder

D. Social anxiety disorder

E. Specific phobia

16.2 A 40-year-old married woman presents with complaints of not being able to leave her house. For the past 5 years, she has had increasing difficulty traveling far from home. She constantly worries that she will not be able to get help if she "freaks out." In fact, when she has ventured out of her neighborhood alone, she has had several episodes of intense fear, associated with shortness of breath, chest pain, diaphoresis, and dizziness, lasting for 20 minutes. She is convinced that if she drives alone or with someone else too far from home, she will have an attack and not be able to obtain help. As a result, she relies on her husband and siblings to do all of her shopping, and when she does travel, she does so with extreme trepidation and anxiety. Which of the following is the most likely diagnosis?

A. Agoraphobia

B. Generalized anxiety disorder

C. Panic disorder

D. Social anxiety disorder

E. Specific phobia

16.3 A 25-year-old single woman describes a lifelong history of being "scared of heights." She becomes uncomfortable when at an elevation higher than three stories, and, whenever traveling or shopping, she becomes preoccupied with knowing the exact heights of buildings. Whenever finding herself at a significant distance from the ground, she has severe anxiety symptoms including trembling, lightheadedness, numbness and tingling, and a fear of dying. Which of the following is the most likely diagnosis?

A. Agoraphobia

B. Generalized anxiety disorder

C. Panic disorder

D. Social anxiety disorder

E. Specific phobia

16.4 A 33-year-old divorced man has the chief complaint of "I'm going to have a heart attack like my father." He explains that his father died of a myocardial infarction at 45 years of age. He is convinced that he is experiencing angina attacks consisting of nervousness, sweating, shortness of breath, palpitations, flushing, and numbness in his hands, each lasting for several minutes. He is anxious about having these symptoms, and, despite negative results from a cardiology workup, remains certain that he will suffer a heart attack. His behavior and lifestyle have not been otherwise affected. Which of the following is the most likely diagnosis?

A. Agoraphobia

B. Generalized anxiety disorder

C. Panic disorder

D. Social anxiety disorder

E. Specific phobia

ANSWERS

16.1 **D.** The most likely diagnosis for this man is social anxiety disorder (social phobia). Although he suffers from panic attacks, they are not unprovoked as in panic disorder because they occur in response to public speaking. His fear is not of having further attacks but rather of being embarrassed or humiliated. His anxiety is related to one specific situation (social situations), not more than one circumstance, as in agoraphobia. Generalized anxiety disorder involves excessive anxiety and worry about a number of events or activities. Specific phobia is characterized by an excessive fear that is cued by the presence or anticipation of a specific object or situation (eg, flying, animals) rather than social or performance situations.

16.2 **A.** This woman most likely has agoraphobia. She avoids driving away from her home for fear of being unable to obtain help in the event of a panic attack. While she does have panic attacks, they are not unprovoked; in other words, they occur in response to her exposure to feared situations (eg, public transportation, being outside her home alone).

16.3 **E.** Specific phobia is the most likely diagnosis for this woman. Although she has panic attacks, they are not unexpected (as in panic disorder) and result from being in an elevated location. Her fears are of a particular situation (heights) rather than of having further panic attacks.

16.4 **C.** The most likely diagnosis for this man is panic disorder. He displays characteristic features of panic attacks, such as recurrent episodes of anxiety associated with physical symptoms. These episodes are spontaneous, and he worries about the consequences of having an additional attack, namely, a myocardial infarction. However, he does not avoid places and his behavior is otherwise unaffected, as in agoraphobia.

CLINICAL PEARLS

▶ Panic disorder is characterized by recurrent, unexpected panic attacks associated with worry about having additional attacks, the consequences of attacks, or a change in behavior because of attacks.

▶ Medical conditions, medications, or substance use that can cause panic attacks should be ruled out.

▶ Major depressive disorder is commonly seen in patients with panic disorder.

▶ Selective serotonin reuptake inhibitors or other antidepressants, as well as cognitive behavioral therapy, are used in the treatment of panic disorder. If benzodiazepines are also administered, they should be used in as low a dose and for as short a time as possible.

REFERENCES

American Psychiatric Association. *Diagnostic and Statistical Manual of Mental Disorders*. 5th ed. Washington, DC: American Psychiatric Publishing; 2013.

American Psychiatric Association. *Treatment Guidelines for Panic Disorder*. 2nd ed. http://www.psychiatryonline.com/pracGuide/pracguideChapToc_9.aspx. Accessed July 22, 2014.

Kessler RC, Chiu WT, Jin R, Ruscio AM, Shear K, Walters EE. The epidemiology of panic attacks, panic disorder, and agoraphobia in the National Comorbidity Survey Replication. *Arch Gen Psychiatry*. 2006;63(4):415-424. doi:10.1001/archpsyc.63.4.415.

Vos SP, Huibers MJ, Diels L, Arntz A. A randomized clinical trial of cognitive behavioral therapy and interpersonal psychotherapy for panic disorder with agoraphobia. *Psychol Med*. Dec 2012; 42(12):2661-2672. Epub Apr 30, 2012.

A 24-year-old single woman is referred to a mental health clinic because of "fear of elevators." She describes being "afraid" of elevators since adolescence, after being stuck in one for over 1 hour. Since that time she has attempted to avoid taking them, either walking stairs or using escalators. However, this has become increasingly difficult given her recent employment on the upper floor of a sky-scraper downtown. She has tried to use the stairs but it takes too long and she is winded by the end. As a result she has been late to meetings and has already been reprimanded. She "forced myself" to ride the elevator several days ago, but felt extremely anxious, with sweating, hyperventilation palpitations, nausea, diz-ziness, and fears that she would suffocate and die. While she realizes this is very unlikely, she is unable to tolerate the elevator. She has decided to come in for help so as to avoid losing her job.

▶ What is the most likely diagnosis?
▶ What are the most appropriate treatment options?

ANSWERS TO CASE 17:
Specific Phobia

Summary: A 24-year-old woman has a long history of being afraid of elevators. She had been able to avoid the situation in the past, but this has now caused impairment at work. When required to take the elevator, she has extreme panic with associated physical symptoms of anxiety. She realizes her fears are out of proportion, but she wishes to get help in order to avoid negatively impacting her job further.

- **Most likely diagnosis:** Specific phobia.

- **Treatment options:** Cognitive behavioral therapy (CBT) with exposure is the treatment of choice for specific phobias. While pharmacologic interventions have not been as studied, benzodiazepines might be useful if CBT is unavailable, or in cases where exposure to the phobic situation will be rare. Selective serotonin reuptake inhibitors (SSRIs) have been shown to be of benefit in only several small studies.

ANALYSIS

Objectives

1. Recognize specific phobia in a patient.

2. Recommend appropriate treatments for this disorder.

Considerations

This patient has had a long-standing **fear of elevators.** She usually handles this fear by avoiding elevators, either walking up/down stairs or using escalators if possible. Her new job has been affected as a result; she arrived late to work and was reprimanded. When taking the elevator, she experiences severe anxiety and physical symptoms of anxiety. Her history and presentation are consistent with a specific phobia.

APPROACH TO:
Specific Phobia

DEFINITION

PHOBIC STIMULUS: Presence of a particular situation or object which promotes fear or anxiety.

DIAGNOSTIC CRITERIA

A. Marked fear or anxiety about a specific object or situation (phobic stimulus).

B. Phobic stimulus almost always provokes fear or anxiety.

C. Phobic stimulus is avoided or endured with fear or anxiety.

D. Fear or anxiety is out of proportion to actual danger.

E. Symptoms last more than 6 months.

F. Symptoms cause significant distress or impairment in social or occupational functioning.

G. Symptoms not better explained by another mental disorder.

CLINICAL APPROACH

Specific phobias are quite common, with the 12-month prevalence rates up to 9% of the population. Specific phobias are more common in women than men (2:1), although rates vary depending on the particular phobia. Common phobias include animal (eg, insects, spiders, dogs), environmental (eg, heights, thunderstorms, water), blood/injection/needles, and situational (elevators, airplanes, enclosed spaces). Patients often (75%) have more than one phobic stimulus. While exposure to most phobic stimuli promote sympathetic nervous system arousal, patients with blood-injection specific phobia demonstrate a vasovagal response immediately, with a brief increase in heart rate and blood pressure, followed by a decrease in both, often with fainting.

DIFFERENTIAL DIAGNOSIS

Individuals with specific phobias are greatly distressed about their anxiety, and they recognize that their fears are out of proportion to any real danger. The main disorders in the differential are the other anxiety disorders. While patients with specific phobia may also suffer from panic attacks, in panic disorder the attacks are unprovoked (*not* in response to a phobic stimulus), and the fear is of having further panic attacks rather than of the specific object or situation. Differentiating specific phobia from agoraphobia can be difficult. In agoraphobia, the fear is of being in at least two situations (eg, public transportation and shopping malls) where escape may be difficult or he/she might have panic or embarrassing symptoms. Patients with social anxiety disorder (social phobia) have anxiety in social situations where they are exposed to possible public scrutiny (eg, public speaking, meeting unfamiliar people) and fear they will act in an embarrassing or humiliating manner.

Generalized anxiety disorder is more global, and the worry is over numerous activities or events.

TREATMENT

Psychotherapy is the treatment of choice for individuals with specific phobias. **CBT with exposure treatment** has demonstrated the most benefit. These strategies involve gradual, repeated confrontation of the phobic stimulus in order to facilitate extinction. Patients are exposed to situations in a hierarchy from least to most feared. This exposure should optimally be in vivo, but can also be imagined or simulated (eg, virtual reality). While efficacy for this treatment is high, the drop-out rate is significant, and long-term gains (greater than one year) are unclear. **Pharmacotherapy** for specific phobia has not been studied as intensely as psychotherapy. However, if a patient refuses or is unable to engage in therapy, medications may have some benefit. **Benzodiazepines** should not be prescribed regularly, although they can be used if a phobic stimulus is anticipated and infrequent. **SSRIs** have also shown benefit in several small trials, but improvement doesn't occur for several weeks. There have not been studies demonstrating benefit from combining psychotherapy and pharmacotherapy.

> ## CASE CORRELATION
>
> - See also Case 19 and Case 22 for presentations of patients who may be fearful of external objects or situations. Social anxiety disorder is a fear of social situations or public speaking; for example, while obsessive compulsive disorder (OCD) might present with anxiety about germs, but be matched by a ritual (a compulsion) to contain the anxiety, which is not present in a specific phobia.

COMPREHENSION QUESTIONS

17.1 A 33-year-old man is self-referred to the clinic with the chief complaint of "stage fright." He is currently a waiter at an Italian restaurant but wishes to be an actor. While he has taken multiple classes, learns his roles easily, and practices at home, during the actual performances he becomes "panicked," worried about forgetting his lines and being laughed at by the audience. This has resulted in his either losing or turning down acting opportunities. Although he enjoys his job at the restaurant, he wishes to eventually be a full-time performer. Which of the following is the most likely diagnosis?

   A. Agoraphobia

   B. Generalized anxiety disorder

   C. Panic disorder

   D. Social anxiety disorder (social phobia)

   E. Specific phobia

17.2 A 38-year-old separated woman is sent to a psychiatrist by her obstetrician-gynecologist. She describes increasing difficulties leaving her home, which stemmed from having a severe panic attack 4 months prior while at the shopping mall. Since that time, although she has not had any further panic attacks, she is "deathly afraid" of having another one. At first she avoided malls, but gradually she has limited her driving, and recently won't even leave her home. In fact, she was "forced" to come in by her sister, who has become very worried about her. During the car ride to the appointment, the patient suffered extreme anxiety, fearful she would have another panic attack while on the highway and be unable to obtain help. Which of the following is the most likely diagnosis?

A. Agoraphobia

B. Generalized anxiety disorder

C. Panic disorder

D. Social anxiety disorder (social phobia)

E. Specific phobia

17.3 A 27-year-old married woman arrives at a community mental health clinic with her husband. She is initially embarrassed and reluctant, but eventually discloses that she has an intense fear of bridges, which has been present since adolescence. While she has rarely needed to drive over bridges, a recent promotion has required her to commute to the corporate headquarters, which are located across the bay past a long bridge. She has only been able to drive with resultant, severe panic, and she has already called in sick and missed work because of her fears. She is now worried about losing her job and wishes to get help "any way I can." Which of the following treatments would be the most appropriate for her condition?

A. Alprazolam

B. Citalopram

C. Cognitive therapy

D. Exposure therapy

E. Psychodynamic therapy

ANSWERS

17.1 **D.** This patient exhibits symptoms of social anxiety disorder or social phobia, characterized by anxiety in social situations (such as performing in public or public speaking) and fears of being embarrassed or humiliated. In agoraphobia the fear is of being in situations where escape may be difficult (eg, public places, malls, crowds) rather than of public scrutiny. Patients with generalized anxiety disorder worry about numerous activities or issues. The hallmark of panic disorder is recurrent, unprovoked panic attacks and fears of having additional attacks, whereas for specific phobia the fear is surrounding a particular object or situation (not being embarrassed or humiliated in public).

17.2 **A.** This woman suffers from agoraphobia, as evidenced by her fears of being in situations (eg, malls, driving) where she will have panic attacks and/or be unable to escape. Generalized anxiety disorder patients have anxiety regarding numerous situations or events, not solely one. While panic attacks, such as the one this patient experienced, are necessary for the diagnosis of panic disorder, they are required to be recurrent and unprovoked. The fears in social anxiety disorder (social phobia) and specific phobia are of embarrassment in social situations and a specific object/situation, respectively.

17.3 **D.** This patient most likely has specific phobia. The treatment of choice for patients with specific phobia is CBT with exposure therapy. While benzodiazepines such as alprazolam can initially help with anxiety, they are not adequate long-term treatments and have addiction potential. Citalopram (an SSRI) may be beneficial in patients with specific phobia, but it is not a first-line treatment. Cognitive therapy alone (without a behavioral component) is not nearly as efficacious as CBT with exposure therapy. Psychodynamic or insight-oriented therapy has not been adequately studied in patients with specific phobia.

CLINICAL PEARLS

▶ Specific phobias involve fear or anxiety about a specific object or situation (phobic stimulus). The fear is out of proportion, and the phobic stimulus is avoided or else endured with significant anxiety.

▶ CBT with exposure is the treatment of choice. Alternatively benzodiazepines or SSRIs may be used.

REFERENCES

Alamy S, Wei Zhang, Varia I, Davidson JR, Connor KM. Escitalopram in specific phobia: results of a placebo-controlled pilot trial. *J Psychopharmacol.* 2008;22(2):157.

American Psychiatric Association. *Diagnostic and Statistical Manual of Mental Disorders.* 5th ed. Arlington, VA: American Psychiatric Publishing; 2013.

Black BW, Andreasen NC. *Introductory Textbook of Psychiatry.* 6th ed. Washington, DC: American Psychiatric Publishing; 2014:164-170, 551-570.

Wolitzky-Taylor KB, Horowitz JD, Powers MB, Telch MJ. Psychological approaches in the treatment of specific phobias: a meta-analysis. *Clin Psychol Rev.* 2008;28(6):1021.

A 10-year-old boy with chronic asthma is brought to a pediatrician for his 6-month checkup. In addition, he has complained of chronic headaches for the past 3 months, as well as increasing gastric upsets, which his family believes are caused by multiple food allergies. The patient has a severe allergy to peanuts, which limits the number of places he can go in public. Thus, he has been homeschooled for a year and is doing well. A review of his history shows that he is a highly articulate, thoughtful child who appears to be at or above the educational level of his peers. The child does not agree to be interviewed separately from his mother, stating, "I don't go anywhere without my mother." The two of them are almost never apart. Two years ago, the mother was hospitalized after a serious bout with lupus. She continues to struggle with her disease, and despite having a thriving career before her illness, she can do very little now. She is home all the time, dealing with her own recovery and the management of her illness. During her hospitalization, the patient was quite worried about her illness and even now believes that if he is not around to monitor her condition, she might get sick and require hospitalization again—or even worse. The mother has difficulty sleeping and is most comfortable on the living room couch. The patient no longer uses his own room but sleeps in a chair next to his mother to continue to keep an eye on her. He has very few friends and can be separated from his mother only briefly, and only if he is in the company of his brother or father. After a short period, he becomes anxious and upset and must be reunited with his mother.

▶ What is the most likely diagnosis?
▶ What is the prognosis for this disorder?
▶ What treatments might be helpful in this disorder?

ANSWERS TO CASE 18:

Separation Anxiety Disorder

Summary: A 10-year-old late latency/early adolescent boy exhibits extreme anxiety when not in the presence of his mother. As a result, he no longer attends school although he seems quite bright and cognitively on target. His anxiety symptoms began after the mother experienced a serious, life-threatening illness. The patient believes that if he is separated from her, something terrible might happen to her. In addition, he reports several somatic complaints that have been difficult to diagnose.

- **Most likely diagnosis:** Separation anxiety disorder (a childhood disorder).

- **Prognosis:** Difficult to treat; the patient is more likely to develop depression and/or an anxiety disorder.

- **Best treatment:** A multisystemic treatment approach is required. Selective serotonin reuptake inhibitors (SSRIs) can be helpful in the management of mood symptoms and anxiety. Relaxation techniques can help, along with a gradual separation program. Home schooling only reinforces the child's fear of separating from the family and should be reconsidered.

ANALYSIS

Objectives

1. Recognize the symptoms of a typical case of separation anxiety disorder.

2. Understand the predisposing factors contributing to the disorder.

3. Understand what other disorders the patient is at a higher risk of developing.

Considerations

The patient has a typical presentation for separation anxiety disorder, which usually begins in the late latency period, peaking at 9 to 10 years of age (Table 18–1). Separation anxiety disorder is more common in girls than boys.

It is often precipitated by the life-threatening disease of a parent—most typically the mother or primary caretaker. Patients become extremely anxious and worried when they are physically separated from the parent. They worry that the

Table 18–1 • DIAGNOSTIC CRITERIA FOR SEPARATION ANXIETY DISORDER
Developmentally inappropriate anxiety about separation from home or from the care taker to which an individual is attached.
Duration of the illness must be at least 4 wk.
Onset of the illness should be prior to 18 y of age.
The disturbance should cause clinically significant impairment in important areas of functioning.

parent will die if they are separated and thus are very difficult to console during these periods. Their beliefs can be quite strong and are minimally amenable to reason or reassurance. These patients often report a number of difficult-to-diagnose somatic complaints themselves. Treatment should always include psychotherapy with exposure-based cognitive behavioral therapy having the most empirical support. These treatments should occur in conjunction with the development of a gradual plan to incrementally separate the patient from the parent, with a final goal of returning the patient to his or her earlier level of school and social functioning. Psychotherapy can be supported with the use of SSRIs to decrease the immediate anxiety the patient is feeling while in therapy. It is important to emphasize that medication without therapy is less likely to produce lasting improvement. There is a small literature suggesting that venlafaxine, tricyclic antidepressants, and buspirone may be effective second-line treatments if SSRIs fail to be of benefit. **Benzodiazepines have not shown efficacy in controlled trials in childhood anxiety disorders.**

Children who have separation anxiety disorder have substantial risk of developing either panic disorder as adults (12.6%), panic with agoraphobia (18.6%) or generalized anxiety disorder (26.2%). In addition, 32.6% will experience an episode of major depression during young adulthood. It is thus important to assure that effective treatment occurs in patients with separation anxiety disorder as children. It is not just a "phase that will pass." Patients with separation anxiety will often resist interventions that cause short-term discomfort, especially efforts to gradually separate them from the parent, and push for parents to drop out of treatment. Parents should be educated regarding the long-term impact of this disorder and the need to complete treatment even under the protests of their child.

APPROACH TO:
Separation Anxiety Disorder

DEFINITIONS

MULTISYSTEMIC TREATMENT: A philosophy of treatment used with children and adolescents. It can involve several specific theories and modalities of treatment, but the essential feature is the involvement of various social systems essential to the life of a child. Examples of the systems involved include school, church, family, and peers.

SOMATIC SYMPTOMS: Vague or diffuse feelings of pain or discomfort for which it is difficult to pinpoint an etiology.

CLINICAL APPROACH

Some degree of anxiety about separation from a parent is normal, and clinical judgment must be used to evaluate the severity of the anxiety and its impact on the functioning of the child. In generalized anxiety disorder, the anxiety does not center exclusively on the issue of separation from a parent but is much more diffuse and occurs in many situations. In major depression, which often coexists with separation anxiety disorder and should be diagnosed concurrently if the criteria for the disorder are met, patients typically have vegetative symptoms including insomnia and anorexia. Panic disorders are rarely seen before the age of 18, and in that case, the fear is of having another panic attack, not of separation.

In childhood, separation anxiety disorder can be very difficult to treat and is resistant to improvement. However, the best prognosis is achieved with a **timely diagnosis and rapid initiation of treatment, usually psychotherapeutic modalities** directed toward the **individual, family, and school.** The SSRIs can be helpful in reducing the anxiety felt by the patient during the behavioral interventions. However, separation anxiety disorder patients should not be treated with medication alone. Family therapy can be necessary to identify and address anxiety triggers and in helping the child develop skills to lessen anxiety symptoms, for example, relaxation techniques. School consultations can be helpful to aid in rapid, assertive reintroduction of the child into the school setting. A **successful transition to gradually longer separations should result in generous praise for the child.**

CASE CORRELATION

- See also Case 20 and Case 53 for presentations of patients who may become anxious when considering being separated from their main attachment figure. However, in GAD the patient is anxious about a whole host of worries, not just separation, and in dependent PD, the patient tends to be indiscriminate about his or her attachment to others, not just one main attachment figure. Personality disorders also cannot be diagnosed before the age of 18, whereas separation anxiety disorder is seen in children.

COMPREHENSION QUESTIONS

18.1 A 10-year-old boy presents with episodes of somatic complaints, anxiety, and crying at school which resolves when he is sent home. He won't go anywhere without his mother. Which of the interventions would be an appropriate part of the plan of treatment?

A. Place on home-bound tutoring to be provided by the school district.

B. Prescribe lorazepam prn for anxiety episodes.

C. Place the patient on fluoxetine in low dose.

D. Immediately restrict access to the mother until anxiety symptoms cease.

E. Reassure the mother that the patient is going through "a phase" and that this will pass with little impact on youth's subsequent life.

18.2 Children or adolescents with separation anxiety disorder are at higher risk for which other psychiatric disorder?

A. Malingering

B. Somatization disorder

C. Bipolar disorder

D. Learning disability

E. Major depression

18.3 When starting an SSRI, such as fluoxetine, in an adolescent patient with separation anxiety disorder, the Food and Drug Administration (FDA) recommends the clinician monitor closely for which of the following?

A. Hypovolemia

B. Hypertension

C. Anorexia

D. Suicidal thoughts

E. Delusions

18.4 In controlled studies, which of the following medications is ineffective for use in childhood anxiety disorders?

A. Venlafaxine

B. SSRIs

C. Buspirone

D. Tricyclic antidepressants

E. Benzodiazepines

ANSWERS

18.1 **C.** This medication is one of several agents in the class collectively called SSRIs. Lorazepam is a benzodiazepine that is habit forming and more likely to disinhibit the child. Home-bound tutoring will only reinforce the patient's dependency on his mother. The separation of the patient should be gradually done in degrees. This disorder is not a phase but an indicator of subsequent risk for psychiatric illness as an adult.

18.2 **E.** Children and adolescents with separation anxiety disorder often present with or later develop symptoms of major depression. In children, this can include a depressed, sad, or irritable mood over an extended period of time.

18.3 **D.** The FDA recently placed a black box warning for the use of antidepressants in children and adolescents. This warning reminds clinicians of some evidence indicating a possible increased incidence of suicidal thoughts among adolescents using antidepressants—particularly SSRIs.

18.4 **E.** Benzodiazepines have not shown efficacy in controlled trials in childhood anxiety disorders.

CLINICAL PEARLS

▶ Separation anxiety disorder is often associated with a severe illness of the caretaker, usually the mother.

▶ Psychotherapy (cognitive behavioral) is the primary treatment of choice with medication having a supportive role.

▶ The earlier separation anxiety disorder is treated, the better the prognosis.

REFERENCES

American Academy of Child and Adolescent Psychiatry. Practice parameter for the assessment and treatment of children and adolescents with anxiety disorders. *J Am Acad Child Adolesc Psychiatry*. 2007;46(2):267-283.

Copeland WE, Angold A, Shanahan L, Costello EJ. Longitudinal patterns of anxiety from childhood to adulthood: the Great Smoky Mountains study. *J Am Acad Child Adolesc Psychiatry*. 2014;53(1): 21-33.

Lewinsohn PM, Holm-Denoma JM, Small JW, Seeley JR, Joiner TE. Separation anxiety disorder in childhood as a risk factor for future mental illness. *J Am Acad Child Adolesc Psychiatry*. 2008;47(5):548-555.

Sadock BJ, Sadock VA, Ruiz P. *Kaplan and Sadock's Synopsis of Psychiatry: Behavioral Sciences/Clinical Psychiatry*. 11th ed. Baltimore, MD: Lippincott Williams & Wilkins; 2014.

A 35-year-old man visits a psychiatrist because he is overwhelmingly anxious about a speech he has to make. The man states that he was recently promoted to a position within his company that requires him to speak in front of an audience of approximately 100 people. He says that the first such speech is coming up in 2 weeks and that worrying about it keeps him from sleeping. He knows that his fear is out of proportion, but he is unable to control it. He explains that he has always had trouble with public speaking because he fears that he might "do something stupid" or otherwise embarrass himself. He has avoided public speaking in the past as much as possible or has spoken in public only before an audience of fewer than 10. Because he knows that he must make the presentation coming up in 2 weeks or he will not be able to keep his new job, he has visited the psychiatrist hoping to find a solution to the problem.

▶ What is the most likely diagnosis?
▶ What are the treatment options open to this patient?

ANSWERS TO CASE 19:

Social Anxiety Disorder

Summary: A 35-year-old man has a long history of being afraid to speak in public. He normally handles his fear by avoiding this activity or by keeping the size of the audience to a minimum. He is required to give a presentation in front of a large audience in 2 weeks and has been extremely anxious about it to the point where he cannot sleep. Although the public speaking event is new, he says he has had similar fears most of his life (> 6 months). The clinician would also want to rule out substance use issues or other medical conditions that may be related to the anxiety. The patient is afraid he will somehow embarrass himself in front of the audience. Not being able to speak in front of this audience will negatively impact his job.

- **Most likely diagnosis:** Social anxiety disorder.

- **Treatment options:** Behavioral or cognitive behavioral therapy (CBT) is the treatment of choice. A typical treatment regimen involves relaxation training followed by progressive desensitization. Pharmacologic interventions include benzodiazepines or beta-blockers over the short term. Currently, two classes of antidepressants are considered for longer-term treatment of social phobia. They include selective serotonin reuptake inhibitors (SSRIs) such as sertraline or fluoxetine and serotonin-norepinephrine reuptake inhibitors (SNRIs) such as venlafaxine.

ANALYSIS

Objectives

1. Recognize social anxiety disorder (SAD) in a patient.

2. Develop an appropriate treatment plan for this patient.

Considerations

This patient has had a long-standing **difficulty speaking in public.** He believes he will look stupid or otherwise embarrass himself. He usually handles this fear by avoiding speaking if possible or by speaking only before a small audience. Since his job promotion, he has been terrified by the thought of speaking to an audience of 100, although it is a necessary requirement of the new position. He has been unable to sleep because of his anxiety. He knows that this level of anxiety about public speaking is abnormal but is unable to quell his fears. His fear of speaking in public is consistent with SAD (Table 19–1).

Table 19–1 • DIAGNOSTIC CRITERIA FOR SOCIAL ANXIETY DISORDER
A marked, persistent fear (at least 6 mo in duration) of at least one social or performance situation in which exposure to unfamiliar people or possible scrutiny of others occurs. The person fears that he or she will act in a way or show anxiety symptoms that will be humiliating or embarrassing.
Exposure to the feared situation(s) invariably provokes anxiety that can take the form of a panic attack.
The person recognizes that the fear is unreasonable.
The avoidance of, anxious anticipation of, or distress in the feared situation(s) interferes with the person's normal routine, or there is marked anxiety about having the phobia.
The fear or avoidance is not related to a substance or due to another medical condition.
If another medical condition is present, the fear is not related to it (eg, the fear of stuttering, or trembling in a patient with Parkinson disease).

APPROACH TO:
Social Anxiety Disorder

DEFINITIONS

ANXIETY: Anxiety is a future-oriented mood state associated with preparation for possible, upcoming negative events. Symptoms include verbal-subjective (worry), overt motor acts (avoidance), and somato-visceral activity (increased heart rate).

PHOBIA: Persistent, irrational, exaggerated, and pathologic fear of a specific situation or stimulus that results in conscious avoidance of the dreaded circumstance.

RELAXATION TRAINING: Exercises to reduce arousal levels and increase one's sense of control; includes progressive muscle relaxation and imaging techniques to obtain this reduction in arousal.

SOCIAL PHOBIA: Dread of being embarrassed in public, fear of speaking in public, or fear of eating in public.

SPECIFIC PHOBIA: Dread of a particular object or situation, such as acrophobia (heights), agoraphobia (open places), algophobia (pain), claustrophobia (closed places), xenophobia (strangers), and zoophobia (animals).

CLINICAL APPROACH

Phobias are the single most common mental disorder in the United States, affecting 5% to 10% of the population. Specific phobias are more common than social phobias, and **women are more often affected** in both categories. Genetics can have a role in predisposing individuals to these disorders. Patients with social phobia may benefit from a number of types of psychotherapy. Cognitive behavioral therapy in both a group and individual format has been studied the most for social phobia. Large studies have shown this to be one of the best choices for improved outcome. **Specific phobias are often treated by exposure therapy,** a type of CBT in which **the individual is slowly desensitized with controlled "doses" of the feared stimulus.**

A large meta-analytic study of SAD showed that brain imaging techniques reflect increased activity in limbic and paralimbic regions. The predominance of evidence implicates the amygdala in the pathophysiology of SAD. The observation of alterations in prefrontal regions and the reduced activity observed in striatal and parietal areas show that much remains to be investigated. The alterations in the medial prefrontal cortex provide additional support for a corticolimbic model of SAD pathophysiology. The dopaminergic and GABAergic hypotheses seem directly related to its physiopathology.

DIFFERENTIAL DIAGNOSIS

Individuals with SAD are **distressed** about their fear, experience **anxiety,** and **recognize that their fright is unreasonable.** The most prominent disorders to rule out are also in the anxiety disorder group. Panic disorder with agoraphobia and agoraphobia without panic attacks are **more generalized** and are not focused just on situations where public scrutiny is possible. Generalized anxiety disorder is more global, and the focus of fear is not just about public performance. If the full criteria for a specific anxiety disorder are not met, anxiety disorder not otherwise specified can be used. Finally, anxiety associated with another major mental illness, performance anxiety, stage fright, or shyness must be considered prior to making a diagnosis.

New changes in the DSM-5 include changing the name of this disorder to **social anxiety disorder** from social phobia as well as some minor criteria changes. Those changes include some duration extension to heighten the severity threshold as well as some new specifiers focusing on performance-related anxiety, as well as mutism when only related to social situations.

TREATMENT

Psychotherapy is helpful in treating social phobia and usually involves a combination of behavioral and cognitive therapy using **desensitization** to the feared situation, **rehearsal** during sessions, and homework assignments in which patients are asked to place themselves in public situations in a graded fashion. Overall, CBT demonstrates both efficacy in randomized controlled trials and effectiveness in naturalistic settings in the treatment of adult anxiety disorders.

In some cases, **psychopharmacotherapy** for severe social phobia has succeeded with the use **of SSRIs, SNRIs, benzodiazepines, venlafaxine, and buspirone.** Buspirone has been shown to augment the treatment of this disorder when used adjunctively with SSRIs. Treating the **anxiety associated with performance situations** can also involve the use **of beta-adrenergic receptor antagonists just before the feared situation. Atenolol and propranolol** have been shown to be helpful in these instances and are the most commonly used. Recently, a meta-analytic study examined the efficacy of second-generation antidepressants in the treatment of social phobia. This study demonstrated more responders to escitalopram, paroxetine, and sertraline than in the placebo groups.

Transcranial magnetic stimulation (TMS) is a nonsystemic direct brain intervention utilizing magnetic pulses to stimulate particular areas of the brain. It has been approved and is helpful for depression. Much research is underway for its use in other psychiatric illness. It has been suggested as a possible treatment for anxiety.

Although positive results have frequently been reported in both open and randomized controlled studies, at present there appears to be no conclusive evidence as to the efficacy of repetitive transcranial magnetic stimulation (rTMS) in the treatment for anxiety.

CASE CORRELATION

- See also Case 16 and Case 20 for presentations of patients who may become anxious in social situations. However, panic disorder patients may sometimes only secondarily become anxious about appearing in public because they are afraid they may experience another panic attack and generalised anxiety disorder (GAD) patients tend to be anxious about a whole host of other worries (not just social situations).

COMPREHENSION QUESTIONS

19.1 Which of the following symptoms might be considered of the somatovisceral type?

A. Worry

B. Obsessions

C. Paresthesia

D. Running away

E. Avoidance

19.2 Which of the following is an area of the brain which appears to be most closely related to anxiety based on functional imaging studies?

A. Nucleus accumbens

B. Left prefrontal cortex

C pituitary gland

D. Amygdala

E. Corpus callosum

19.3 There is well accepted evidence that which of the following treatments is effective in social anxiety disorder?

A. Cognitive behavioral therapy

B. TMS

C. Haloperidol

D. Clozapine

E. St. John's wort

ANSWERS

19.1 **C.** These are feelings of prickling or tingling in the fingers or extremities commonly associated with anxiety and panic attacks. The other basic symptoms of anxiety include those of the verbal subjective which include worry, and motor, which includes behaviors such as avoidance or running away.

19.2 **D.** Functional imaging studies have consistently showed the amygdala playing a central role in the area of anxiety. The amygdala is an almond-shaped mass of gray matter located as part of the limbic system.

19.3 **A.** CBT is a specific psychotherapy that has the greatest and most accepted evidence base behind it supporting its utility in anxiety disorders. Although other treatments may also be useful, this should be the psychotherapy of first choice in the area of anxiety.

CLINICAL PEARLS

▶ Social anxiety disorder is one of the most common anxiety disorders, affecting approximately 3% of the general population. Onset usually occurs in late childhood or early adulthood, and the course is often chronic.

▶ Anxiety disorders have a high degree of comorbidity.

▶ Cognitive behavioral therapy, a form of psychotherapy, is the treatment of choice for social phobia.

▶ New criteria for social anxiety disorder include a duration criteria of typically 6 months or longer

▶ Beta-blockers such as propranolol and atenolol are the agents of choice for treatment of the anxiety provoked by performance situations. SSRIs and SNRIs may also be useful for longer-term treatment.

▶ Panic attacks can be part of the presentation of social phobia but this does not mean an individual has panic disorder.

REFERENCES

Craske MG, Rauch SL, Ursano R, Prenoveau J, Pine DS, Zinbarg RE. What is an anxiety disorder? *Depress Anxiety*. 2009;26:1066-1085.

Freitas-Ferrari MC, Hallak JE, Trzesniak C, et al. Neuroimaging in social anxiety disorder: a systematic review of the literature. *Prog Neuropsychopharmacol Biol Psychiatry*. May 30, 2010;34(4):565-80. doi: 10.1016/j.pnpbp.2010.02.028. Epub Mar 4, 2010.

Hansen RA, Gaynes BN, Gartlehner G, Moore CG, Twari R, Lohr KN. Efficacy and tolerability of second-generation antidepressants in social anxiety disorder. *Int Clin Psychopharmacol*. May 2008;23(3):170-179.

Jorstad-Stein EC, Heimberg RG. Social phobia: an update on treatment. *Psychiatr Clin North Am.* 2009;32:642-663.

Otte C. Cognitive behavioral therapy in anxiety disorders: current state of the evidence. *Dialogues Clin Neurosci.* 2011;13(4):413-421.

Paes F, Machado S, Arias-Carrión O, et al. The value of repetitive transcranial magnetic stimulation (rTMS) for the treatment of anxiety disorders: an integrative review. *CNS Neurol Disord Drug Targets.* Aug 2011;10(5):610-620.

Sadock BJ, Sadock VA. *Kaplan & Sadock's Synopsis of Psychiatry.* 10th ed. Baltimore, MD: Lippincott Williams & Wilkins; 2007:674-677.

Sadock BJ, Sadock VA, Ruiz P. *Kaplan and Sadock's Synopsis of Psychiatry: Behavioral Sciences/Clinical Psychiatry.* 11th ed. Baltimore, MD: Lippincott Williams & Wilkins; 2014.

A 34-year-old woman presents to the family medicine clinic for evaluation of insomnia and muscle tension. She has been experiencing these symptoms chronically, but notes that they have worsened lately. On further questioning, she admits to increased stress because of trying to balance work as a lawyer and raising her first child. While at the office, she finds herself distracted by worry about her little girl's safety. The patient was a victim of molestation as a child and fears that someone might take advantage of her daughter at day care. She worries that she will get fired and the family will lose their home. As her parents get older, she has increasing concern about their health. She denies any other psychiatric symptoms, past psychiatric history, or medical diagnoses. The patient does not use any alcohol or illicit substances. She denies any formal psychiatric diagnoses in her family but states, "they could have used some professional help."

On mental status examination, the patient is well groomed and dressed in a business suit. She is cooperative, but she often looks down at her hands when she speaks. She grips her purse tightly and fidgets with the zipper. She crosses and uncrosses her legs, and repeatedly taps her high heels on the floor. The patient talks quickly, but is not pressured. She describes her mood as "worn out;" her affect is anxious. Her thought process is linear, logical, and goal directed, although she perseverates on her worries. Her thought content focuses on all the possibilities of what could go wrong in her life and the lives of her loved ones. She denies SI, HI, and AVH.

▶ What is the most likely diagnosis?
▶ What is the most effective treatment?

ANSWERS TO CASE 20:

Generalized Anxiety Disorder

Summary: A 34-year-old woman with no psychiatric or medical history presents with an exacerbation of somatic symptoms of chronic anxiety. When probed, she admits to generalized anxiety with a host of worries regarding various aspects of her life. Her anxiety has become clinically significant and is interfering with her ability to work.

- **Most likely diagnosis:** Generalized anxiety disorder (GAD).

- **Treatment:** The most effective treatment regimen encompasses therapy and medication, typically selective serotonin reuptake inhibitors (SSRIs).

ANALYSIS

Objectives

1. Understand the diagnostic criteria for GAD (Table 20–1).

2. Be aware of the medications used to treat GAD and the problems associated with each.

Considerations

This clinical scenario depicts a typical case of GAD. Like many patients, she presents to her primary care physician with insomnia and muscle tension. This patient has a long history of generalized anxiety but recently her symptoms have become clinically significant. Although she has a history of trauma, which intensifies worries regarding her daughter's safety, she denies any posttraumatic stress disorder (PTSD) symptomatology. She denies medical or substance problems.

Table 20–1 • DIAGNOSTIC CRITERIA FOR GENERALIZED ANXIETY DISORDER
Persistent, excessive, uncontrollable anxiety/worry ≥ 6 mo.
The person struggles to control the worry.
At least three of these symptoms: • Restlessness • Fatigue • Impaired concentration • Irritability • Muscle tension • Disrupted sleep
Symptoms are not better accounted for by another psychiatric disorder. Not caused by the direct effects of a substance or medication or medical illness.
Clinically significant distress or impairment of psychosocial functioning.

APPROACH TO:
Generalized Anxiety Disorder

DEFINITIONS

ANXIETY: Worry about a future threat accompanied by physical symptoms, typically muscle tension.

FEAR: Emotional response with autonomic hyperarousal (in preparation for fight or flight) triggered by a perceived impending threat.

PANIC ATTACKS: Brief episode of intense fear or discomfort accompanied by somatic symptoms. Panic attacks are not limited to panic disorder, or even anxiety disorders, and may be seen in other psychiatric illnesses, such as mood and psychotic disorders.

CLINICAL APPROACH

Generalized anxiety disorder (GAD) involves persistent, excessive, uncontrollable anxiety about various domains of life for the majority of a 6-month time period. Associated symptoms may include irritability, restlessness, fatigue, insomnia, impaired concentration, and muscle tension. These symptoms cause significant distress and/or impairment in the patient's social life, academics, or career.

GAD typically is **a chronic condition** that can worsen with life stressors. Like most anxiety disorders, GAD occurs more frequently in women than in men. There is a great degree of overlap of symptoms between the various anxiety disorders and depressive disorders, and high comorbidity among them.

Although effective treatments are available, only one-third of those suffering receive help. Anxiety disorders cost the US billions of dollars a year, with the majority of the cost consisting of repeated use of health care services and working days lost.

Changes from *DSM-IV-TR* to *DSM-5*: None

DIFFERENTIAL DIAGNOSIS

Prior to diagnosing a primary anxiety disorder, one must rule out substance intoxication/withdrawal, a substance/medication-induced anxiety disorder, and an anxiety disorder due to another medical condition. A candid history regarding substances, current medications, the temporal relationship between symptoms and use, collateral information, vital signs, physical examination, blood alcohol level, and urine drug screen will help to determine if substances contribute to or cause the patient's anxiety. Explicitly ask about over-the-counter (OTC) drugs and herbal supplements. A medical etiology may be revealed through a medical history, a timeline of symptoms in relation to exacerbation or amelioration of medical illness, and vital signs, physical examination, and laboratory test results.

When establishing a diagnosis of GAD versus other anxiety disorders, look for a broad base of anxiety generalized across various domains. Other anxiety disorders typically have a specific focus or trigger, such as social anxiety disorder in which the worry stems from the judgment of others. GAD patients will worry regardless of social evaluation. Anxiety commonly occurs with other disorders such as PTSD, obsessive-compulsive disorder (OCD), adjustment disorders, mood disorders, and psychotic disorders. A diagnosis of GAD should only be made if the symptoms are not better accounted for by another disorder.

TREATMENT

The most effective treatment for GAD entails a two-pronged approach combining both pharmacotherapy and psychotherapy. Cognitive behavioral therapy (CBT) has been studied and proven effective in many disorders, including GAD. CBT focuses on identifying and changing dysfunctional thought patterns in order to positively impact one's emotions and behaviors. CBT can be beneficial in targeting the anxiety-ridden cognitions in GAD. Psychodynamic psychotherapy can be helpful in understanding the maladaptive patterns and unconscious reasons for the anxiety and working through those to ultimately attain mastery over the symptoms. Psychotherapy helps patients develop coping skills for life with longer-lasting treatment gains compared to medications.

From the armamentarium of agents, SSRIs are a first-line medication for many disorders, including GAD. If there is no response after an adequate trial, then switch to another SSRI. If symptoms continue without abating, selective serotonin-norepinephrine reuptake inhibitors (SNRIs) or tricyclic antidepressants (TCAs) can be tried. The full benefits of SSRI/SNRI treatment should be seen in 4 to 8 weeks. If no response occurs, then switch agents. If a partial response is observed, then augment with another agent. Other second-line medications, often used as augmentation, include benzodiazepines, hydroxyzine, buspirone, and mirtazapine.

Benzodiazepines should be used only as an adjunct until the SSRI or other medication has become therapeutic, except in rare cases. Use caution when choosing to prescribe benzodiazepines because of the potential for addiction, oversedation, and cognitive impairment. In the elderly, benzodiazepines contribute to fall risk. Patients quickly develop a tolerance to benzodiazepines and may experience withdrawal or rebound anxiety when benzodiazepines are discontinued. Benzodiazepine withdrawal, similar to alcohol withdrawal, can lead to serious medical sequela such as seizures. During rebound anxiety, patients reexperience their initial symptoms to a greater degree. This can increase a patient's resistance to stopping the benzodiazepine.

Consider likely comorbidities when developing a treatment plan so that all disorders can be targeted. For example, with comorbid depression, SSRIs would be useful in managing both disorders, whereas benzodiazepines would not be effective.

> ## CASE CORRELATION
>
> • See also Case 19 and Case 22. In social anxiety disordered patients, concern about being in public or speaking in public are the prominent symptoms; GAD patient have much more far-reaching varieties of worry. In OCD, patients have obsessional thoughts, but the focus of the thoughts is not about upcoming problems, but rather inappropriate ideas that take the form of intrusive and unwanted thoughts, urges, or images.

COMPREHENSION QUESTIONS

20.1 A 28-year-old female medical student is brought to the physician by her boyfriend because of unremitting headaches and always "worrying about everything." The patient admits that she has been even more "stressed out" than usual over the last year about interview season, the couples match, getting married, moving out of state, and student loans. Her headaches have increased in frequency and intensity. She reports difficulty sleeping through the night and constant fatigue. The patient's boyfriend complains that lately, "she freaks out about every little thing. I can't deal with this anymore. I don't even know if matching together is still a good idea." Which of the following is the most likely diagnosis?

A. Anxiety disorder due to another medical condition

B. Substance/medication-induced anxiety disorder

C. Somatic symptom disorder

D. Generalized anxiety disorder

20.2 A 37-year-old male college professor with a history of GAD and major depressive disorder (MDD) has been referred to psychiatry by his primary care physician. His symptoms have been relatively well controlled up until last semester when he received negative reviews from his students. Since this time, he has started to doubt his ability to teach, worry about his career, and ruminate on each lesson plan. He worries that his reputation among the students has been irrevocably damaged, which makes him feel despondent. The professor desperately wants to get help, but is hesitant to try any medication that will impair his intellectual prowess. Which of the following is the most effective treatment approach?

A. CBT

B. CBT and escitalopram

C. Psychoeducation and lorazepam

D. Psychodynamic psychotherapy

E. Pregabalin

20.3 The college professor described in the previous question follows up with the psychiatrist in 4 weeks after starting the indicated treatment. He reports a decrease in symptoms, but states that he does not want to take the medication any longer. When asked why, he blushes and stammers, "*it's* not working right." Which SSRI side effect is the most common with long-term treatment and often results in nonadherence?

A. GI upset

B. Insomnia

C. Sexual dysfunction

D. Weight gain

E. Emotional numbing

ANSWERS

20.1 **D.** The patient most likely suffers from generalized anxiety disorder. This case demonstrates the key symptoms of GAD: worrying about "everything" excessively and physical symptoms associated with the anxiety. The patient's worries interfere with her ability to function, particularly in her relationship. Ruling out an anxiety disorder due to another medical condition is important, especially for a patient who presents with prominent physical symptoms. In this case, the temporal picture of increasing headaches, fatigue, and insomnia correlate with interview season and its aftermath. Inquire about any medications or OTC and investigate if these could contribute to or exacerbate the anxiety. Adjustment disorder could be on the differential given an identifiable stressor followed by an impairment of functioning, but this patient's symptoms are better accounted for by GAD. Although the patient suffers from distressing somatic symptoms, she does not have anxiety about these somatic symptoms or her health in general.

20.2 **B.** The patient would benefit most from combination therapy involving both evidence-based treatments of CBT and an SSRI. Escitalopram is FDA-approved specifically for GAD. CBT alone would help the patient, but adding an SSRI at this time would be recommended given the severity of the symptoms and the co-occurrence of MDD. Psychodynamic psychotherapy may be helpful, but CBT has more evidence at this time and combination treatment with medication is warranted. Psychoeducation is helpful for all patients in understanding their psychiatric condition and treatment options. Benzodiazepines may be useful for controlling anxiety symptoms short term, but they can exacerbate depressive symptoms and cause cognitive impairment. Although there has been some evidence to demonstrate that pregabalin can be effective in treating GAD, it remains a second-line agent.

20.3 **C.** Sexual dysfunction is the most common with long-term treatment and may be underreported. Make sure to inquire about it and modify as needed. The other side effects listed are bothersome, but resolve and are more tolerable.

CLINICAL PEARLS

▶ Anxiety disorders are the most common psychiatric disorder encountered in primary care. Many patients will present with the somatic complaints of GAD.

　▶ Many medical conditions can mimic GAD, thus a full medical workup is necessary.

　▶ Algorithm for approaching anxiety disorders:

　　▶ Step 1. Rule out substance or medication induced:

　　　▶ Adverse effect, toxicity, or withdrawal

　　　▶ Look for common offenders, including Rx and OTC medications, herbals/supplements, illicit substances

　　　▶ Work up: BAL, urine drug screen, serum drug levels

　　▶ Step 2. Rule out identifiable medical disorders:

　　　▶ Screen for endocrinopathies, neurologic diseases, etc

　　　▶ Work up: blood glucose, UA, CBC, CMP, ammonia, TSH, pregnancy test

　　▶ Step 3. Characterize the anxiety disorder.

▶ Generalized anxiety disorder is highly comorbid with other anxiety disorders and depressive disorders. Consider comorbidities when deciding on a treatment plan.

▶ SSRIs are a first-line medication for treating GAD.

▶ As with many psychiatric disorders, using a two-pronged approach with psychopharmacology and psychotherapy has the best results.

REFERENCES

American Psychiatric Association. *Diagnostic and Statistical Manual of Mental Disorders*. 5th ed. Washington, DC: American Psychiatric Association; 2013.

Gabbard G. *Gabbard's Treatments of Psychiatric Disorders*. 5th ed. Arlington, VA: American Psychiatric Association; 2014.

Sadock BJ, Sadock VA, Ruiz P. *Kaplan & Sadock's Synopsis of Psychiatry*. 11th ed. Baltimore, MD: Lippincott Williams & Wilkins; 2014.

A 55-year-old female schoolteacher with coronary artery disease and recent myocardial infarction presents to the emergency room (ER) complaining of heart palpitations, chest discomfort, and shortness of breath. She appears very anxious and asks repeatedly, "Am I having another heart attack?!" The patient denies any triggers to her symptoms and reports, "it all started out of nowhere." Since her heart attack 6 months ago, she has suffered from several of these episodes. Subsequently, she asked for an extended medical leave of absence. She denies any substance use but states that she quit smoking after the myocardial infarction.

Mental status examination reveals an obese, anxious woman who speaks hurriedly between breaths. Vital signs are significant for tachypnea and tachycardia. Cardiac examination also demonstrates a rapid rate with an irregular rhythm. The remainder of the physical examination is unremarkable.

▶ What is the most likely diagnosis?
▶ What is the best diagnostic test?
▶ What is the best treatment approach for this disorder?

ANSWERS TO CASE 21:
Anxiety Disorder Due to Another Medical Condition

Summary: A 55-year-old woman with coronary artery disease (CAD) and recent myocardial infarction (MI) presents to the ER experiencing symptoms indicative of an arrhythmia and anxiety. She appears to be experiencing a panic attack. Her physical examination is significant for tachypnea and tachycardia with an irregular rhythm. The symptoms have been occurring for the last several months since the patient's MI.

- **What is the most likely diagnosis?** Anxiety disorder due to another medical condition, in this case an arrhythmia.

- **What is the best diagnostic test?** Electrocardiogram (ECG).

- **What is the treatment approach for this disorder?** The treatment should address the underlying cause, the arrhythmia in this case. If anxiety remains despite stabilizing the arrhythmia or if the arrhythmia could not be adequately controlled, then the therapeutic approach would be essentially identical to treating a primary anxiety disorder, namely selective serotonin reuptake inhibitors (SSRIs). Avoid medications that could worsen the underlying medical etiology.

ANALYSIS

Objectives

1. Recognize anxiety disorder due to another medical condition (Table 21−1 for the diagnostic criteria).

2. Conduct an appropriate workup to determine the diagnosis.

3. Understand how the initial treatment approach may differ compared to the treatment of primary anxiety disorders.

Considerations

This patient presents with anxiety and panic attacks caused by a medical condition. She has CAD and recently suffered from a MI. She likely developed an arrhythmia

Table 21–1 • DIAGNOSTIC CRITERIA FOR ANXIETY DISORDER SECONDARY TO A MEDICAL CONDITION
Anxiety or panic attacks are the predominant symptoms.
The history, physical examination, and/or laboratory findings strongly suggest that the symptoms are a direct physiologic consequence of a medical condition.
The symptoms are not better explained by another psychiatric disorder.
Does not occur only during delirium.
The symptoms cause clinically significant distress and/or impairment in functioning.

after the heart attack. Evidence from the history and physical examination lead to the conclusion that her anxiety and panic attacks are pathophysiologic sequelae of the arrhythmia. An abnormal ECG would help to confirm this diagnosis.

APPROACH TO:
Anxiety Disorder Due to Another Medical Condition

DEFINITIONS

ANXIETY: Worry about a future threat accompanied by physical symptoms, typically muscle tension.

PANIC ATTACKS: Brief episodes of intense fear or discomfort accompanied by somatic symptoms. Panic attacks are not limited to panic disorder, or even anxiety disorders, and may be seen in other psychiatric illnesses, such as mood and psychotic disorders.

CLINICAL APPROACH

Many medical conditions can manifest with symptoms that resemble anxiety disorders, including panic disorder and generalized anxiety disorder. In anxiety due to another medical condition, prominent anxiety or panic attacks predominate coupled with clinical data indicating a medical etiology. The medical condition has an established physiologic mechanism for inducing anxiety. Examine the timing of the anxiety or panic attacks with respect to onset, exacerbation, and remission of the medical problem. The disease state occurs prior to the onset of anxiety symptoms, although anxiety may be the harbinger. Anxiety disorders due to another medical condition follow the course of the condition's pathophysiology. When the medical illness is treated, the anxiety usually improves. The presentation often includes salient physical symptoms and may be atypical in nature, such as older age of initial presentation. There is less likelihood of personal or family history of anxiety disorders. As with all psychiatric disorders, the symptoms must impair the patient's ability to function.

    Changes from *DSM-IV* to *DSM-5*: Obsessions and compulsions were removed from the criteria as obsessive-compulsive disorder (OCD) was removed from the anxiety disorders. With the elimination of Axis III, the medical condition should be listed followed by the diagnosis of anxiety disorder due to the medical condition (eg, arrhythmia, anxiety disorder due to arrhythmia).

DIFFERENTIAL DIAGNOSIS

Multiple medical illnesses can induce anxiety, including systemic conditions, endocrinopathies, metabolic disturbances, immune system disorders, and neurologic diseases. In fact, major neurocognitive disorders (dementia) may cause anxiety. Anxiety can be the initial or prominent symptom in Graves disease, hypothyroidism, hypoparathyroidism, carcinoid syndrome, and B_{12} deficiency. Pheochromocytoma, seizure disorders, and chronic obstructive pulmonary disease (COPD) can cause panic attacks. Patients can have independent, coexisting psychiatric and medical illness. Various medical problems have increased rates of comorbid anxiety disorders. Primary anxiety disorders may develop in the context of chronic medical problems but would not be diagnostically and physiologically linked to the medical condition. Carefully tease out the patient's psychiatric history, course of illness, and current symptoms to determine the diagnosis. The standard psychiatric laboratory workup should include complete blood count with leukocyte differential, comprehensive metabolic panel (electrolytes, blood urea nitrogen [BUN], creatinine, blood glucose, and hepatic markers), urinalysis, thyroid stimulating hormone, urine drug screen, medication levels, and a pregnancy test. As with other psychiatric disorders, the symptoms cannot occur exclusively in the context of delirium.

Carefully screen for substance intoxication/withdrawal and substance/medication-induced anxiety disorder to determine if substances contribute to or cause the patient's anxiety. Obtain a thorough personal history and collateral information regarding any substance use or medication misuse. Similar to screening for a medical etiology, investigate the temporal relationship between anxiety onset and substance/medication use. Look for anxiety that appears cyclically or during a particular time of day. Obtain vitals signs, perform a physical examination, and check a blood alcohol level and urine drug screen. Explicitly ask about over-the-counter (OTC) drugs and herbal supplements. Medications known to cause anxiety include steroids, anticholinergics, and sympathomimetics. Ironically, even SSRIs—the first-line treatment for anxiety—can induce feelings of anxiety temporarily.

Other possible diagnoses include psychiatric disorders, such as mood and psychotic disorders, which can cause anxiety. Inquire about relevant symptom clusters that meet the criteria for other psychiatric disorders and past history of psychiatric illness. Adjustment disorder could present with anxiety as the stress response to having a medical disease. In this disorder, the anxiety would correlate with coping with the medical condition. Illness anxiety disorder should also be considered. This disorder presents with anxiety about health and medical issues—regardless of whether or not the patient has an actual disease process. If a medical condition does co-occur, determine if a physiologic relationship exists between the medical disease and the anxiety.

TREATMENT

Treatment of an anxiety disorder due to another medical condition begins with targeting the underlying illness. When the medical condition is treated, the anxiety symptoms will likely also improve. If anxiety symptoms remain after addressing the medical condition, use the same treatment strategy as with primary anxiety disorders. Begin with SSRIs and utilize benzodiazepines sparingly for a limited duration. Psychotherapy can help patients develop adaptive ways of coping with stressors.

> ## CASE CORRELATION
>
> - See also Case 16 and Case 24 for diagnoses that may also present with anxiety. These three disorders (panic disorder, substance/medication-induced anxiety disorder, and anxiety due to another medical condition) must be teased apart by a careful history into the patient's medical condition, medications or substances used/abused, and a time course of the anxiety symptoms. Adjustment disorders may also present with anxiety, but this anxiety is a maladaptive response to the stress of the illness itself, not an anxiety which is the direct physiological cause of the medical illness.

COMPREHENSION QUESTIONS

21.1 A 23-year-old male medical student with a history of hypothyroidism presents to his primary care provider for an annual examination. He has been studying intensely for Step I and trying new methods to stay focused. He started drinking an herbal tea that claims to "boost intelligence" several times a day over the past month. He reports feeling more anxious and jittery than ever, but has been able to study for longer hours. He has had heart palpitations after he drinks the tea and has had more difficulty sleeping. His hypothyroidism has been well controlled on a consistent medication regimen over the last year. Which of the following is the most likely diagnosis?

A. Anxiety disorder due to another medical condition

B. Generalized anxiety disorder

C. Obsessive-compulsive disorder

D. Specific phobia

E. Substance/medication-induced anxiety disorder

21.2 A 45-year-old man with a history of schizophrenia and Type II diabetes presents to the emergency department after drinking alcohol and snorting cocaine. He states that he feels anxious and "just can't calm down." He is diaphoretic and tremulous. Which of the following tests should be ordered STAT?

A. Abdominal ultrasound

B. Accucheck

C. B_{12} level

D. Thyroid-stimulating hormone level

E. Urine toxicology

21.3 A 36 year-old woman with a history of generalized anxiety disorder is brought to the emergency department by her husband due to sudden onset of dyspnea, heart palpitations, and intense anxiety. She pants, "I feel like I'm going to die." She has no significant past medical history or family medical history. Her only medications are oral contraceptives and venlafaxine. She smokes one pack of cigarettes daily. On examination, she appears to be in acute distress with a pulse of 160 beats/min, a blood pressure of 84/44 mm Hg, and a respiratory rate of 32 breaths/min. An ECG shows sinus tachycardia. After initial stabilization of the patient, what is the most appropriate next step?

A. Administer IV lorazepam.

B. Inquire about current social stressors.

C. Order a high-resolution chest CT.

D. Prescribe oral buspirone.

E. Recommend cognitive behavioral therapy.

ANSWERS

21.1 **E.** The most likely diagnosis is substance-induced anxiety disorder because the student's symptoms developed during a month of heavy tea ingestion. The symptoms include anxiety, insomnia, and heart palpitations, all of which could be caused by caffeine, a common ingredient of tea. Caffeine is known to induce or contribute to anxiety. Treatment consists of reducing or gradually eliminating caffeine from the diet. Anxiety due to another medical condition should also be considered, especially given the patient's known history of hypothyroidism. Although the patient's thyroid function has been well controlled over the last year, it would be important to check his thyroid-stimulating hormone (TSH) and T4 levels to investigate if the patient is being overtreated or undertreated with thyroid medication. Levothyroxine may cause anxiety or even panic attacks when dosed too high, essentially causing iatrogenic hyperthyroidism. The patient does not exhibit generalized anxiety, obsessions, or compulsions. He is concerned about his academic success, but this worry has not led to impaired functioning. He does not exhibit a specific fear, even with the upcoming Step I test.

21.2 **B.** A STAT accucheck is critical in the ER setting, especially for symptomatic patients with diabetes. Hypoglycemia should be high on the list of possible causes for the patient's anxiety, diaphoresis, and tremulousness. The patient's anxiety could be caused by alcohol withdrawal or cocaine intoxication. The urine toxicology is an essential part of any psychiatric workup, but this would not be a STAT laboratory. Given that the patient endorses substance use, there is high likelihood the results would confirm recent cocaine. If there were clinical suspicion for thyrotoxicosis, TSH and T4 should be ordered immediately. A blood glucose level would still be ordered acutely. Folate and B_{12} may be low due to heavy alcohol use and require replacement. Although important to obtain, B_{12} and TSH are not likely urgent orders. At this time, there is no indication for an abdominal ultrasound.

21.3 **C.** This patient's symptoms are concerning for a pulmonary embolus: dyspnea, tachypnea, tachycardia, and hypotension. Her daily use of cigarettes and oral contraceptives puts her at greater risk for PE than the general population. Thus, a high-resolution chest CT is indicated. Although she has a psychiatric history, dismissing her complaints as primary anxiety/panic attacks would be negligent. Lorazepam may result in respiratory depression and clinical deterioration. Inquiring about social stressors is not the appropriate next step in the setting of hemodynamic instability.

CLINICAL PEARLS

▶ Many medical illnesses produce prominent anxiety symptoms. Complete a thorough history, physical examination, and diagnostic workup to determine a causal relationship.

▶ Look for a pattern of anxiety or panic presenting in relation to onset or exacerbation of medical illness and resolving when the medical problem remits.

▶ Screen for atypical aspects of the presentation, which decrease the likelihood of a primary anxiety disorder: older age of onset, salient somatic symptoms, and lack of personal and family psychiatric history.

▶ A prior diagnosis of psychiatric illness should not preclude careful evaluation for a medical cause of symptoms.

REFERENCES

American Psychiatric Association. *Diagnostic and Statistical Manual of Mental Disorders*. 5th ed. Washington, DC: American Psychiatric Association; 2013.

Kaufman D, Milstein M. *Clinical Neurology for Psychiatrists*. 7th ed. London, England: Elsevier; 2013.

Sadock BJ, Sadock VA, Ruiz, P. *Kaplan & Sadock's Synopsis of Psychiatry*. 11th ed. Baltimore, MD: Lippincott Williams & Wilkins; 2014.

A 13-year-old adolescent girl is brought to a psychiatrist by her mother. The patient states that for the past 6 months she has been showering for long periods, up to 5 hours at a time. She says she is unable to stop this behavior although it is distressing to her and causes her skin to crack and bleed. She reports that the symptoms started after she began to have recurrent thoughts of being dirty or unclean. These thoughts occur many times a day. She states that she grows increasingly anxious until she is able to take a shower and clean herself. The patient claims that the amount of time she spends in the shower is increasing because she must wash herself in a particular order to avoid getting the "clean suds" mixed up with the "dirty suds." If this happens, she must start the whole showering process over again. The patient states that she knows that she "must be crazy," but she seems unable to stop herself. The patient's mother verifies the patient's history. She claims that her daughter has always been popular in school and has many friends. She emphatically states that her daughter has never used drugs or alcohol. The patient's only medical problem is a history of asthma, which is treated with an albuterol inhaler. The patient's mental status examination is otherwise unremarkable except as noted earlier.

▶ What is the most likely diagnosis for this patient?
▶ What would be the best type of psychotherapy for this condition?
▶ What would be the best type of pharmacotherapy for this patient?

ANSWERS TO CASE 22:
Obsessive-Compulsive Disorder (Child)

Summary: A 13-year-old girl has a 6-month history of excessive showering, up to 5 hours at a time. This showering is preceded by recurrent thoughts of being dirty or unclean. The patient becomes increasingly anxious because of these thoughts unless she is able to shower. She has a particular order of showering that must be followed or she must start over again. The patient is aware of the abnormal nature of her thoughts and behavior and is distressed by them.

- **Most likely diagnosis:** Obsessive-compulsive disorder (OCD).

- **Best psychotherapy:** Behavioral therapy involving exposure and response prevention.

- **Best pharmacotherapy:** A selective serotonin reuptake inhibitor (SSRI).

ANALYSIS

Objectives

1. Understand the diagnostic criteria of OCD.

2. Know the psychotherapeutic treatment of choice for this disorder.

3. Know the pharmacologic treatment of choice for this disorder.

4. Know what other conditions can mimic OCD.

Considerations

This patient has a classic history of OCD. She has recurrent thoughts of being dirty or unclean (obsessions) and must shower (the compulsion), or she becomes increasingly anxious. The thoughts she has are not simply excessive worries about real-life problems. She has tried to ignore these thoughts but is unable to do so and is distressed by them. (Note that the ability to see that the obsessions and/or compulsions are unreasonable is a prerequisite for the diagnosis in adults, although not in children.) There is no evidence that this patient is abusing drugs or alcohol or has a medical disorder that might be causing her symptoms. However, these could still be a possibility and ruling them out should be part of a good workup. New-onset OCD symptoms have also been associated with streptococcal infections and from abuse of stimulant medications (methylphenidate, amphetamines).

APPROACH TO:

Obsessive-Compulsive Disorder (Child)

DEFINITIONS

CLOMIPRAMINE: A serotonin and dopaminergic neurotransmitter inhibitor in the class of tricyclic and tetracyclic agents that is effective in the treatment of OCD. The main adverse effects are sedation, anticholinergic side effects, and at toxic levels, cardiac dysrhythmias. (Because of the side effects, many clinicians use SSRIs for this disorder; higher doses than those used for depression are required.)

COMPULSIONS: Repetitive behaviors or mental acts that a person feels driven to perform in response to an obsession according to a rigid set of rules. These behaviors or mental acts are aimed at preventing or reducing distress or preventing a feared event or situation. Typically, there is no realistic connection between the feared event or situation and the behavior or mental act.

EXPOSURE: Presenting the patient with the feared object or situation. Exposure to the feared object or situation, coupled with relaxation training and response prevention, constitutes a behavior modification program proven successful in patients with OCD.

OBSESSIONS: Recurrent and persistent thoughts or images that are experienced as intrusive and inappropriate and cause marked anxiety or distress. They are not simply excessive worries about real-life problems.

PANDAS: Pediatric autoimmune neuropsychiatric disorders associated with streptococcal infections—a group of disorders, including OCD, that have been demonstrated to occur after a streptococcal infection.

CLINICAL APPROACH

According to the *Diagnostic and Statistical Manual of Mental Disorders, 5th edition* (*DSM-5*), the hallmark of **OCD** is recurrent obsessions and/or compulsions (Table 22–1). The obsessions are persistent in the conscious awareness of the patient, who typically recognizes them as being absurd and irrational and often has a desire to resist them. However, half of all patients offer little resistance

Table 22–1 • DIAGNOSTIC CRITERIA FOR OBSESSIVE-COMPULSIVE DISORDER
The presence of either obsessions or compulsions.
The person realizes that the obsessions or compulsions are excessive and unreasonable; this requirement need not apply to children.
The obsessions or compulsions cause marked distress, are time consuming, or interfere with the person's normal routine.
If another major mental illness is present, the contents of the obsessions or compulsions are not restricted to it.

to compulsions. Overall, OCD is a disabling, time-consuming, distressing disorder that interferes with one's normal routine, occupational function, social activities, and/or relationships.

Obsessive-compulsive disorder is now grouped into the *DSM-5* category of obsessive-compulsive-related disorders. These were regrouped in the most recent version because of similarities regarding phenomenology, familial expression, and etiological mechanisms. Included now in this category are body dysmorphic disorder, hoarding disorder, trichotillomania, and excoriation (skin-picking) disorder.

The lifetime prevalence of OCD is approximately 2% to 3% across all ethnicities. Obsessive-compulsive disorder accounts for up to 10% of outpatient psychiatric clinic visits, making it the fourth most common psychiatric diagnosis after phobias, substance-related disorders, and major depressive disorder. Men and women are affected equally; however, adolescent males are more commonly affected than adolescent females. The mean age of presentation is 20 years of age. Onset can occur in childhood, and case reports describe children as young as 2 years old with the disorder. Individuals affected with OCD often have additional psychiatric disorders; these include major depressive disorder, social phobia, generalized anxiety disorder, alcohol use disorders, specific phobia, panic disorder, and eating disorders. Interestingly, 20% to 30% of OCD patients have a history of tics, with Tourette disorder comorbid in 5% to 7% of patients. A functional study of patients with OCD and major depressive disorder (MDD) showed that altered anterior cingulate glutamatergic neurotransmission may be involved in the pathogenesis of OCD and MDD. A recent study also showed that pediatric patients with OCD showed MRI changes in the dorsolateral prefrontal and parietal areas that normalized after successfully completing a course of cognitive behavioral therapy.

DIFFERENTIAL DIAGNOSIS

The differential diagnosis for OCD must include other anxiety disorders that could cause a person to behave outside his or her normal behavior patterns. Persons with obsessive-compulsive personality disorder do not meet the criteria for the disorder, and they have a lesser degree of impairment. Patients with phobias (specific phobia or social phobia) attempt to avoid the feared object but do not obsessively ruminate about it unless directly presented with it. Patients with generalized anxiety disorder worry excessively, and their anxiety is spread across many areas, not on just one aspect of the obsession. They also do not develop compulsions. Care must be taken to rule out any medical conditions or the use of any substances with effects that can mimic symptoms of OCD. Abuse of stimulant medication in adolescents and young adults is growing. A significant side effect to stimulant use can be obsessions and compulsions, especially in higher doses. In addition, care should be taken to look for a history of recent streptococcal infections. Childhood-onset OCD has been associated with these infections and is referred to as pediatric autoimmune neuropsychiatric disorder associated with streptococcal infections (PANDAS). Thoughts and behavior must be carefully evaluated to ensure that they are not overtly bizarre or psychotic and thus indicating that the patient is suffering from a psychotic disorder such as schizophrenia.

TREATMENT

The treatment of OCD in children and adolescents can involve psychotherapeutic and psychopharmacologic interventions. Both have been shown to be helpful in controlled clinical trials. **The greatest efficacy can be seen when psychotherapy is combined with SSRIs.** The primary psychotherapeutic treatment involves cognitive behavioral therapy referred to as **exposure/response prevention.** In this type of treatment, the therapist and patient develop a list of triggers for the compulsive behavior. The items on this list are arranged into a hierarchy, which is the key to the treatment. The **child is exposed to the least anxiety-provoking trigger first and then, using anxiety-reducing techniques, is gradually moved to higher levels** of the hierarchy until tolerance is developed. Repeated exposure to the triggers is associated with decreased anxiety. This type of treatment requires a good relationship with the therapist as well as a moderate to high degree of motivation on the part of the patient. Additionally, cognitive behavioral family therapy for OCD has been shown to provide long-term relief that is equally as effective as individual and group-based therapy.

The second type of treatment shown to be effective for OCD in clinical trials is psychopharmacologic intervention. The class of medications found to be most effective in treating OCD includes **SSRIs.** The first medication used was the **nonselective agent, clomipramine.** In appropriate doses, it has been found to be significantly superior to a placebo in reducing OCD symptoms. It can require several weeks to become effective at appropriate dose levels. The more recent and specific **SSRIs (fluoxetine, sertraline, and fluvoxamine)** have been shown to significantly reduce both obsessions and compulsions in children and adolescents compared to a placebo.

The above treatments are often delivered in a relatively low-intensive outpatient setting to motivated recipients. In some resistant or nonadherent patients, a residential setting to deliver the treatment has been shown quite effective.

CASE CORRELATION

- See also Case 17 and Case 20 for disorders which may also present with excessive worry or fear. OCD might present with anxiety about germs, but be matched by a ritual (a compulsion, a shower in the case presented above) to contain the anxiety, which is not present in a specific phobia. In OCD, patients have obsessional thoughts, but the focus of the thoughts are not about upcoming problems, such as seen in GAD, but rather inappropriate ideas that take the form of intrusive and unwanted thoughts, urges, or images.

COMPREHENSION QUESTIONS

22.1 A 17-year-old high school senior is referred to a psychiatrist by his counselor because of academic difficulty. Although he had always been an honors student, this past year his grades have dropped, especially in mathematics. When questioned, he reveals the new onset of "superstitions" involving numbers. When presented with certain numbers, he feels compelled to count forward and then backward to and from that number. He becomes anxious about not completing this task, although he is unable to state a particular consequence. If interrupted, he must begin all over again. He realizes that there is "no good reason" for his behavior, but is unable to stop it. Because of this, he not only feels "tortured," but he may need to repeat a year in school. He denies any past psychiatric history. You begin treating him with sertraline and cognitive therapy to address the obsessions. He misses appointments with his therapist, feels therapy will not be helpful, and the parents believe he is not taking his medications regularly. What interventions should be considered next?

A. Change the medication to fluoxetine.

B. Electroconvulsive therapy.

C. Residential setting to deliver treatment.

D. Adding an augmenting neuroleptic.

E. Psychodynamic psychotherapy plus pharmacotherapy.

22.2 The patient in Question 22.1 begins treatment for his condition. As treatment develops, the parents inform you that he had an episode of glomerulonephritis treated with antibiotics several weeks ago prior to developing these symptoms. What other possible issue might be related to his current symptoms?

A. Sydenham chorea

B. Asperger syndrome

C. Passive-aggressive personality disorder

D. Pediatric autoimmune neuropsychiatric disorders associated with streptococcal infections

E. Huntington disease

22.3 The patient in Questions 22.1 and 22.2 is started on sertraline. What is the most common side effect to this medication?

A. Neuroleptic malignant syndrome

B. Suicidal ideations

C. Tardive dyskinesia

D. Serotonin syndrome

E. Nausea and diarrhea

ANSWERS

22.1 **C.** This individual suffers from OCD with symptoms of obsessions, compulsions, significant anxiety, and interference in his academic functioning. Whereas behavioral therapy and medications such as clomipramine and SSRIs are helpful in treating OCD, there is evidence that a combination of the two provides the greatest efficacy. However, if the patient is nonadherent or resistant to treatment in an outpatient setting a more structured environment might ensure success. There is an absence of studies documenting improvement in OCD solely with psychodynamic psychotherapy.

22.2 **D.** Pediatric autoimmune neuropsychiatric disorders associated with streptococcal infections (PANDAS) have been specifically associated with development or exacerbation of OCD in children and adolescents. The symptoms will develop temporally after a demonstrated streptococcal infection.

22.3 **E.** Nausea and diarrhea are the most common side effects to Sertraline in patients with OCD (30% and 24% respectively).

CLINICAL PEARLS

▶ Some children with OCD do not understand that the symptoms are unreasonable because they have not yet achieved the necessary developmental capacity.

▶ Individual and family cognitive behavioral therapy has proven effective for the treatment of OCD.

▶ SSRIs such as fluvoxamine, sertraline, and fluoxetine are commonly used for pharmacologic intervention in childhood OCD. In addition, although more side effects may be present, clomipramine has also been used effectively.

▶ The combination of medication with behavior therapy can provide the best outcomes for treating OCD.

  ▶ Residential treatment should be considered for nonadherent or otherwise resistant patients.

REFERENCES

Björgvinsson T, Hart AJ, Wetterneck C, et al. Outcomes of specialized residential treatment for adults with obsessive-compulsive disorder. *J Psychiatr Pract.* Sep 2013;19(5):429-437.

Garcia AM, Sapyta JJ, Moore PS, et al. Predictors and moderators of treatment outcome in the Pediatric Obsessive Compulsive Treatment Study (POTS I). *J Am Acad Child Adolesc Psychiatry.* Oct 2010;49(10):1024-1033.

Huyser C, Veltman DJ, Wolters LH, de Haan E, Boer F. Functional magnetic resonance imaging during planning before and after cognitive-behavioral therapy in pediatric obsessive-compulsive disorder. *J Am Acad Child Adolesc Psychiatry.* Dec 2010;49(12):1238-1248.

Leslie DL, Kozma L, Martin A, et al. Neuropsychiatric disorders associated with streptococcal infection: a case-control study among privately insured children. *J Am Acad Child Adolesc Psychiatry*. Oct 2008;47(10):1166-1172.

Rosenberg DR, Mirza Y, Russell A, et al. Reduced anterior cingulate glutamatergic concentrations in childhood OCD and major depression versus healthy controls. *J Am Acad Child Adolesc Psychiatry*. 2004;43(9):1146-1153.

Sadock BJ, Sadock VA, Ruiz P. *Kaplan and Sadock's Synopsis of Psychiatry: Behavioral Sciences/Clinical Psychiatry*. 11th ed. Baltimore, MD: Lippincott Williams & Wilkins: 2014.

A 34-year-old married woman comes to an intake appointment with a psychiatrist with a chief complaint of "I've been depressed recently." One year ago she was raped by an unknown assailant in the parking lot of a grocery store, and, since that time, "things just have not been the same." She describes becoming irritable and angry with her spouse for no apparent reason and feels disconnected from him emotionally. In fact, she feels "numb" most of the time, having "lost the joy from life." Her sleep is restless, and she is having trouble focusing on her work as a laboratory technician. She has nightmares about the rape in which the event is replayed. The patient admits that she has told very few people about the rape and tries "not to think about it" as much as possible. She avoids going anywhere near the location where the event occurred and remains anxious when shopping at a supermarket.

On mental status examination, her appearance, behavior, and speech are all unremarkable. Her mood is "depressed," and her affect is congruent and restricted. Her thought process is linear and logical. She denies suicidal or homicidal ideation, although wishes her attacker would "die a horrible death." She denies paranoia, delusions, or perceptual disturbances. Her cognition is grossly intact. Her judgment and impulse control are not impaired.

▶ What is the most likely diagnosis?
▶ Should this patient be hospitalized?

ANSWERS TO CASE 23:

Posttraumatic Stress Disorder

Summary: A 34-year-old woman suffered a traumatic event 1 year ago. Since that time, she has been depressed, irritable, angry, and disconnected emotionally. She feels "numb" and has significant anhedonia. She has trouble sleeping and concentrating. She has nightmares about the rape and tries not to think about it. She avoids going near the place where it occurred and has anxiety when going to the grocery store. On mental status examination, she shows a depressed mood that is congruent with her affect, which is also restricted. She has violent fantasies toward her attacker but no overt homicidal or suicidal ideation.

- **Most likely diagnosis:** Posttraumatic stress disorder (PTSD).

- **Should this patient be hospitalized:** No. She is not currently suicidal and has a support system, housing, and employment. Although she has vague, homicidal fantasies (which are not uncommon in this type of presentation), she has no specific plan or intent to kill her attacker, nor does she know him or his location. This patient is not committable at this time. Admission to the hospital should not be offered on a voluntary basis either, as she could be adequately treated on an outpatient basis.

ANALYSIS

Objectives

1. Describe the diagnostic criteria of PTSD and how to make the diagnosis in a patient.

2. Understand the indications for psychiatric hospitalization in a patient with PTSD.

Considerations

This patient shows many of the characteristic signs and symptoms of PTSD. After a significant traumatic event, she finds herself responding emotionally (depression, anger, and irritability) but having anhedonia and withdrawing from those she cares about. She is reexperiencing the event through nightmares and recurrent intrusive thoughts. She tries not to think about it (by pushing it out of her mind) and avoids the location where she was raped, as well as suffers anxiety when shopping at a grocery store. She has trouble sleeping and concentrating, which is interfering with her ability to work. The results of her mental status examination are consonant with this picture too.

APPROACH TO:

Posttraumatic Stress Disorder

DEFINITION

POSTTRAUMATIC STRESS DISORDER: A syndrome that develops after a person is exposed to a traumatic event, with ongoing symptoms of reexperiencing,

Table 23–1 • DIAGNOSTIC CRITERIA FOR POSTTRAUMATIC STRESS DISORDER
Exposure to actual or threatened death, serious injury, or sexual violence in at least *one* of the following ways: directly experiencing or witnessing event(s), learning of event(s) occurring to a close family member, or experiencing repeated exposure to aversive details of traumatic event(s).
Presence of at least *one* of the following: recurrent, intrusive, distressing memories of the event(s); recurrent distressing dreams related to the event(s); dissociative reactions (eg, flashbacks) of the event(s) recurring; psychological distress at exposure to cues that symbolize or resemble the event(s); or marked physiological reactions to cures that symbolize or resemble an aspect of the event(s).
Persistent avoidance of or efforts to avoid distressing memories, thoughts, or feelings about the event(s) and/or avoidance of or efforts to avoid external reminders that arouse distressing memories, thoughts, or feelings about the event(s).
Negative alterations in thinking and mood associated with the event(s) as evidenced by at least *two* of the following: inability to remember an important aspect of the event(s); persistent and exaggerated negative beliefs about oneself, others, or the world; inappropriate blaming of oneself or others; persistent negative emotional state; anhedonia; feelings of detachment from others; persistent inability to experience positive emotions.
Alterations in arousal associated with the event(s), as evidenced by at least *two* of the following: irritability or angry outbursts; reckless or self-destructive behavior; hypervigilance; pronounced startle response; problems concentrating; or sleep disturbance (eg, difficulty falling/staying asleep or restless sleep).
The symptoms cause significant distress or impairment in social or occupational functioning. Duration is > 1 mo.

avoidance of reminders, negative alterations of thoughts and mood, and symptoms of increased arousal (Table 23–1).

CLINICAL APPROACH

The identification of PTSD in a patient involves understanding the traumatic event and the patient characteristics. The trauma itself can be a single event or multiple events occurring over several weeks, months, or even years (such as in cases of domestic violence). The context and type of trauma are also important (eg, motor vehicle accident, combat, torture, rape). If the trauma occurs when the individual is very young or very old, the effects can be much more severe. Risk factors for developing PTSD include female gender, childhood emotional problems and/or adversity, previous psychiatric illness, lower educational level, lower socioeconomic status, exposure to prior trauma, lower intelligence, dissociation during the trauma, and a family psychiatric history. Resilience in the face of trauma is increased by the presence of strong social support.

DIFFERENTIAL DIAGNOSIS

The vast majority (80%) of individuals with PTSD also have another comorbid psychiatric illness, such as major depressive disorder, another anxiety disorder, or substance use disorder(s); this must be kept in mind when reviewing the differential diagnosis. Patients can suffer injuries during traumatic events, especially traumatic brain injuries (especially in combat veterans). Some sequelae, particularly partial complex seizures, may mimic symptoms of PTSD. If the patient is not asked about the occurrence of a trauma, many symptoms of PTSD resemble those of generalized anxiety or panic disorder. The social withdrawal and numbing exhibited by individuals with PTSD may be confused with depressive symptoms. Patients with borderline personality disorder can also have a history of trauma, especially related to events occurring in early childhood, and they may also exhibit posttraumatic symptoms such as intrusive memories and hyperarousal. Many patients with dissociative disorders have a history of trauma and can experience posttraumatic symptoms; however, the symptoms are limited to prominent dissociation, such as episodes of amnesia. An individual with acute intoxication or undergoing withdrawal can display many of the symptoms of PTSD. In addition, continued alcohol or drug use can exacerbate chronic PTSD symptoms. Malingering is rare, but when compensation is involved, there is a potential for false claims of illness.

TREATMENT

The **treatment of PTSD** is usually **multimodal, including pharmacotherapy, psychotherapy, and social intervention.** Selective serotonin reuptake inhibitors (SSRIs), such as **sertraline and paroxetine,** and (less studied) serotonin-norepinephrine reuptake inhibitors (SNRIs) are very effective in reducing the symptom clusters (reexperiencing, avoidance, alterations in cognition/mood, hyperarousal) in PTSD. Tricyclic antidepressants and monoamine oxidase inhibitors (MAOIs) are not as effective. Antidepressants are usually first administered at a low dose and titrated upward, as tolerated by the patient. Some response can be noted by 2 to 4 weeks, but a full response to medication can take up to 24 weeks. Initially, a hypnotic medication (such as trazodone) can be used at night to facilitate sleep.

Prazosin, an alpha-1 adrenergic antagonist, is also very effective in treating PTSD, especially the reexperiencing and arousal symptom clusters. Atypical (or second-generation) antipsychotics are often used to augment treatment with antidepressants, although they have not consistently demonstrated efficacy, nor have mood stabilizers. Benzodiazepines should be avoided given the significant comorbidity of PTSD with substance use disorders. The psychotherapies that have been used most successfully in PTSD include various forms of cognitive behavioral therapy (CBT). Some examples of CBT used in PTSD are cognitive processing therapy and prolonged exposure therapy; most of these therapies involve both exposure, in which the patient is encouraged to relive the traumatic event(s) in his or her imagination, coupled with cognitive therapy, in which various thoughts and beliefs generated by the trauma are explored and reframed. These therapies often have significant overlap but require significant training and should be conducted only by experienced clinicians.

Social intervention can be of significant importance following a traumatic event: providing shelter, food, clothing, and housing can be immediate and necessary tasks. Restoring a sense of safety and security is crucial after a traumatic event. For example, increasing social support to individuals and groups who have suffered a natural or accidental disaster can be the first order of business. For many individuals, joining a support group of fellow survivors (rape, combat) is also very helpful.

> ## CASE CORRELATION
>
> - See also Case 24 and Case 25 for diagnoses that may also present with symptoms compatible with that of PTSD. However, adjustment disordered patients are reacting to a stressor that does not meet PTSD criteria, or have symptoms themselves that do not meet all the PTSD criteria. Acute stress disorder may appear identical to PTSD, but the duration of the disorder is 3 days to 1 month following exposure to the traumatic event, not longer.

COMPREHENSION QUESTIONS

23.1 A 36-year-old businessman who survived a serious car accident 4 months ago complains of "jitteriness" when driving to work and is currently using public transportation because of his anxiety. He has found himself "spacing out" for several minutes at a time and having difficulty concentrating on his job. He has felt "sad" much of the time, has trouble sleeping at night, has lost 4 lb because of a decreased appetite, and admits that his job performance is slipping. Which of the following is the most likely diagnosis?

A. Major depressive disorder

B. Panic disorder

C. Social anxiety disorder (social phobia)

D. Specific phobia

E. Temporal lobe epilepsy

23.2 A patient is referred to a therapist to begin psychotherapy for his PTSD. Which of the following has been shown to be the most efficacious treatment for his condition?

A. Cognitive behavioral therapy

B. Dialectical-behavioral therapy

C. Hypnotherapy

D. Insight-oriented therapy

E. Psychoanalysis

23.3 Despite a course of psychotherapy, the above patient in Question 23.2 continues to suffer from recurrent nightmares, flashbacks, hypervigilance, and emotional numbing. Which of the following medications is most likely to be helpful as monotherapy in this patient?

A. Alprazolam

B. Buspirone

C. Prazosin

D. Risperidone

E. Valproic acid

ANSWERS

23.1 **A.** This patient exhibits the features of major depressive disorder, which commonly occurs with PTSD. While he experienced a traumatic event prior to his presentation and he exhibits several symptoms of PTSD, he does not meet full criteria for PTSD. It would be unlikely for this patient to suddenly develop an anxiety disorder such as panic disorder, social anxiety disorder, or specific phobia. While the "spacing-out" periods are likely to be episodes of dissociation occurring because of the trauma, possible neurologic injury should be considered, especially because of his history and the change in his job performance. In addition, the patient might be using alcohol to aid in sleeping or to decrease the hypervigilance he has experienced since the accident, so this should be explored.

23.2 **A.** While different types of psychotherapy have been found to be effective in PTSD, various forms of cognitive behavioral and exposure therapy have been the best studied and found to be the most useful. Dialectical-behavioral therapy is a specific therapy developed for the treatment of borderline personality disorder. Hypnotherapy, insight-oriented therapy, and psychoanalysis have not been adequately studied in the treatment of PTSD patients.

23.3 **C.** Individuals with PTSD often respond to SSRIs or SNRIs. Additionally, alpha-1 antagonists such as prazosin have demonstrated efficacy in significantly reducing the symptom clusters of PTSD. However, benzodiazepines such as alprazolam, buspirone, second-generation (atypical) antipsychotics (such as risperidone), and mood stabilizers (such as valproic acid) are not recommended as monotherapy for the treatment of PTSD. Although alprazolam might assist in decreasing the patient's general anxiety, the incidence of substance abuse is high among patients with PTSD. Addictive medications should be avoided in these individuals.

CLINICAL PEARLS

▶ Stress symptoms exist along a continuum. The milder forms require only a "tincture of time" to resolve; symptoms that persist 3 months after the trauma are unlikely to resolve without treatment.

▶ Establishing safety should be the first treatment intervention in trauma-related disorders.

▶ A diagnosis of PTSD rests on exposure to a traumatic event, as well as symptoms of reexperiencing, avoidance of reminders, negative alterations in thoughts and mood, and symptoms of increased arousal.

▶ Selective serotonin reuptake inhibitors are very beneficial in the treatment of PTSD, and alpha-1 adrenergic antagonists have also demonstrated efficacy in reducing symptoms.

REFERENCES

DSM-5, APA.

Ipser JC, Stein DJ. Evidence-based pharmacotherapy of post-traumatic stress disorder (PTSD). *Int J Neuropsychopharmacol.* 2012;15:825-840.

Jonas DE, Cusack K, Forneris CA, et al. Psychological and pharmacological treatments for adults with posttraumatic stress disorder (PTSD). Comparative Effectiveness Reviews. RTI International–University of North Carolina Evidence-based Practice Center. Rockville, MD: Agency for Healthcare Research and Quality (US); Apr 2013. Report No.: 13-EHC011-EF.

Krystal JH, Rosenheck RA, Cramer JA, et al. Adjunctive risperidone treatment for antidepressant-resistant symptoms of chronic military service–related PTSD: a randomized trial. *JAMA.* 2011;306(5):493-502.

Raskind MA, Peterson K, Williams T, et al. A trial of prazosin for combat trauma PTSD with nightmares in active-duty soldiers returned from Iraq and Afghanistan. *Am J Psychiatry.* 2013;170(9):1003.

A 17-year-old young woman is brought to her primary care physician by her mother because of frequent complaints of headaches and stomachaches for the past 3 to 4 weeks. The mother tells the doctor that the girl has also been doing worse in school during this same time period and believes it is because of the chronic aches. The girl has missed many days of school because of her complaints. Mother has already taken her to have her vision and hearing checked, neither of which is a problem. On further questioning, it is found that the young woman's father is enlisted in the military and left for a 6-month overseas combat assignment 5 weeks ago. He e-mails her several times a week, but the mother notes how much the daughter worries about him and his safety. When interviewed, the girl also notes that in addition to her worries about her father, she sometimes cries frequently but feels better when she talks to her friends. She occasionally has a bad dream about her father and feels she sleeps more uneasily as a result.

▶ What is the most likely diagnosis for this patient?
▶ What is the treatment of choice for this disorder?

ANSWERS TO CASE 24:

Adjustment Disorder

Summary: A 17-year-old young woman presents to her primary care physician with a number of short-term (3-4 weeks) somatic complaints. In addition, she also has some mild symptoms related to mood and anxiety because of her father's service commitment. She is able to maintain general functioning, but there does seem to be some decline. She shows evidence of good strengths in that she can express these feelings to others and feels better as a result.

- **Most likely diagnosis:** Adjustment disorder with mixed anxiety and depressed mood.

- **Treatment of choice:** Psychotherapy (supportive).

ANALYSIS

Objectives

1. Recognize adjustment disorder in a patient.

2. Understand the best treatment recommendation for patients with this disorder.

Considerations

A few weeks after her father was sent overseas to fulfill an armed services obligation, the patient begins to have some difficulties. These showed up first in terms of somatic complaints. This is a common presentation for anxious or depressed feelings in children. These should be worked up to reassure both the parents and the patient that there is nothing seriously wrong physically. When further investigated, we find that the patient has additional, more classically psychiatric symptoms in the areas of mood and increased worry. She is functioning adequately, but there does seem to be some significant decline, more than one might expect under the circumstances. The symptoms have been short in duration (< 6 months) and occurred within 4 months of the stressor (father going overseas). Her prognosis is good, given her supportive environment and responsiveness to talking about her feelings. (See the diagnostic criteria in Table 24–1.) Supportive therapy would be indicated in this situation as well as an evaluation of the mother to see how she is managing.

APPROACH TO:

Adjustment Disorder

DEFINITIONS

CLINICALLY SIGNIFICANT SYMPTOMS: Distress in excess of what might be expected in response to the particular stressor in question. To be considered clinically significant, these symptoms must include a marked impact on functioning in a variety of settings.

Table 24–1 • DIAGNOSTIC CRITERIA FOR ADJUSTMENT DISORDER WITH MIXED ANXIETY AND DEPRESSED MOOD
Development of an emotional response to a specific stressor within 3 mo of the onset of that stressor.
Clinically significant symptoms developed as a response to the stressor.
The symptoms do not persist longer than 6 mo after the stressor is resolved.
Six different subtypes of adjustment disorder are recognized: • With depressed mood • With anxiety • With mixed anxiety and depressed mood • With disturbance of conduct • With depressed mood • Unspecified

SUPPORTIVE PSYCHOTHERAPY: A type of therapy in which individuals are taught how to confront issues such as phobias and stressors.

CLINICAL APPROACH

Differential Diagnosis

Adjustment disorder with depressed mood can difficult to distinguish from major depression. The difference between the two is a matter of degree. Patients with major depression can see its onset following the onset of a stressor, although even after the stressor is removed, the major depression continues. Also, in major depression, marked difficulties involving sleep, appetite, concentration, and energy level are noted, and nontransient suicidal ideation and psychotic symptoms can occur. In children or adolescents, irritable mood is often seen rather than the classic depressed mood seen in adults.

Mood disorders arising secondary to the use of a substance or a general medical condition must always be ruled out. Clinicians should exclude any symptom complexes characteristic of other stress-induced disorders as well (such as in acute stress disorder or posttraumatic stress disorder [PTSD]) before diagnosing adjustment disorder. With PTSD, the stressor is usually actual or threatened death or serious injury. Finally, normal grief reactions or bereavement can be difficult to differentiate from adjustment disorders, but if the stressor is within expected and/or culturally acceptable ranges, adjustment disorder should generally not be diagnosed.

In *DSM-5*, adjustment disorders have been reclassified in a grouping of trauma- and stressor-related disorders. More controversially, in the diagnostic criteria for major depressive disorder, the bereavement exclusion has been removed. Although response to a significant loss may closely resemble a depressive episode, *DSM-5* advises consideration of a major depressive episode overlying such a normal response upon consideration of the individual's history and the cultural norms at hand. The category of "other specified trauma- and stressor-related disorder" includes a description of persistent complex bereavement disorder, which is "characterized by severe and persistent grief and mourning reactions."

TREATMENT

The treatment of choice for adjustment disorder is psychotherapy. Group psychotherapy can often be helpful, especially if the group members all have similar stressors, for example, patients with breast cancer or individuals who have experienced a similar trauma. Individual therapy gives patients an opportunity to work through the meaning of the stressor in their lives and the impact it has on their emotional well-being. Medications are not generally indicated, although short-term medications to induce sleep can be helpful if sleep disturbance is part of the symptom presentation. Finally, in the case of extremely acute stressors, for example, a specific traumatic event such as a car accident or an incidence of violence, supportive techniques such as relaxation training, reassurance, and environmental modification (eg, changing the locks on an apartment door, or moving, if a patient has been the victim of an in-home rape) can be helpful.

CASE CORRELATION

- See also Case 13 and Case 23 for diagnoses that may also present with emotional or behavioral symptoms of distress following a traumatic event. Patients with a major depressive disorder have a different symptom profile than those with an adjustment disorder, though the major depressive disorder may occur in response to a stressor. Adjustment disordered patients are reacting to a stressor that does not meet PTSD criteria, or have symptoms that do not meet all the PTSD criteria.

COMPREHENSION QUESTIONS

24.1 Adjustment disorder is diagnosed in a 45-year-old woman who was fired from a job she held for 20 years. She undergoes supportive psychotherapy. Nine months later, she is seen by her physician, but none of her symptoms have resolved. During this time, she has found another job that is similar to her first position in duties and salary. Which of the following is the most likely diagnosis?

A. Adjustment disorder

B. Posttraumatic stress disorder

C. Major depressive disorder

D. Bipolar disorder

E. Schizoaffective disorder

24.2 A 52-year-old man presents to his primary care physician after the death of his wife from breast cancer 2 months ago. He complains of depression, inconsolable sadness, frequent crying, and an inability to focus upon his work and usual activities. Which of the following treatments would likely be most helpful for him?

   A. Supportive psychotherapy

   B. Family therapy

   C. A selective serotonin reuptake inhibitor antidepressant

   D. Psychoanalysis

   E. Behavioral modification therapy

24.3 A 27-year-old woman and her 7-year-old son present to a mental health center for treatment. The patients were passengers in the back of the family car, when they were struck by a semitractor trailer, which killed the father and an older sister. Both mother and son endorse significant depressive symptoms. Which of the following symptoms would most likely differ between the presentations of these two patients?

   A. Irritability

   B. Suicidal thoughts

   C. Flashbacks

   D. Insomnia

   E. Inattention

24.4 Which of the following scenarios is most consistent with an adjustment disorder?

   A. A depressed 62-year-old man experiences a variety of auditory hallucinations which include his mother, who died when he was a child.

   B. A 37-year-old man who recently lost his wife to ovarian cancer expresses a wish that he could be "with her again."

   C. A 19-year-old marine experiences intrusive memories, sleep disturbance, and hypervigilance after he was the only member of his platoon to escape an ambush unharmed.

   D. A 70-year-old woman with metastatic renal cancer refuses further treatment and tells her treatment team that she is ready to die.

   E. A 30-year-old woman who has a history of multiple suicide attempts and self-mutilation, cuts her wrist and presents to the emergency department after being told that her psychiatrist will be going on an extended vacation.

ANSWERS

24.1 **C.** The duration requirement for symptoms occurring *after* the stressor is resolved is met for a major depression in this case. Because the stressor has been removed, an ongoing adjustment disorder would be an incorrect answer. There is no evidence for psychosis or manic moods, so options relating to bipolar or schizoaffective disorder would be incorrect. PTSD would not be a viable option because the patient has not had a life-threatening stressor occur.

24.2 **A.** Supportive psychotherapy is indicated to help the patient deal with his response to his loss, either in an individual or a group setting. Medications are not indicated for bereavement, except perhaps a mild sleep aid if insomnia is a problem. Behavioral modification and/or psychoanalysis are both unnecessary in this setting, because a much more acute problem which is not behavioral in nature is at issue. The patient does not indicate familial problems (other than his wife's death), so supportive therapy is the best option.

24.3 **A.** In the clinical presentation of children and adolescents, one will often find evidence of irritability or short temper rather than a feeling of sadness or depression. The ability to understand the concept of depression seems to be developmentally mediated. All the other options might well be present in both the mother and child.

24.4 **B.** Scenario A suggests a primary psychotic disorder. In scenario B, the individual is not expressing a clear wish to die, but rather a longing to be with his recently deceased loved one. Scenario C is consistent with acute stress disorder. Scenario D does not suggest any mental disorder. Scenario E is suggestive of borderline personality disorder.

CLINICAL PEARLS

▶ Adjustment disorder has several different subtypes of symptoms: depressed mood, anxiety, or disturbance of conduct.

▶ Children often feel irritable rather than depressed.

▶ The chronology of the symptoms is very important in making the correct diagnosis.

▶ The most important treatment modality for adjustment disorder involves psychotherapy and not a somatic intervention.

REFERENCES

American Psychiatric Association: *Diagnostic and Statistical Manual of Mental Disorders*. 5th ed. Washington, DC: American Psychiatric Publishing; 2013.

Black BW, Andreasen NC. *Introductory Textbook of Psychiatry*. 6th ed. Washington, DC: American Psychiatric Publishing; 2014:164-170, 551-570.

Sadock BJ, Sadock VA, Ruiz P. *Kaplan and Sadock's Synopsis of Psychiatry: Behavioral Sciences/Clinical Psychiatry*. 11th ed. Baltimore, MD: Lippincott Williams & Wilkins; 2014.

A 35-year-old man is brought to see a psychiatrist by his friend because "ever since the disaster that killed his wife, he has been out of it." The patient states that 1 week previously the town in which he lived was hit by a tornado. His house was destroyed, and his wife of 2 years was killed. The patient states that he feels as if "I'm living in a fog—this just can't be real." He says that he feels disconnected from everything and everyone—he knows they are trying to help him, but he just feels numb. He claims that when he closes his eyes, all he sees is an image of his wife being buried under rubble, and he hears the loud roar of the tornado. The patient says that since that time he has isolated himself from others as much as possible so that he does not have to talk about what happened. He has not slept well for several days, and when he hears a loud noise, he thinks the tornado is coming back, which makes him very anxious and jumpy. He has been unable to work and has not called any of his insurance companies to tell them about the disaster. The patient states that he has never been to a psychiatrist before and came today only because his friend insisted.

▶ What is the most likely diagnosis for this patient?
▶ What should be the next step in his treatment?

ANSWERS TO CASE 25:

Acute Stress Disorder

Summary: A 35-year-old man presents to a psychiatrist 1 week after living through a tornado that killed his wife. Since that time he has been "in a daze," and he describes feelings of numbness and derealization. He sees recurrent intrusive images of the event and tries to avoid thinking about it. He does not sleep well and becomes anxious when he hears a loud noise. His ability to function has been impaired (he is not able to work or call his insurance companies).

- **Most likely diagnosis:** Acute stress disorder.

- **Next step in treatment:** The major initial approach is support, especially facilitating and strengthening family and community support. Prior spiritual or religious affiliation, which can lend meaning to the event and loss, can be very helpful to the individual. Educating the patient and family about expected symptoms and a variety of coping techniques (such as relaxation training) can be very helpful. The use of sedatives or hypnotics in the short term can also be useful.

ANALYSIS

Objectives

1. Recognize acute stress disorder (ASD) in a patient.

2. Understand the recommended treatment approaches for patients with this disorder.

Considerations

This patient suffered an acute traumatic episode 1 week prior to his appearance at the psychiatrist's office. The response to the trauma has lasted more than 3 days but less than 4 weeks. The patient experiences several dissociative symptoms (feeling in a daze, derealization, numbing). He relives the event over and over in his mind (seeing his wife killed and hearing the tornado). The patient avoids talking about the trauma to avoid arousing recollections of it. He has symptoms of anxiety (insomnia, anxiety when hearing loud noises) that prevent him from functioning well (not working, failing to call his insurance companies to report the losses).

APPROACH TO:

Acute Stress Disorder

DEFINITIONS

DEREALIZATION: A perception that the environment is somehow different or strange, although the individual cannot account for the changes.

DISSOCIATIVE AMNESIA: Memory loss of some component of an event, which in the case of ASD is usually traumatic.

CLINICAL APPROACH

Acute stress disorder (ASD) is a syndrome that develops shortly after an individual is exposed to a traumatic event. It is characterized by intense fear and feelings of helplessness, as well as a number of dissociative symptoms. The traumatic events are usually frightening enough to cause strong reactions in anyone; examples are war (as a combatant, civilian survivor, or refugee), torture, political violence, terrorism, natural or accidental disasters, and sexual or physical assault. The fear response is activated via the hypothalamic-pituitary-adrenal axis and locus ceruleus/norepinephrine system, resulting in a cascade of further physiologic events. Acute stress disorder is defined as occurring within the first 4 weeks after a traumatic event because research indicates that in many individuals this syndrome can resolve without progressing to posttraumatic stress disorder (PTSD).

DIAGNOSTIC CRITERIA

Acute stress disorder occurs within 4 weeks of the traumatic event and lasts for a minimum of 3 days. The diagnosis requires the presence of at least 9 of 14 symptoms in any of the five categories:

I. **Intrusion symptoms**

   1. Recurrent, involuntary, and intrusive distressing memories of the traumatic event

   2. Recurrent distressing dreams related to the event

   3. Dissociative reactions in which the individual feels or acts as if the event were reoccurring

   4. Intense or prolonged psychological distress or marked physiological reactions to internal or external cues that symbolize or resemble an aspect of the event

II. **Negative mood**

   5. Persistent inability to experience positive emotions

III. **Dissociative symptoms**

   6. An altered sense of reality of one's surroundings

   7. Inability to remember an important aspect of the traumatic event

IV. **Avoidance symptoms**

   8. Efforts to avoid distressing memories, thoughts, or feelings associated with the event

   9. Efforts to avoid external reminders that arouse distressing memories, thoughts, or feelings associated with the event

V. **Arousal symptoms**

   10. Sleep disturbance

   11. Irritable or angry outburst

   12. Hypervigilance

   13. Problems with concentration

   14. Exaggerated startle response

If the symptoms persist for more than 1 month and meet criteria for PTSD, the diagnosis must be changed from ASD to PTSD.

DIFFERENTIAL DIAGNOSIS

An individual involved in an accident or assault is likely to have suffered a **head injury**, which can produce a postconcussion clinical picture resembling the dissociative symptoms of ASD. A patient can have an **independent substance abuse** or dependence problem and drinks and uses street drugs to "self-treat" the symptoms of ASD, complicating the diagnosis. **Cocaine** intoxication can resemble the hypervigilance and hyperarousal of ASD. Other anxiety disorders such as **panic disorder** can resemble ASD; the occurrence of a traumatic event and the reliving of it, along with avoidance symptoms, differentiate the disorders. **Dissociative disorders** can resemble ASD because of the dissociative symptoms associated with the latter. In order to make the correct diagnosis, the clinician must ask about the other symptom clusters present in ASD; patients with dissociative disorders do not have the trauma history or display the avoidance behavior of patients with ASD. **Malingering** should be in the differential diagnosis for patients pursuing financial gain as compensation for a traumatic event; this is especially true considering recent publicity about the disorder. Experienced clinicians should be able to detect genuine symptoms of hyperarousal and reexperiencing of an event in a patient with ASD.

TREATMENT

Treatment of a patient with ASD consists of supportive intervention. There is a wide range of possibilities based on the type of trauma, the patient's culture, and the presence or absence of a social network. The clinician should attempt to mobilize all active social supports, including family, religious groups, and the community, to assist the individual. Education about the symptoms and coping skills can be very helpful. Research on critical incident stress debriefing (CISD), in which the individual is encouraged to talk about and process thoughts about the event, is inconclusive regarding its effectiveness. When insomnia and marked hypervigilance are problematic, hypnotics and anxiolytics can be used on a short-term basis. There is emerging research that suggests that beta-blockers, such as propranolol, started directly following the traumatic event, are effective in preventing the development of PTSD.

CASE CORRELATION

- See Case 6 and Case 23 for diagnoses that may also present with perceptual disturbances. In schizophrenia the perceptual disorders may be hallucinations or delusions, while acute stress disorder patients may suffer from flashbacks, which are perceptual disturbances directly related to the traumatic event. Acute stress disorder is of a shorter time course than PTSD, 3 days to 1 month.

COMPREHENSION QUESTIONS

25.1 A 21-year-old woman comes in for treatment after developing symptoms a few days after she was raped at a college dorm party. She says she has been very anxious, fears returning to school, and is thinking about dropping out. She is also experiencing insomnia, poor concentration, intrusive flashback of the event, nightmares, and her mood is constantly depressed. She has refused to talk to her family about the event because, "she just wants it to go away." What is the most likely diagnosis?

   A. Acute stress disorder

   B. Adjustment disorder

   C. Factitious disorder

   D. Generalized anxiety disorder

   E. Posttraumatic stress disorder

25.2 Treatment of ASD should focus primarily on which of the following?

   A. Biofeedback

   B. Debriefing the individual about the event

   C. Mobilizing social supports

   D. Pharmacologic treatments such as selective serotonin reuptake inhibitors

   E. Psychotherapy

25.3 Acute stress disorder is diagnosed in a 32-year-old woman who witnessed her fiancé being shot to death in a robbery attempt. She has difficulty sleeping and feels that she is not emotionally attached to anything around her. She also has repetitive flashbacks of the event and avoids going near the location where the incident occurred. Which of the following medications might be helpful to this patient over the short term?

   A. Buspirone

   B. Paroxetine

   C. Risperidone

   D. Valproate

   E. Zolpidem

ANSWERS

25.1 **A.** The most likely diagnosis is ASD, because this patient's symptoms occurred within 4 weeks of the event and have lasted at least 3 days. If the symptoms had lasted longer than 4 weeks, the diagnosis for a patient with these symptoms would become PTSD. An adjustment disorder is characterized by mood disturbances (anxiety, depression) in response to a difficult situation, but adjustment disorders do not present with the avoidance symptoms (avoiding talking about the incident) and/or reexperiencing of the traumatic event. Generalized anxiety disorder presents with the patient constantly worrying about a wide variety of imagined problems, not connected to an individual traumatic event. Factitious disorder is the feigning of mental or physical illness for secondary gain.

25.2 **C.** Pharmacologic treatments, psychotherapy, and biofeedback are primarily interventions for PTSD; the results of research are currently unclear regarding the benefits of debriefing for those with ASD. Mobilizing social supports is the most effective intervention in treating patients with ASD.

25.3 **E.** The use of a hypnotic for insomnia is likely to be helpful to this patient in the short term. Buspirone is used for those patients diagnosed with generalized anxiety disorder, while paroxetine is used in the treatment of major depression. Risperidone is an antipsychotic, and valproate is used for mood stabilization of patients with bipolar disorder.

CLINICAL PEARLS

▶ Acute stress disorder occurs within 4 weeks of a traumatic event and lasts at least 3 days to a maximum of 4 weeks.

▶ When symptoms of ASD persist beyond 4 weeks, PTSD must be considered.

▶ Individuals with ASD feel detached, feel "unreal," and can have dissociative amnesia.

▶ Mobilizing social support is the first intervention in treating patients with ASD; most symptoms resolve without pharmacologic treatment.

▶ There are many resilience and risk factors in the development of PTSD or ASD, but most individuals develop symptoms given a traumatic stressor of sufficient magnitude.

REFERENCES

American Psychiatric Association. *Diagnostic and Statistical Manual of Mental Disorders*. 5th ed. Arlington, VA: American Psychiatric Publishing; 2013.280-286.

Black BW, Andreasen NC. *Introductory Textbook of Psychiatry*. 6th ed. Washington, DC: American Psychiatric Publishing; 2014:252-254.

Hales RE, Yudofsky SC, Roberts LW. *The American Psychiatric Publishing Textbook of Psychiatry*. 6th ed. Washington, DC: American Psychiatric Publishing; 2014:480-482.

A 22-year-old woman is brought to the clinic by her brother who voices concern about the patient's strange behavior. He states that his sister struggles with depression which acutely worsened after a painful breakup with her abusive boyfriend. She did not return home for several days, after which he finally found her at a bar across town. She had facial bruising and appeared disheveled. His sister acted like a "completely different person" and spoke with a French accent. He was unaware of his sister ever learning French. He finally convinced her to come back home with him that night. Since returning home, the woman has "been her normal self." The brother admits that they had a rough childhood, often suffering from physical abuse at the hands of their father. He states that despite an unstable upbringing, "We have done pretty well for ourselves. Both of us are clean and employed."

The patient denies any recollection of the past few days. Her last memory before the episode was her boyfriend yelling at her and his fist flying at her face. She felt herself disconnect from her body and cannot recall what happened next. She states that her boyfriend been increasingly jealous and possessive of her. He accused her of cheating on him, which she adamantly denies. The patient reports that her boyfriend became abusive over the past few months when she began receiving late night phone calls from strange men asking "for the French girl" to "meet up again." She denies straying in her relationship and feels bewildered about these phone calls. The patient does not remember much of her childhood and has "blocked out" the abuse. On memory testing, the patient is oriented to person, place and time and does not exhibit any gross impairment.

▶ What is the most likely diagnosis for this patient?
▶ What could be a causal factor and is highly associated with this disorder?

ANSWERS TO CASE 26:

Dissociative Identity Disorder

Summary: The patient is a 22-year-old woman with a history of childhood trauma and chronic depression with reported dissociative symptoms triggered by domestic violence. She felt a sense of depersonalization—disconnected from her body—in the face of her attacker. She had an episode of amnesia after the physical abuse and similarly had amnestic episodes surrounding childhood abuse. Her brother found the patient acting like a different person after she disappeared for several days. She has recently had strange men tell her they have met her before as a French woman. Currently, her symptoms have resolved and she has returned to baseline functioning. Her memory testing did not reveal any gross impairment.

- **Most likely diagnosis:** Dissociative identity disorder (DID).

- **Causal factor:** Most DID patients have experienced **significant physical and sexual trauma, often during their childhood**. Creation of an alternate identity can be conceptualized as a protective but maladaptive mechanism for the core personality. The fragmentation of a patient's identity results in a splitting off of an alternate to take the abuse while the core personality escapes. This allows for a compartmentalization of the traumatic experience encased within the alternate personality that experienced it.

ANALYSIS

Objectives

1. Learn the criteria for DID (Table 26–1 for diagnostic criteria).

2. Understand management of this disorder.

Considerations

Like most patients with DID, this woman suffered from severe abuse during her childhood. She experienced amnestic episodes as a child, often triggered by trauma. When faced again with the onslaught of an attack, she felt herself leaving her body behind. **Depersonalization** was a vehicle to escape and disconnect from the pain. She had an amnestic episode over the course of several days. The patient relocated

Table 26–1 • DIAGNOSTIC CRITERIA FOR DISSOCIATIVE IDENTITY DISORDER
Loss of integrative abilities leading to a fragmented identity with two or more independent personalities dominating at different times.
Pathologic **possession** involves experiences **outside cultural/religious practice.**
The symptoms may be **observed by others or are self-reported.**
Extensive memory lapses in autobiographical information, daily occurrences, and/or traumatic events.
The symptoms are not due to a medical condition or substance use.
The condition causes distress or impairs social/occupational functioning.

across town, the result of **dissociated travel or a dissociative fugue.** She presented with an alternate personality when her brother found her, speaking with a French accent. In corroboration with the possibility of an alternate, the patient has been receiving numerous late-night phone calls from seemingly unknown men, asking for a French girl. As this alternate personality, the patient could live through the trauma. Dissociation represents a **disruption in the patient's sense of self as an unconscious coping strategy** to deal with further abuse. As with this patient, distinct losses of autobiographical information may occur, often from childhood.

APPROACH TO:
Dissociative Identity Disorder

DEFINITIONS

AMNESIA: Extensive lapses in autobiographical memory.

DEPERSONALIZATION: Sense of detachment from one's self; feeling as if an outside observer of one's own being (eg, out-of-body experience).

DEREALIZATION: Sense of detachment from one's surroundings (eg, familiar people and environments seem unreal).

DISSOCIATION: Discontinuity of mental state due to splitting off from memory/ self which may involve depersonalization, derealization, or amnesia. Unconscious defense mechanism to protect one's self against the memory of overwhelming trauma.

CLINICAL APPROACH

Working with these patients can be challenging. The diagnosis is controversial and challenging to conceptualize. Over the course of treatment, clinicians likely witness switches in DID patients' identities. Longer sessions may be helpful in capturing the broader clinical picture. Clinicians need to be very careful when attempting to recover memories, as these patients are particularly vulnerable to suggestion.

DID, formerly known as multiple personality disorder (MPD), involves **subjectively experiencing fragmentations of the self into distinct identities.** The core personality of the individual remains, but may undergo an amnestic state while the alters predominate. The core personality typically lacks awareness of the alters, but the other personalities maintain awareness of each other. Identity switches may be triggered by the trauma itself, subsequent microtraumas, removal from the abusive environment, or death of an abuser.

Dissociative symptoms can be conceptualized as both additions and negations of experience. The *addition* of unusual experiences or "positive" symptoms encompasses unwanted intrusions into one's state of awareness along with derealization and depersonalization. "Negative" symptoms refer to the inability to access information, that is, amnesia. Patients may be told about skills unbeknownst to them or find items they do not recall obtaining. Many report dissociative flashbacks during which they reexperience the trauma with subsequent amnesia regarding the flashback content.

Most patients with DID **develop posttraumatic stress disorder (PTSD).** Many have **comorbid depressive disorders, personality disorders, and conversion disorders.**

Changes from *DSM-IV* **to** *DSM-5*: **Symptoms may now be reported** in addition to being observed. Extensive memory lapses involve nontraumatic experiences in addition to traumatic events. **Pathological possession** has been added as a potential part of dissociation, involving unwanted, involuntary, and distressing experiences outside one's culturally sanctioned practice.

DIFFERENTIAL DIAGNOSIS

DID may exhibit various presentations and thus may be confused with other disorders. Patients with delirium or major neurocognitive disorders (dementia) suffer from memory impairment and changes in behavior. Patients with seizure disorders experience postictal confusion. To rule out an underlying medical or neurologic condition, clinicians need to perform a physical examination, including neurologic examination and cognitive testing, as well as order appropriate laboratory workup, electroencephalography (EEG), and brain imaging. Intoxication with different substances can cause amnesia: alcohol, hallucinogens, barbiturates, benzodiazepines, and steroids. Alcohol intoxication or blackouts can lead to lapses in memory. To rule out an issue caused by substance use, clinicians need to order a urine drug screen in addition to history and physical examination.

DID encompasses all the features of the other dissociative disorders: depersonalization/derealization disorder and dissociative amnesia disorder. When episodes of extensive memory lapses occur regarding vital autobiographical information, dissociative amnesia may be diagnosed. The inaccessible memories usually involve a traumatic or stressful event and exceed typical forgetfulness. During dissociative amnesia, patients may experience a fugue or "flight" during which they travel. Individuals experiencing dissociative fugue suddenly and unexpectedly travel far away from their homes and cannot recall their previous identity or past. The person usually adopts a new identity in the course of the fugue. Although now considered a subtype of dissociative amnesia disorder, dissociative fugue more commonly occurs in DID. Depersonalization/derealization disorder involves recurrent feelings of detachment from one's own physical or mental processes while maintaining an intact sense of reality. These patients often feel like they are observing their bodies and thoughts from a distance.

Patients with complex PTSD can experience dissociative states during which they relive past traumas. The intensity may vary from intrusive sensations to complete disconnection from surroundings, that is, flashbacks. These patients may be vulnerable to involvement in relationships which recapitulate past childhood trauma and result in revictimization.

Distinguish bipolar spectrum disorders from DID by delineating the course of mood swings. Rapid mood swings commonly occur because of dissociative symptomatology, whereas discrete, cyclic mood episodes are more representative of bipolar mood disorder.

Schizophrenia and other psychotic disorders may present similarly, for example, with the perception of hearing voices or delusions of inhabitation by someone else. Unlike psychotic patients, individuals with DID maintain intact reality testing when not dissociating.

Borderline personality disorder (BPD), often arising after a history of trauma, may present with dissociative experiences and identity issues. The other maladaptive pervasive personality traits help distinguish BPD from DID. Patients with personality disorders may enthusiastically display their "identities" versus true DID patients who typically disavow dissociative experiences.

Similarly, factitious or malingered presentations will typically be an ostentatious, flamboyant showcase of dissociative symptoms. Factitious disorder describes the conscious production of symptoms to attain and maintain the sick role, whereas malingering involves intentional production of symptoms for secondary gain. Maintain suspicion if symptoms appear fabricated along with an obvious motivating factor, such as obtaining disability/compensation.

TREATMENT

Psychodynamic psychotherapy can help develop healthier coping strategies for dealing with the underlying stressor. The goal of treatment is to facilitate integration between the separated identities and memories which precipitated the dissociation. Management ranges from symptom containment to reshaping cognitive distortions. Hypnotic interventions can reduce symptoms and assist in accessing different personality states. Of note, DID patients have higher levels of hypnotizability compared to other individuals. Pharmacotherapy, although not first-line DID treatment, may target associated symptoms of comorbid disorders, such as PTSD and major depressive disorder. Selective serotonin reuptake inhibitors (SSRIs) are often used to help treat comorbid depression and PTSD.

CASE CORRELATION

- See Case 23 and Case 60 for patients who may present with dissociative symptoms. PTSD patients may present with dissociative symptoms that are related to the traumatic event (amnesia for part of the event, dissociative flashbacks), but patients with DID will have symptoms like those, but unrelated to any traumatic event; that is, amnesia for everyday events for example. Patients who are malingering may report dissociative symptoms but tend to be relatively undisturbed by or "enjoy" having the disorder, as opposed to dissociative identity disordered patients.

COMPREHENSION QUESTIONS

26.1 A 38-year-old barista presents to her primary care physician with concern about memory problems. She has had trouble recalling significant personal information and life events. The patient reports that dating has been problematic because during intimate encounters, "I just disconnect. I feel so scared and ashamed. I'm floating above my body, looking down on what's happening." Her current boyfriend has described that sometimes she talks like a "little girl" and other times like a "sophisticated southern belle." He finds it endearing, but news of this behavior frightened the patient as she has no recollection. Her boyfriend has said he loves the way she plays piano, but she cannot remember ever touching the instrument. She drinks socially on the weekends, but denies heavy use, black outs, or withdrawal symptoms. Which of the following is the most likely diagnosis?

A. Alcohol use disorder

B. Borderline personality disorder

C. Dissociative amnesia

D. Dissociative identity disorder

E. PTSD

26.2 A 12-year-old girl with a history of complex trauma is admitted to the inpatient child psychiatry unit for the management of disruptive behaviors. On the unit, she has a verbal altercation with a staff member. She stops responding directly to the staff member and appears very frightened. She turns away and begins wailing, "Don't hurt me, daddy. Please, please don't…" If the patient is forcibly placed into physical restraints, what would be the most likely result?

A. Mortality

B. Psychotic break

C. Retraumatization

D. Symptom resolution

26.3 A 22-year-old woman is referred for neuropsychological testing after reporting confusion and amnestic episodes. She has received bills in the mail for credit cards she does not remember opening. The woman has found clothing in her closet that she does not recall purchasing. She has been tagged in numerous pictures on Facebook with people she does not know and has been checked into venues unfamiliar to her. What is the most likely diagnosis?

A. Borderline personality disorder

B. Dissociative identity disorder

C. Factitious disorder

D. Malingering

E. PTSD

ANSWERS

26.1 **D.** The patient presents with symptoms consistent with dissociative identity disorder. She describes amnestic episodes and depersonalization during intimate encounters. This history may be indicative of past sexual trauma which has been compartmentalized and "forgotten." Her boyfriend has observed what may be different alter identities dominating at various times. She has no recollection of this or her ability as a pianist. Although the woman works at a bar, she denies heavy alcohol use or history of blackouts. Dissociative amnesia does not capture the patient's spectrum of symptoms, which goes beyond extensive memory gaps. As the patient may also be exhibiting fragmentations in her identity and depersonalization, DID better accounts for the clinical picture. Borderline personality disorder may be associated with dissociative symptoms, but there are various character pathology traits which the patient does not exhibit. Patients with PTSD will have amnestic events related to the trauma they have experienced, but these occur around traumatic memories, not during everyday events. The patient appears genuinely concerned and confused about her symptoms, which would be more consistent with DID.

26.2 **C.** The girl appears to be having a flashback or reexperiencing a traumatic event. Forcibly placing her in physical restraints would most likely cause retraumatization. Consider more supportive approaches, particularly if a patient is not putting herself or others in danger. Symptom exacerbation would be a more likely outcome than symptoms resolution. Although mortality is a low risk, proper restraint checks along with frequent reassessments are essential for any patient who is being restrained. Use of restraints would not cause a psychotic break.

26.3. **B.** This patient presents with symptoms that could be explained by dissociative identity disorder. She is experiencing distinct lapses in memory with unexplained occurrences in her personal life. Borderline personality disorder patients may dissociate, but there is no history in this patient of other associated characterologic traits such as pervasive affective instability, impulsivity, and self-injurious behavior. Patients with PTSD will have amnestic events related to the trauma they have experienced, but these occur around traumatic memories, not during everyday events. For factitious and malingered symptoms, the patient intentionally produces symptoms. This patient has no known motivating factor to be in the sick role, as in factitious disorder, or for secondary gain, as in malingering.

CLINICAL PEARLS

▶ DID is almost universally associated with a history of significant trauma, but patients may not want to disclose this information or they may not remember.

▶ Routinely ask patients about experiences of blackouts, time loss, and lapses in memory.

▶ Utilize restraints judiciously in patients with a significant trauma history.

REFERENCES

American Psychiatric Association. *Diagnostic and Statistical Manual of Mental Disorders*. 5th ed. Washington, DC: American Psychiatric Association; 2013.

Sadock BJ, Sadock VA, Ruiz, P. *Kaplan & Sadock's Synopsis of Psychiatry*. 11th ed. Baltimore, MD: Lippincott Williams & Wilkins; 2014.

A 24-year-old man is admitted to the neurology service with new-onset blindness. The patient awoke on the morning of his admission entirely unable to see. A detailed workup by the neurology service, including physical, laboratory studies, and imaging revealed no clear medical reason for this abnormality—the patient was found to be otherwise healthy. A psychiatric consultation was subsequently ordered.

The patient tells the psychiatrist that he does not know why he is blind. He emigrated from Mexico several years ago, coming to the United States to make money in order to support his sick mother. She remained ill for several years, but he was unable to send her money because he lost the money gambling. She died recently, and he became despondent because he would never see her again.

On mental status examination, the patient is alert and oriented to person, place, and time. His appearance and hygiene are good, and he does not seem to be overly concerned with his blindness. His mood is described as "Okay," and his affect is congruent and full range. He has normal thought processes and denies having suicidal or homicidal ideation, delusions, or hallucinations.

▶ What is the most likely diagnosis for this patient?
▶ What is the most appropriate treatment for this patient?

ANSWERS TO CASE 27:

Conversion Disorder (Functional Neurological Symptom Disorder)

Summary: A 24-year-old man presents with new-onset blindness for which there is no physiologic or anatomic explanation. The patient says that his mother died recently, after he was unable to send her money because he lost it gambling. He does not seem to be bothered by his blindness.

- **Most likely diagnosis:** Conversion disorder (functional neurological symptom disorder).

- **Best therapy:** Education about the illness, when presented to the patient, often results in resolution of symptoms. Cognitive behavioral therapy (CBT) and/or physical therapy (PT) can also be useful.

ANALYSIS

Objectives

1. Recognize conversion disorder (functional neurological symptom disorder) in a patient (Table 27–1 for diagnostic criteria).

2. Be able to describe the most appropriate treatment of patients with this disorder.

Considerations

This patient presents with a new onset of blindness following his mother's death, when he (unconsciously) realizes that he will never be able to "see" her again. A component of guilt is involved because the patient came to the United States to earn money to help his mother but could not fulfill this obligation because he gambled away the money. There is no physiologic or anatomic explanation for his blindness, and the patient seems to be unconcerned about it, displaying *la belle indifference*.

Table 27–1 • DIAGNOSTIC CRITERIA FOR CONVERSION DISORDER (FUNCTIONAL NEUROLOGICAL SYMPTOM DISORDER)
One or more symptoms of altered voluntary motor or sensory function.
Evidence of incompatibility between the symptoms and recognized neurological or medical conditions.
The symptom or deficit is not better explained by another medical or mental disorder.
The symptom or deficit causes significant distress or impairment in functioning or warrants medical evaluation.

APPROACH TO:

Conversion Disorder (Functional Neurological Symptom Disorder)

DEFINITION

LA BELLE INDIFFERENCE: Inappropriate lack of concern about one's disability.

CLINICAL APPROACH

Ensuring that the symptoms are not explained by an underlying medical or neurologic condition is very important when considering a diagnosis of conversion disorder (functional neurological symptom disorder). It is not unheard of for this disorder to be misdiagnosed in patients who are later found to have multiple sclerosis, for example. However, it is not always a case of either/or. As listed in the criteria, **the symptom or deficit must be incompatible with a recognized neurological or medical condition.** It is not uncommon for individuals with underlying neurologic diseases to also develop conversion symptoms that do not conform to anatomic or physiologic parameters. For example, a patient with a diagnosed seizure disorder can display additional seizure-like movements (the so-called "pseudoseizures" or psychogenic nonepileptic seizures) without corresponding epileptic discharges appearing on an electroencephalogram. In such cases, conversion symptoms occurring in addition to an established illness may function as a mode of communication that expresses unconscious conflict.

The main diagnoses in the differential include somatic symptom disorder, illness anxiety disorder (hypochondriasis), as well as factitious disorder and malingering. Somatic symptom disorder is a chronic disorder that includes multiple physical symptoms that are distressing or result in significant disruption in functioning. Illness anxiety disorder (hypochondriasis) is a chronic preoccupation with having or acquiring a serious illness, coupled with anxiety about health and performing excessive health-related behaviors. Factitious disorders involve the intentional production or falsification of physical or psychological signs or symptoms in order to present as ill or impaired (assume the sick role). **Malingering** is not a mental illness but involves the intentional production or exaggeration of symptoms motivated by external incentives (eg, avoiding a jail sentence, military duty, or work, or obtaining financial compensation). There is often misunderstanding about the differences among conversion disorder, factitious disorder, and malingering. In the first, there is an *unconscious* or *unintentional* production of symptoms because of conflicts or stressors, whereas in the latter two, there is a *conscious* or *intentional* production of symptoms.

CLINICAL COURSE AND TREATMENT

In most cases, conversion symptoms resolve on their own, without treatment. However, it is not at all unusual for the same or similar problems to recur, especially in the presence of a new stressor or conflict. Patients with conversion disorder tend to be responsive to suggestion. Reassurance coupled with education regarding their illness can often quickly result in resolution of the symptom(s). This may include a comment such as, "Under stress, the body can react in unusual ways; this will likely get better soon on its own." It is essential to not to imply that patients are exaggerating, faking, or consciously producing their symptoms or that their problems are "all in their heads." This approach only tends to alienate the patient, create more stress, and possibly worsen the deficit. CBT and/or PT have also been shown to be helpful in conversion disorder, and may be employed in those patients where reassurance and education do not result in remission of symptoms. Hospitalization for conversion disorder is usually not necessary, except in cases where the disability is so severe as to preclude the activities of daily living. In such cases, the patient is usually discharged within several days, after symptoms have resolved.

CASE CORRELATION

- See also Case 16 and Case 30 for patients that may present with symptoms consistent with a conversion disorder. Panic disordered patients may present with episodic neurological symptoms (paresthesias and trembling) but these are typically transient and acutely episodic (ie, during panic attacks). Factitious disordered patients may present with conversion symptoms, but there may be evidence that the loss of function is being deliberately feigned (eg, present during the examination but not at home).

COMPREHENSION QUESTIONS

27.1 A 17-year-old boy presents with a complaint of his "legs giving out" for 1 week. During each episode he experiences a generalized weakness and is unable to move his arms and legs. The episodes last a few minutes. He is currently in the 11th grade earning Bs and Cs. Further questioning reveals that his parents have recently separated after a long period of verbal abuse toward each other. His physical examination and neurologic workup are unremarkable. Laboratory studies are also within normal limits. Which of the following is the most likely diagnosis?

A. Body dysmorphic disorder

B. Conversion disorder (functional neurological symptom disorder)

C. Factitious disorder

D. Illness anxiety disorder

E. Malingering

27.2 Which of the following approaches would be the most effective for the patient in the above Question 27.1?

A. Confrontation about intentionally producing symptoms

B. Explaining that the symptoms are not real

C. Reassurance that a cause will be found

D. Suggestion that symptoms will improve with time

E. Suggestion that the family begins therapy

27.3 A 42-year-old man returns to his internist for the fourth time in 5 months with the same complaints of intermittent numbness of his fingers and indigestion. Although his medical workup has been unremarkable, this has failed to reassure him. He remains anxious and is now concerned that he has celiac disease and requests a gastrointestinal (GI) consultation. Which of the following is the most likely diagnosis?

A. Body dysmorphic disorder

B. Conversion disorder (functional neurological symptom disorder)

C. Factitious disorder

D. Illness anxiety disorder

E. Malingering

27.4 A 32-year-old divorced woman is admitted for second- and third-degree burns of her right hand, which she attributes to accidentally spilling hot oil while she was cooking dinner. Upon evaluation, the surgeon recognizes the patient as someone he had treated for a similar burn on the same hand 3 months ago. Further detailed review of her medical records reveals that this is her sixth burn-related injury in 2 years. Which of the following is the most likely diagnosis?

A. Body dysmorphic disorder

B. Conversion disorder (functional neurological symptom disorder)

C. Factitious disorder

D. Illness anxiety disorder

E. Malingering

ANSWERS

27.1 **B.** This patient most likely has conversion disorder (functional neurological symptom disorder), as evidenced by his altered sensory and motor functioning. Patients with body dysmorphic disorder have a preoccupation with an imagined defect in appearance. There is no evidence that he is intentionally producing the symptoms in order to assume the sick role as in factitious disorder, or for "secondary gain" (avoid jail, military duty, work, or obtain financial compensation), consistent with malingering. Illness anxiety disorder (hypochondriasis) is a preoccupation with having a serious illness.

27.2 **D.** Although the deficits often remit spontaneously, education about the illness and suggesting that the symptoms will improve can facilitate the process. These patients do not intentionally produce their symptoms (as in factitious disorder or malingering), and explaining that their deficits are not real may aggravate the situation and worsen their problems. Whereas reassurance about their likely *improvement* is appropriate, implying that their symptoms are caused by a neurologic illness (assuming that this has been ruled out) would be inaccurate and may serve to reinforce their use of physical symptoms.

27.3 **D.** Illness anxiety disorder (hypochondriasis) is characterized as an individual's preoccupation with having or acquiring a serious illness, along with performing excessive health-related behaviors. Their anxiety often stems from a misinterpretation of physical symptoms or functions. In contrast, patients with body dysmorphic disorder are preoccupied with an imagined defect in appearance. As the patient is not consciously producing symptoms in order to present as ill or impaired, this would not be considered a factitious disorder. Unlike conversion disorder (functional neurological symptom disorder), illness anxiety disorder (hypochondriasis) is not limited to sensory or motor symptoms or deficits. If the patient were malingering there would be obvious secondary gain.

27.4 **C.** Patients with factitious disorders consciously produce symptoms to present as ill or impaired (maintain the "sick role"). In factitious disorder, there is no obvious secondary gain such as monetary compensation or avoidance of work as seen in malingering.

CLINICAL PEARLS

▶ Conversion disorder (functional neurological symptom disorder) involves one or more sensory or motor deficits.

▶ Conversion disorder symptoms are not intentionally produced.

▶ It is important to rule out an underlying medical or neurologic illness because a significant proportion of individuals initially presenting with conversion symptoms eventually develop a recognized illness.

▶ In most cases, educating the patient, coupled with suggestion that the symptoms or deficits will improve quickly results in remission of symptoms.

REFERENCES

American Psychiatric Association. *Diagnostic and Statistical Manual of Mental Disorders*. 5th ed. Arlington, VA: American Psychiatric Publishing; 2013.

Duncan R, Razvi S, Mulhern S. Newly presenting psychogenic nonepileptic seizures: incidence, population characteristics, and early outcome from a prospective audit of a first seizure clinic. *Epilepsy Behav*. Feb 2011;20(2):308-311.

Goldstein LH, Chalder T, Chigwedere C, et al. Cognitive-behavioral therapy for psychogenic nonepileptic seizures: a pilot RCT. *Neurology*. 2010;74:1986.

Nielsen G, Stone J, Edwards MJ. Physiotherapy for functional (psychogenic) motor symptoms: a systematic review. *J Psychosom Res*. Aug 2013;75(2):93-102.

Sharpe M, Walker J, Williams C, et al. Guided self-help for functional (psychogenic) symptoms: a randomized controlled efficacy trial. *Neurology*. 2011;77:564.

Stone J. The bare essentials: functional symptoms in neurology. *Pract Neurol*. 2009;9:179.

A 54-year-old woman is seen in her family doctor's office. She has seen her doctor more than 20 times over the last year. She believes that she has some kind of serious medical disease because she "just doesn't feel right." The patient occasionally complains of vague stomach rumblings, aches and pains in her ankles and wrists, and occasional headaches but the intensity of these symptoms are mild. She scours the Internet for articles about serious, life-threatening diseases and brings these articles in when she visits her physician, convinced that she has a variety of the diseases listed. She frequently checks her heart rate, pulse, and blood pressure looking for any signs of illness. She states that she feels relieved and "safe" for a short period of time after every negative test result but then becomes convinced that she is ill again and makes another doctor's appointment. In the past year, she has taken off so much time from work for doctors' visits that she was put on probation. Other than noting that she is very concerned about having a serious disease, the results of her mental status examination are unremarkable. She has no symptoms suggesting a severe depression, and there is no evidence of thought disorder or psychosis. She becomes insulted when the primary care physician suggests she sees a psychiatrist and refuses a referral.

▶ What is the most likely diagnosis for this patient?
▶ What should the primary care practitioner do for this patient?

ANSWERS TO CASE 28:

Illness Anxiety Disorder

Summary: A 54-year-old woman is referred to a psychiatrist by her physician. She complains of numerous, mild vague symptoms and believes that they are caused by a serious illness. These concerns resulted in her scheduling numerous appointments with the physician in the past year. She is concerned about the prospect of having a serious disease, although she is temporarily relieved when test results come back negative. Her behavior has had serious ramifications in her work life.

- **Most likely diagnosis:** Illness anxiety disorder.

- **Best approach:** Schedule frequent, regular clinic appointments with the patient to assure her that her complaints are being taken seriously. The goal is to have contact with the patient before the relief she gets from reassurance fades to the point where she is convinced she has a new disease. Invasive diagnostic techniques or procedures should be avoided unless there is convincing objective evidence that they are necessary. The patient is unlikely to follow up with referrals to a psychiatrist or other mental health professional. The primary care physician is going to have to do the supportive counseling.

ANALYSIS

Objectives

1. Recognize illness anxiety disorder in a patient.

2. Understand the treatment recommendations for the primary physician treating the patient.

Considerations

This patient clearly meets the criteria for illness anxiety disorder (formerly hypochondriasis) (Table 28–1). It should be noted that patients with significant somatic complaints that would have been diagnosed with hypochondriasis in the past would now be diagnosed as having a somatic symptom disorder in DSM-5. She is preoccupied with the idea that she has a serious medical illness. Despite appropriate medical evaluation, the fear persists, although it is temporarily alleviated when test results come back negative. Her preoccupation with illness is impairing other aspects of her life. There are no other signs or symptoms suggesting another psychiatric disorder that might account for this behavior (such as generalized anxiety disorder [GAD] or panic disorder).

The DSM-5 criteria for this disorder includes preoccupation with having or acquiring a serious illness that has been present for at least 6 months where any somatic symptoms that are present are only of mild intensity. The patient should either engage in excessive behaviors (like frequent checking of the body for illness or seeking reassurance from the Internet) or exhibit maladaptive avoidance (like avoiding people who are even mildly sick or refusing to travel far from the doctor).

Table 28–1 • DIAGNOSTIC CRITERIA FOR ILLNESS ANXIETY DISORDER
Preoccupation with fears of having a serious illness and has large degree of anxiety about health.
Bodily symptoms are minor in nature and not the predominant problem.
Preoccupation persists despite medical evaluation and reassurance.
Either engages in excessive activities to monitor health status or conversely attempts to avoid monitoring health status to not feel the excessive alarm that the anxiety produces.
Belief is not delusional or limited to a specific concern about appearance.
Preoccupation causes distress or impairment in functioning.
Duration of 6 mo.
Preoccupation is not better accounted for by another mental disorder.

The psychiatric symptoms should not be better attributed to other psychiatric disorders.

APPROACH TO:
Illness Anxiety Disorder

DEFINITIONS

DYSMORPHIA: A condition in which one body part is perceived to be out of proportion to the rest of the body (eg, the nose is much too large or an arm is much too small).

SOMATIC SYMPTOM DISORDER: A condition in which physical symptoms seem as if they are part of a general medical disorder although no general medical condition, other mental disorder, or substance is present. In this case, psychological conflicts can be translated into physical problems or complaints. With the number one complaint of patients being about some type of physical symptom, it is no wonder that this disorder is often observed in a general medical setting.

CLINICAL APPROACH

Differential Diagnosis

As in other somatoform disorders, it is important to rule out medical conditions that can be the cause of chronic complaints, especially those that do not present an obvious diagnosis, for example, autoimmune diseases, occult malignancies, neurodegenerative diseases, and human immunodeficiency virus (HIV) disease. On the *initial* presentation of a patient suspected of having illness anxiety disorder, obtaining a thorough history, review of systems, and performing a physical examination are necessary in order to assure both clinician and patient that a serious illness is not likely present. In the absence of clear, objective clinical evidence that a test is needed, testing should be avoided; instead, ensure that all past medical records and testing results are obtained, and assure the patient you are watching her closely.

Given the degree of preoccupation with having an illness, the symptoms of illness anxiety disorder can be mistaken for the delusions present in a psychotic disorder such as schizophrenia or delusional disorder, somatic type. In psychotic disorders such as schizophrenia and schizoaffective disorder, however, other associated symptoms and signs are part of the picture, including hallucinations, paranoia, ideas of reference, a flat affect, social isolation, lack of motivation, loose associations, and disorganized behavior. In delusional disorder, somatic type, the specific illness is always the same, and the patient cannot be reassured and will *not* consider other alternatives. In **illness anxiety disorder,** however, the **bodily complaints or disease can change over time; these complaints are mild in nature,** and the **patient can usually be reassured,** albeit temporarily, when presented with medical evidence. In individuals with poor insight, making this distinction can be quite difficult. Research suggests that these patients have a psychosocial communication style in which patients focus on the psychosocial consequences of their illness and the restrictions to their lives rather than on the symptoms' implications on their health.

Finally, other somatic symptom disorders should be considered in the differential diagnosis. In illness anxiety disorder, the focus is on the fear of having a serious illness. In somatic symptom disorder, the focus is on having multiple physical complaints involving several different systems rather than an actual disease. In conversion disorder, a sensory or motor deficit is present and is usually transient. The *DSM-IV* pain disorder would be classified in *DSM-5* as somatic symptom disorder with predominant pain and is a chronic illness where the symptoms are limited to the sensation of pain. In body dysmorphic disorder, the preoccupation is not with having a serious illness but with an imagined defect in appearance or excessive concern about a minor physical anomaly. In malingering, the patient is manufacturing symptoms for secondary gain. In factitious disorder (sometimes called Munchausen syndrome), the patient has an overwhelming need to be cared for as a patient and will not only have numerous physical complaints but will often do things to themselves to produce illness.

The median age of onset of hypochondriasis is 25 years of age, and it may be expected that a similar pattern will hold true for illness anxiety disorder.

TREATMENT

There is no *treatment* for illness anxiety disorder per se, although if comorbid depressive or anxiety disorders are present, they should be treated appropriately. The primary care physician needs to realize that illness anxiety disorder is a chronic disorder with about 42% of patients having symptoms for 4 to 5 years and 25% having symptoms for 10 years or more.

Management of illness anxiety disorder is a more realistic goal, and this is usually accomplished by the primary care physician, as patients are often reluctant to see a psychiatrist given their belief about having a *medical* illness. **Regularly scheduled appointments** are much more helpful than "as needed" visits, as this establishes a trusting relationship, minimizes doctor shopping, and avoids repeated and unnecessary tests and procedures. **The complaints and concerns of patients should be taken seriously,** and they should be assured that they will be well cared for. **Inappropriate or unnecessary tests should not be performed in order to reassure**

a patient. Instead, testing should be done only when there is a high level of suspicion or a clear clinical indication of a disease. Studies which have trained primary care physicians to provide either cognitive behavioral therapy or relaxation training to these patients produced equal outcomes with a 15% decrease in ambulatory visits and associated costs.

Although individuals with illness anxiety disorder can be reassured when presented with evidence, the effect is usually only temporary, and they usually return with the same fear or the belief that they have a different disease. One placebo-controlled randomized study showed that both cognitive behavioral therapy and paroxetine were equally effective in producing short-term improvement in illness anxiety disorder.

CASE CORRELATION

- See Case 20 and Case 29 for patients that may also present with worries about their health. However, in GAD, individuals have excessive worry about a number of situations, not just their health, and somatic symptom disorder patients have significant somatic symptoms present, not just a primary concern that they are ill.

COMPREHENSION QUESTIONS

28.1 A 42-year-old woman describes a 20-year history of numerous physical complaints, including joint pain, dysuria, headaches, chest pain, nausea, vomiting, irregular menses, and double vision. Although they do not all occur at the same time, she has been suffering from one or more of these problems throughout her adult life. Many workups have been done for her, and she has undergone repeated hospitalizations, but no specific cause has yet been found. She is extremely anxious and has become significantly disabled as a result. Which of the following is the most likely diagnosis?

A. Body dysmorphic disorder

B. Illness anxiety disorder

C. Somatic symptom disorder with predominant pain

D. Somatic symptom disorder

E. Conversion disorder

28.2 A 26-year-old woman presents to her physician with the chief complaint of, "I have epilepsy." She states that for the past 3 weeks she has had seizures almost daily. She describes the episodes as falling on the ground, followed by shaking her arms and legs uncontrollably. These events last for approximately 10 minutes. She is unable to otherwise move during the time, although she denies any loss of consciousness, bladder, or bowel functions. She has never injured herself during these, but as a result she has been unable to continue her job. She is somewhat bothered as she received a promotion 1 month ago. Which of the following is the most likely diagnosis?

A. Body dysmorphic disorder

B. Conversion disorder

C. Illness anxiety disorder

D. Seizure disorder

E. Somatic symptom disorder

28.3 A 36-year-old man is referred to a primary care physician for evaluation of his complaints. He is convinced that he has colon cancer despite being told that it is unlikely because of his young age. He occasionally notices traces of red blood on the toilet paper which has been attributed to hemorrhoids and has abdominal cramps when he eats too much. A review of the records demonstrates numerous prior appointments in connection with the same or similar complaints, including repeatedly negative results from tests for occult fecal blood and normal results from colonoscopies. He continues to be worried about dying of cancer and requests another colonoscopy. Which of the following is the most likely diagnosis?

A. Body dysmorphic disorder

B. Illness anxiety disorder

C. Somatic symptom disorder with predominant pain

D. Somatic symptom disorder

E. Conversion disorder

28.4 Which of the following strategies by the primary care doctor would be the most effective in treating the patient in Question 28.3?

A. Antianxiety medication

B. Extensive medical workups to provide reassurance

C. Referral for psychotherapy

D. Regularly scheduled appointments with reassurance

E. An antipsychotic medication

ANSWERS

28.1 **D.** The most likely diagnosis for this woman is somatic symptom disorder. She presents with numerous somatic complaints, related to several body areas, which are not fully explained by a medical cause. The focus is on the *symptoms* themselves, **not** on a perceived physical defect (as in body dysmorphic disorder), on the fear of having a specific disease (as in illness anxiety disorder), or on symptoms of pain (as in somatic symptom disorder with predominant pain).

28.2 **B.** The most likely diagnosis in this woman is conversion disorder ("pseudo-seizures"). Conversion disorder patients present with neurological symptoms (eg, sensory deficit, motor weakness, seizures) that are felt to be unconsciously produced and believed to be caused by a psychological conflict or stressor. It is unlikely a seizure disorder given her retention of consciousness and lack of incontinence or injury. Her focus is not on an imagined defect in appearance, on the fear of having a serious illness caused by misperceived body sensations, or on multiple physical complaints.

28.3 **B.** The most likely diagnosis for this man is illness anxiety disorder. His chief complaint is a concern that he has colon cancer. He remains focused on this illness despite prior evaluations with negative results and reassurance from his physician. Although he has several gastrointestinal symptoms (blood in stools due to hemorrhoids and abdominal cramps), he is probably misinterpreting them. His worry is caused by fears of having colon cancer, not about a distorted body image, pain sensations, or numerous physical symptoms.

28.4 **D.** The most effective strategy for treating individuals with illness anxiety disorder is to schedule regular appointments. In this way, any physical complaints are addressed, and reassurance is provided, albeit temporarily. This approach also minimizes both doctor shopping and unnecessary testing. Treatment with an antianxiety (or antidepressant) agent is not helpful in illness anxiety disorder, unless a comorbid anxiety (or depressive) disorder is present. Because individuals with this disorder are fearful of having a medical illness, they usually resist seeing a psychiatrist.

CLINICAL PEARLS

▶ The distinctive feature of illness anxiety disorder is a fear of having a serious illness based on a misinterpretation of bodily sensations.

▶ Extensive, repetitive, or invasive tests or procedures should be avoided in individuals with illness anxiety disorder unless a clear clinical indication is present.

▶ Antidepressants and antianxiety medications are not indicated unless comorbid depressive or anxiety disorders are present.

▶ The most effective treatment for patients with illness anxiety disorder is to schedule frequent, regular appointments with the same primary care physician, coupled with education and reassurance.

REFERENCES

Barsky AJ, Ahren DK, Bauer MR, Nolido N, Orav EJ. A randomized trial of treatments for high-utilizing somatizing patients. *J Gen Intern Med*. 2013;28(11):1396-1404.

Greevan A, van Balkom AJLM, Visser S, et al. Cognitive behavior therapy and paroxetine in the treatment of hypochondriasis: a randomized controlled trial. *Am J Psychiatry*. 2007;164(1):91-99.

Sadock BJ, Sadock VA, Ruiz P. *Kaplan and Sadock's Synopsis of Psychiatry: Behavioral Sciences/Clinical Psychiatry*. 11th ed. Baltimore, MD: Lippincott Williams & Wilkins; 2014.

A 42-year-old woman presents to her primary care physician with a chief complaint of back pain for the past 6 months that began after she was knocked down by a man attempting to elude the police. She states that she has extreme pain on the right side of her lower back, near L4 and L5. The pain does not radiate, and nothing makes it better or worse. She says that since the injury she has been unable to function and spends most of her days lying in bed or sitting up, immobile, in a chair. Immediately after the accident, she was taken to an emergency department where a workup revealed back strain but no fractures. Since then, the patient has repeatedly sought help from a variety of specialists, but the ongoing pain has been neither adequately explained nor relieved. She denies other medical problems, although she mentions a past history of domestic violence that resulted in several visits to the emergency department for treatment of bruises and lacerations.

On mental status examination, the patient is alert and oriented to person, place, and time. She is cooperative and maintains good eye contact. She holds herself absolutely still, sitting rigidly in her chair and grimacing when she has to move even the smallest amount. Her mood is depressed, and her affect is congruent. Her thought processes are logical, and her thought content is negative for suicidal or homicidal ideation, delusions, or hallucinations.

- ▶ What is the most likely diagnosis of this patient?
- ▶ What is the best approach to this patient?

ANSWERS TO CASE 29:

Somatic Symptom Disorder with Predominant Pain

Summary: A 42-year-old woman has unremitting back pain for 6 months since she was knocked down. The pain is right sided, located near L4 and L5. There are no exacerbating or alleviating factors, and the pain does not radiate. The patient is nonfunctional since the event. No fractures were found at the time of the accident—a diagnosis of back strain was made. Further workups over the past 6 months show no anatomic or physiologic reason for continued pain. The patient has a history of domestic violence and on multiple occasions was treated in the emergency department for bruises and lacerations. The results of her mental status examination are noncontributory to the diagnosis.

- **Most likely diagnosis**: Somatic symptom disorder with predominant pain.

- **Best approach**: Validate the patient's experience of pain. Explain the role of psychological factors as a cause and consequence of pain. Consider antidepressants and referral to a pain clinic.

ANALYSIS

Objectives

1. Recognize somatic symptom disorder with predominant pain in a patient.

2. Understand the chronicity, approach, and treatment options for patients with somatic symptom disorder with predominant pain.

Considerations

This patient has **back pain** that is unaccounted for by a general medical condition. As a result, she is distressed and unable to function. There are no data suggesting that the condition was produced intentionally or is being feigned. It is possible (based on her history of domestic violence) that the accident **triggered memories of the psychological trauma** she experienced and thus has a role in the severity of her current pain. The patient does not exhibit signs or symptoms of any other disease that might better account for the pain. Table 29–1 lists the diagnostic criteria for somatic symptom disorder with predominant pain.

APPROACH TO:

Somatic Symptom Disorder with Predominant Pain

DEFINITIONS

BIOFEEDBACK: A relaxation technique by which patients are trained to induce physiologic changes (most frequently the induction of alpha waves on an electroencephalogram [EEG] or vasodilatation of peripheral capillaries) that result in a relaxation response.

> **Table 29–1 • DIAGNOSTIC CRITERIA FOR SOMATIC SYMPTOM DISORDER WITH PREDOMINANT PAIN**
>
> One or more somatic symptoms that are distressing or result in significant disruption of daily life.
>
> Excessive thoughts, feelings, or behaviors related to the somatic symptoms or associated health concerns as manifested by at least one of the following:
> • Disproportionate and persistent thoughts about the seriousness of one's symptoms
> • Persistently high levels of anxiety about health or symptoms
> • Excessive time and energy devoted to these symptoms or health concerns
>
> Although any one somatic symptom may not be continuously present, the state of being symptomatic is persistent (typically > 6 mo).
>
> Predominate pain is a specifier for individuals whose symptoms predominately involve pain.

*Specify if persistent: A persistent course is characterized by severe symptoms, marked impairment, and long duration (> 6 mo). Also specify if mild, moderate, or severe.

DYSPAREUNIA: Painful sexual intercourse.

SOMATIC SYMPTOM DISORDER WITH PREDOMINENT PAIN: One of several somatic symptom and related disorders listed in the *DSM-5*. All the disorders share a common feature: the predominance of somatic symptoms associated with significant stress and impairment. Somatic symptom disorder with predominant pain is diagnosed in individuals whose somatic complaints involve pain. Pain is a very common complaint in medicine and occurs more often in older patients (fourth and fifth decades of life) and in those who are likely to have job-related physical injuries. A number of psychodynamic factors can be involved, including inability to express emotions verbally, an unconscious need to obtain attention by suffering physical pain, or an unconscious need for punishment. Individuals also learn this form of help-seeking in a family that models and reinforces the behavior.

CLINICAL APPROACH

Differential Diagnosis

Pain is a very common complaint in medicine. It is important that the patient undergo an evaluation for all medical or surgical illnesses that could cause the pain. Patients with depression and/or anxiety can sometimes present with a primary complaint of pain; however, on evaluation, the depressive symptoms predominate. Patients with hypochondriasis can complain of pain symptoms, but the main clinical feature is a conviction that they have a serious medical illness. Patients with factitious disorder falsify an injury or illness. Patients who are malingering can consciously present false reports of pain in order to achieve secondary gain (such as financial compensation, or evading the police by being hospitalized). Patients with pain disorders often use substances to relieve distress, which can mask the pain disorder or some other medical or surgical illness.

TREATMENT

In treating a patient with pain disorder, the clinician must accept that the **condition is often chronic** and that the goal of pain relief can be unrealistic; providing **gradual**

improvement of functioning is a more reasonable approach. Although the physician must validate the existence of the patient's pain, education about the contributing effect of psychological factors and constant reassurance is important. The use of antidepressants can be an effective pharmacologic approach; **both tricyclics and selective serotonin reuptake inhibitors (SSRIs) have been shown to be helpful.** These agents work by decreasing comorbid depression or by exerting an independent analgesic effect. **Analgesic medications are generally not helpful,** and the patient has usually tried this approach before seeking treatment. Narcotic analgesics should be avoided given their abuse and withdrawal potential. Biofeedback is helpful in certain pain disorders, specifically headaches and muscle tension. Hypnosis and nerve stimulation are also used. Psychodynamic psychotherapy focused on the impact of the disorder on the patient's life can be helpful. For treatment-resistant individuals, comprehensive pain clinics (either inpatient or outpatient) should be considered.

CASE CORRELATION

- See Case 20 and Case 28 for patients who may also present with worries about their health. However, in generalized anxiety disorder (GAD), individuals have excessive worry about a number of situations, not just their health, and illness anxiety disorder patients have no significant somatic symptoms present, just a primary concern that they are ill.

COMPREHENSION QUESTIONS

29.1 A 63-year-old woman returns to her family physician with continuing headaches for 9 months. She describes the pain as "constant … always with me," around her entire scalp. She does not appreciate much variation throughout the day, and she cannot name any aggravating or alleviating factors. Although she occasionally feels light-headed when in severe pain, she denies photophobia, visual changes, nausea, or vomiting. She is especially upset about the headaches as she retired in the past year and has been unable to visit her infant granddaughter. Complete neurologic examination, computerized tomography, magnetic resonance imaging, laboratory studies, and lumbar punctures have been unremarkable. Which of the following is her most likely diagnosis?

    A. Factitious disorder

    B. Conversion disorder (functional neurological symptom disorder)

    C. Illness anxiety disorder

    D. Malingering

    E. Somatic symptom disorder with predominant pain

29.2 Which of the following is the most useful approach for the patient in Question 29.1?

A. Confrontation regarding the psychological nature of her pain.

B. Prescribe non-narcotic pain medication.

C. Reassurance that there is no evidence of pain.

D. Referral to a mental health professional.

E. Validation of her experience of pain.

29.3 The patient in Questions 29.1 and 29.2 feels that her headaches are now unbearable. Which of the following treatments is the most appropriate?

A. Acetaminophen

B. Biofeedback

C. Lorazepam

D. Nonsteroidal anti-inflammatory medication

E. Oxycodone

ANSWERS

29.1 **E.** This patient presents with criteria for somatic symptom disorder with predominant pain. She has unremitting headaches that are the focus of her complaints. They have interfered with her ability to travel, and the onset seems to coincide with her retirement and new grandchild. Her condition is not intentionally produced as in factitious disorder or malingering, nor is there any appreciable secondary gain (avoidance of work, financial compensation, etc). The concern is not on having a serious medical illness as in illness anxiety disorder, and she does not have altered voluntary motor or sensory function as in conversion disorder.

29.2 **E.** One of the most important aspects in management of this disorder is to validate and reassure the patient's experience of pain. An empathic response will serve to strengthen the therapeutic alliance. Conversely, implying that the symptoms are "not real" or denying that there is anything wrong will only cause the patient further distress and can actually worsen the pain. Although referral to a mental health professional can be indicated and helpful given the psychological factors present in pain disorder, this subject should first be gently broached with the patient in order to avoid the appearance of not taking the pain seriously. Analgesic medication is generally not helpful, and narcotic analgesics should be avoided given their abuse and withdrawal potential.

29.3 **B.** Biofeedback and relaxation techniques have demonstrated efficacy in patients with somatic symptom disorder with predominant pain, particularly with headaches. Analgesics are often not helpful in these patients. Potentially addicting medications such as benzodiazepines and opiates should especially be avoided in these individuals given the chronic nature of this illness.

CLINICAL PEARLS

▶ Patients with somatic symptom disorder with predominant pain actually feel pain; it does not help to tell them that "it's all in your head."

▶ Somatic symptom disorder with predominant pain tends to be a chronic condition. Patience, acceptance, reassurance, and regular visits can promote amelioration of the intensity and frequency of complaints. The patient's therapeutic relationship with the clinician is very important in the management of this condition.

REFERENCES

American Psychiatric Association. *Diagnostic and Statistical Manual of Mental Disorders*. 5th ed. Arlington, VA: American Psychiatric Publishing; 2013:309-315.

Black BW, Andreasen NC. *Introductory Textbook of Psychiatry*. 6th ed. Washington, DC: American Psychiatric Publishing; 2014:263-265, 268.

Hales RE, Yudofsky SC, Roberts LW. *The American Psychiatric Publishing Textbook of Psychiatry*. 6th ed. Washington, DC: American Psychiatric Publishing; 2014:532-537.

A 41-year-old nurse presents to the emergency department with concerns that she has hypoglycemia from an insulinoma. She reports repeated episodes of headache, sweating, tremor, and palpitations. She denies any past medical problems and only takes nonsteroidal anti-inflammatory medications for menstrual cramps. On physical examination, she is a well-dressed woman who is intelligent, polite, and cooperative. Her vital signs are stable except for slight tachycardia. The examination is remarkable for diaphoresis, tachycardia, and numerous scars on her abdomen, as well as needle marks on her arms. When asked about this, she says that she feels confused because of her hypoglycemia.

The patient is subsequently admitted to the medical service. Laboratory evaluations demonstrate a decreased fasting blood sugar level and an increased insulin level, but a decreased level of plasma C-peptide, which indicates exogenous insulin injection. When she is confronted with this information, she quickly becomes angry, claims the hospital staff is incompetent, and requests that she be discharged against medical advice.

▶ What is the most likely diagnosis?
▶ How should you best approach this patient?

ANSWERS TO CASE 30:

Factitious Disorder

Summary: A 41-year-old female health care worker presents to the emergency department with symptoms typical of an insulinoma, including headache, diaphoresis, palpitations, and tremors. She denies a medical history, although her physical examination demonstrates prior surgeries and injections. Laboratory evaluation points to exogenously administered insulin. When confronted with this evidence, she becomes hostile and asks to leave the hospital.

- **Most likely diagnosis:** Factitious disorder.

- **Best approach:** In order to engage the patient in psychiatric treatment, attempt to ally with her. Working in conjunction with the patient's primary care physician is often more effective than working with the patient alone. Focus on patient management versus curing the patient. Personal awareness of one's own feelings toward the patient must be maintained, because it is often very easy to get angry with such patients and behave punitively.

ANALYSIS

Objectives

1. Recognize factitious disorder (Table 30–1).

2. Differentiate factitious disorder from conversion disorder and malingering.

3. Understand the best approach to patients with factitious disorder.

Considerations

Although this patient initially presents with classic symptoms of hypoglycemia, perhaps caused by an insulinoma, discrepancies are noted in her story, especially her **denial of a medical history in light of the numerous scars.** Her laboratory evaluations are consistent with the use of insulin, with which she undoubtedly injects herself. Specifically, although her insulin levels are increased, her serum C-peptide levels are decreased. **When confronted, she becomes hostile and defensive and asks to leave the hospital. No obvious external incentives** are present. The fact that the patient consciously created the hypoglycemia rules out the diagnosis of a somatic symptom or conversion disorder. The absence of a secondary gain differentiates

Table 30–1 • DIAGNOSTIC CRITERIA FOR FACTITIOUS DISORDER
Falsification of physical or psychological signs or induction of injury or disease with identified deception.
The individual presents himself or herself to others as ill, impaired, or injured.
External incentives for the behavior (as in malingering) are absent.
The behavioral is not better explained by another mental disorder, such as delusional or another psychotic disorder.

factitious disorder from malingering. It is useful to note that she is an intelligent woman who works in the health care field, a common scenario for this disorder.

APPROACH TO:
Factitious Disorder

DEFINITIONS

PSEUDOLOGIA PHANTASTICA: The telling of "tall tales," or lying, commonly seen in factitious disorder.

MUNCHAUSEN SYNDROME: Factitious disorder, especially involving repeated episodes, seeking admission at different hospitals, and pseudologia phantastica.

MUNCHAUSEN SYNDROME BY PROXY: Factitious disorders induced in children by parents, who are usually very cooperative after taking them to the hospital.

CLINICAL APPROACH

Although the true incidence of this disorder is unknown, it seems to be more common in hospital and health care workers. The etiology is unclear and may have to do with poor parent–child relationships during childhood. Affected individuals usually have average to above-average intelligence, poor self-identity, and strong dependency needs. They feign physical symptoms so convincingly that they are hospitalized or operated upon.

DIFFERENTIAL DIAGNOSIS

The possibility of an authentic underlying medical cause with an unusual presentation should be ruled out. In addition, given the self-inflicted nature of the symptoms, it is essential that the patient be examined for any legitimate complications as well. Examples include adhesions resulting from frequent (unnecessary) abdominal surgeries leading to obstruction, serious infections produced by the injection of urine or feces into the veins, and coma caused by hypoglycemia.

Differentiating factitious disorder from conversion and other somatic disorders, as well as malingering, can be difficult. The essential feature of factitious disorder is the falsification of medical or psychological signs and symptoms in oneself or others that are associated with an identified deception. This behavior is in contrast to that seen in conversion and other somatic disorders, in which both the underlying conflicts and the production of the symptoms are *unconscious*. In malingering, both the motivation (an external incentive) and the fabrication are *conscious*.

Patients with factitious disorder can also meet criteria for borderline personality disorder. Patients with both disorders frequently have histories of childhood mistreatment such as physical, sexual, or emotional abuse.

TREATMENT

There is no treatment per se for factitious disorders. If there is an underlying psychiatric disorder such as major depression or an anxiety disorder, it should be treated as indicated. Like patients with somatic disorders, these individuals are extremely resistant to mental health treatment. When discovered, they usually flee the hospital, frequently repeating the same or a similar cycle at another facility. *Managing* this disorder is more appropriate than *treating* it. Liaison with a psychiatric consultation service is helpful in engaging the patient in psychiatric treatment, as is working with the hospital staff to cope with the feelings of anger, betrayal, and mistrust that frequently come to the forefront. Treatment team meetings are recommended to help coordinate care between providers. It also allows team members to articulate and manage feelings they may have toward the patient. It is useful to keep in mind that individuals with factitious disorder are very ill and that, like other "genuine" patients, they require help and caring.

CASE CORRELATION

- See also Case 57 and Case 60 for patients who cause injuries to themselves. Borderline personality disordered patients may cause deliberate self-harm, but this is not usually done in conjunction with deception. Malingering patients intentionally report symptoms for personal gain (escape from military obligation, time off work), while factitious disorder patients lack an obvious reward for their symptoms.

COMPREHENSION QUESTIONS

30.1 Which of the following is most likely the motivation behind the behavior displayed in factitious disorder?

    A. The motivation is unconscious and thus the patient is unaware of it.

    B. Desire to avoid jail.

    C. Desire to take on the patient role.

    D. Desire to obtain compensation.

    E. Desire to obtain narcotics.

30.2 Which type of personality disorder is most likely to occur comorbidly with factitious disorder?

    A. Antisocial

    B. Avoidant

    C. Borderline

    D. Obsessive-compulsive

    E. Schizoid

30.3 Which of the following scenarios is most consistent with factitious disorder?

    A. Feigning psychosis to avoid criminal charges

    B. Lying about back pain to receive time off from work

    C. Pseudoseizures in the context of a family conflict

    D. Placing feces in urine to receive treatment for a urinary tract infection

    E. Recurrent fears of having a serious illness

30.4 Which of the following is the most useful approach for patients with factitious disorder?

    A. Confronting their feigning of symptoms

    B. Discharging them from the hospital

    C. Establishing a therapeutic alliance

    D. Pharmacotherapy

    E. Referring them to legal authorities

ANSWERS

30.1 **C.** While it is not a criterion, it is thought the primary desire in factitious disorder is to assume the sick role and be taken care of (primary gain). In contrast, in malingering, the motivation is to achieve a tangible gain (such as avoiding work, school, or a prison sentence) or to obtain narcotics or financial compensation (secondary gain). If the motivation is unconscious, conversion and other somatic disorders need to be considered.

30.2 **C.** Borderline personality disorder is not uncommon in patients with factitious disorder. Individuals with either of these disorders often have similar histories of abuse, molestation, and emotional neglect. Patients with borderline personality disorder also act out their internal psychological conflicts on an interpersonal level, and they display the chaotic, labile, affective state seen in factitious disorder.

30.3 **D.** The hallmark of factitious disorder is intentional feigning of a physical or psychiatric illness. Examples include injecting oneself with insulin to create hypoglycemia, taking anticoagulants to fake a bleeding disorder, and contaminating urine samples with feces to simulate a urinary tract infection. Lying about back pain in order to avoid work or feigning psychosis to avoid criminal charges is an example of malingering. Pseudoseizures are an example of a conversion disorder. Fear of having a serious disease caused by misinterpretation of bodily sensations is characteristic of illness anxiety disorder.

30.4 **C.** Although there is no specific treatment for factitious disorder, the best way to help these patients is to attempt to establish a therapeutic alliance and a working relationship. Although this can be difficult, only then can the patient's need to feign illness be addressed and dealt with in a psychotherapeutic environment. Confrontation is necessary in some circumstances, but if an accusatory or a judgmental manner is employed, patients flee care and begin the cycle again at another hospital. The premature discharge of such patients from the hospital or referral to legal services has the same result, although in cases of factitious disorder by proxy (where a caretaker simulates illness in a child), referral to child protective services is necessary because this behavior is considered a form of child abuse. Pharmacotherapy use should be limited unless the patient has a comorbid axis I disorder. Because of abuse potential, medications should be used with caution.

CLINICAL PEARLS

▶ The essential feature of factitious disorder is the falsification of medical or psychological signs and symptoms in oneself or others that are associated with an identified deception.

▶ Factitious disorder is more common in women and in those in the health care professions.

▶ The course of factitious disorder is usually chronic, with a pattern of lying, self-inflicted injuries, repeated hospitalizations, and premature discharges.

▶ The best management of factitious disorder involves early identification, avoidance of unnecessary tests and treatments, empathic understanding of the need to be sick, establishment of a therapeutic working relationship, and potential referral to a mental health professional.

REFERENCES

American Psychiatric Association. *Diagnostic and Statistical Manual of Mental Disorders*. 5th ed. Arlington, VA: American Psychiatric Publishing; 2013:324-326.

Black BW, Andreasen NC. *Introductory Textbook of Psychiatry*. 6th ed. Washington, DC: American Psychiatric Publishing; 2014:277-279.

Hales RE, Yudofsky SC, Roberts LW. *The American Psychiatric Publishing Textbook of Psychiatry*. 6th ed. Washington, DC: American Psychiatric Publishing; 2014:547-552.

A 19-year-old woman is referred to a psychiatrist after her roommates become concerned about her behavior. The patient tells the psychiatrist that for the past 2 years, since beginning college, she has been making herself vomit by sticking her fingers down her throat. This behavior occurs regularly, as many as three or four times a week, and worsens when she is stressed out at school. The patient says that she regularly gorges herself with food and is worried that she will become overweight if she does not vomit it up. She describes her gorging episodes as "eating whatever I can find" in large quantities and mentions one incident in which she ordered three large pizzas and ate them all by herself. The patient states that she feels out of control when she is gorging herself but is unable to stop. She is ashamed of this behavior and goes to great lengths to hide how much she eats. She notes that her sense of self-esteem seems to be very dependent on her weight and whether or not she sees her body image as fat. She agreed to see a psychiatrist after her roommates found out about the self-induced vomiting.

A physical examination shows a young woman, 5 ft 6 in tall and weighing 135 lb. Her vital signs are blood pressure 110/65 mm Hg, respiration 12 breaths/min, temperature 98.2°F (36.8°C), and pulse rate 72 beats/min (bpm). The results of the rest of her physical examination are within normal limits.

▶ What is the most likely diagnosis for this patient?
▶ What treatment modalities should the psychiatrist recommend?
▶ What areas of the physical and laboratory evaluation should receive special attention?

ANSWERS TO CASE 31:

Bulimia Nervosa

Summary: A 19-year-old woman has been binging on large quantities of food, above and beyond what most people would eat under similar circumstances. She is embarrassed about the binging and worries that it will make her obese. She then engages in purging behavior, as often as three or four times a week. This behavior accelerates when she is under stress, and the patient feels she has no control over it. The results of her physical examination are normal, and she is of normal weight.

- **Most likely diagnosis:** Bulimia nervosa.

- **Best treatment modalities:** Nutritional rehabilitation, cognitive behavioral psychotherapy, and treatment with an antidepressant (selective serotonin reuptake inhibitor [SSRI]).

- **Physical examination and laboratory tests:** Parotid glands, mouth, teeth for caries, abdominal examination for esophageal or gastric injury, dehydration from laxative use, ipecac-associated hypotension, tachycardia, and arrhythmias. Serum electrolytes, magnesium, and amylase levels should also be checked.

ANALYSIS

Objectives

1. Diagnose bulimia in a patient (Table 31–1).

2. Understand the most effective treatment regimens that should be recommended.

3. Be aware of the laboratory tests that most commonly show abnormalities in patients with this disorder.

Considerations

This patient has all the cardinal signs of bulimia. She binges on food, and during these binges she eats more than a normal person would under the same circumstances. She is extremely ashamed of this behavior and goes to great lengths to hide it. It occurs at least weekly for at least 3 months. She feels her behavior is out of control and by purging she is engaging in inappropriate behavior (in this case vomiting) so that she will not gain weight because of her excessive intake of food. These patients use inappropriate ways of controlling weight including fasting, excessive

Table 31–1 • DIAGNOSTIC CRITERIA FOR BULIMIA NERVOSA
Recurrent episodes (at least once a week for 3 mo) of binge eating and inappropriate compensatory behavior such as purging, fasting, or excessive exercise.
Self-evaluation is largely (and unduly) based on body shape and weight.
The behavior does not occur only during an episode of anorexia nervosa.

exercise, and misuse of laxatives, diuretics, or enemas along with the often-seen vomiting. It is a common finding that binging episodes increase during times of stress. **Patients with bulimia are usually normal or near normal in weight.** However, their self-evaluation of themselves is often very dependent on their weight and perception of their body shape. It should be noted that resent studies show that a growing proportion of patients with bulimia nervosa are obese or significantly overweight. Being both overweight and bulimic may require a substantially different approach to the treatment of the patient.

Frequent exposure to gastric juices from vomiting can result in severe dental erosion. The parotid glands can enlarge, and the patient can have elevated serum amylase levels. The self-induced vomiting can cause acute gastric dilatation and esophageal tears. Severe abdominal pain in these patients requires nasogastric suction tubes, x-ray studies, and possible surgical consultation. Electrolyte abnormalities, especially low magnesium and potassium, are common. Laboratory abnormalities found in individuals with bulimia nervosa demonstrate hypochloremic-hypokalemic alkalosis resulting from repetitive emesis. If they use ipecac to cause vomiting, they can have ipecac intoxication with pericardial pain, dyspnea, and generalized muscle weakness associated with hypotension, tachycardia, and electrocardiogram (ECG) abnormalities. Ipecac intoxication can cause a toxic cardiomyopathy that can lead to death.

According to American Psychiatric Association practice guidelines, individuals with bulimia nervosa should have a three-pronged approach to treatment:

1. There should be a plan developed for nutritional rehabilitation in which the patient has regular, nutritionally balanced meals to replace the pattern of fasting then binging with vomiting often seen in this population. This should be supplemented with nutritional counseling.

2. Cognitive behavioral psychotherapy on an individual basis to deal with the underlying cognitive patterns that drive bulimia combined with group therapy (often based on an addiction-model 12-step program) is the best way for dealing with the immediate issues. If the patient moves back in with her parents, this should be supplemented with family therapy.

3. Treatment with an antidepressant, usually an SSRI, can produce a decrease in vomiting and binging behavior, but it is important to realize that without psychotherapy, purging behaviors can return. Fluoxetine has the most evidence for efficacy and should be the first medication tried with sertraline being the only other SSRI demonstrated as being effective in bulimia. Medication should be continued for 9 to 12 months after symptoms have gone into remission.

APPROACH TO:
Bulimia Nervosa

DEFINITIONS

BINGE EATING: Eating an amount of food definitely larger than most people would eat during a similar period of time and experiencing a sense of lack of control.

NONPURGING TYPE: Type of bulimia where fasting and excessive exercise is utilized without frequent purging.

PURGING: Self-induced vomiting, and/or misuse of laxatives, diuretics, or enemas for the purpose of preventing weight gain.

CLINICAL APPROACH

Differential Diagnosis

Bulimia nervosa is estimated to occur in 1% of adolescent and young adult females, but eating-disorder-like behavior (brief times of purging) can affect up to 5% to 10% of young women. Its onset is usually later in adolescence than that of anorexia nervosa, and it can also start in adulthood. Like individuals with anorexia, bulimic patients tend to be high achievers, have a family history of depression, and respond to social pressures to be thin. In contrast to patients with anorexia, those with bulimia often exhibit coexisting alcohol dependence and emotional lability but more readily seek help. Binge eating and purging are the hallmarks of the disease.

One of the main disorders in the differential diagnoses is anorexia nervosa, binge-eating/purging type. Although binging and purging behavior can be seen in anorexia as well as in bulimia, **anorexia is distinguished by the** requirement **of being underweight and amenorrheic. Bulimic patients can be underweight, of normal weight, or even overweight.** Despite their purging, the sheer amount of high-caloric food eaten more than compensates for the amount purged.

Patients with binge-eating disorder have the binge eating without inappropriate compensatory behaviors and are often overweight.

Another concern is individuals who present with **purging behavior** who do not necessarily meet the criteria for bulimia nervosa. It is not uncommon for adolescents and young adults (especially women) to engage in purging behavior in order to lose weight. This behavior is usually learned from peers and is distinguished from bulimia by being **short lived, infrequent, and unassociated with physical sequelae.**

Binging behavior can be seen with central nervous system tumors, Klüver-Bucy syndrome, and Klein-Levin syndrome as well.

CLINICAL COURSE

Typical onset is in females during adolescence or early adulthood with the peak onset at ages 18 to 19. It has a mortality rate of up to 3%. After 5 to 10 years of treatment, approximately 50% of bulimic patients will be recovered, 30% will be partially recovered, and 20% will meet full criteria for active bulimia. One-third of recovered bulimic patients will have a relapse within 4 years of recovery.

TREATMENT

Cognitive behavioral psychotherapy to resolve cognitive distortions is the most effective type of psychotherapeutic intervention. Adolescents living at home often benefit from family-based therapy that includes parents in an effort to disrupt pathological eating and weight control behaviors. After this initial work, the responsibility for maintenance of remission then transitions to the adolescent. Group therapy is effective because bulimic patients often feel ashamed of their symptoms and have difficulty dealing with interpersonal problems. Groups show them that they are not alone and give them opportunities to practice interpersonal problem-solving skills. Generally, studies of the effects of medication alone show that they are not as effective as when given in combination with psychotherapy. In cases of effective treatment, a reduction of the purging rate by more than 50% over the first 4 weeks of treatment is often seen.

Studies have shown that cognitive behavioral therapy as usually practiced (focused on cognitive distortions of body image) in bulimia nervosa is ineffective in reducing weight and may result in overweight patients with this disorder dropping out of treatment. In overweight patients with bulimia, appetite awareness training and a structured behavioral weight loss program along with a modified type of cognitive behavioral therapy that is appetite-focused is preferable.

CASE CORRELATION

- See also Case 32 and Case 57 for patients who present with eating abnormalities. Binging and purging behavior may be a part of anorexia, but these patients must have a significantly low body weight in addition. Binge eating is part of the impulsive behavior common to borderline personality disordered patients, but they have a long history of other impulsive behaviors, including self-harm, as well.

COMPREHENSION QUESTIONS

31.1 Bulimia differs from anorexia nervosa in which one of the following ways?

A. Patients with bulimia tend to be low achievers in academics compared to patients with anorexia.

B. Patients with bulimia may not have any symptoms until early adulthood while anorexia typically begins in early adolescence.

C. Patients with bulimia are less likely to abuse alcohol and have less emotional lability than patients with anorexia.

D. Bulimic patients tend to be overweight, whereas anorexic patients are underweight.

E. Patients with bulimia are more resistant to receiving help and often must be forced to see a therapist.

31.2 A 34-year-old woman presents with a 10-year history of episodes in which she eats large quantities of food, such as eight hamburgers and three quarts of ice cream, at a single sitting. Because of her intense feelings of guilt, she then repeatedly induces vomiting. This cycle repeats itself several times a week. She is extremely ashamed of her behavior but says, "I can't stop doing it." On examination, which of the following physical findings is most likely to be seen?

A. Dental caries

B. Lanugo

C. Muscle wasting

D. Alopecia

E. Body weight at less than the 10th percentile of normal

31.3 Which of the following laboratory abnormalities would most likely be found in the patient in Question 31.2?

A. Hypermagnesemia

B. Hypoamylasemia

C. Hypochloremic-hypokalemic alkalosis

D. Elevated thyroid indices

E. Hypercholesterolemia

31.4 Which of the following treatment options would be a contraindicated treatment option for the patient in Questions 31.2 and 31.3?

A. Nutritional rehabilitation

B. Cognitive behavioral psychotherapy

C. Careful use of SSRIs

D. Group psychotherapy

E. Atypical antipsychotic medications

ANSWERS

31.1 **B.** Patients with both disorders tend to be high achievers but patients with bulimia tend to be less resistant to getting help, have more alcohol abuse, and have more emotional lability than patients with anorexia, who tend to be more emotionally constricted. Bulimia often has a later onset than anorexia.

31.2 **A.** The most likely diagnosis for this woman is bulimia nervosa. Physical findings can include dental caries, a round face caused by enlarged parotid glands, or calluses on the fingers resulting from recurrent self-induced vomiting. Lanugo and muscle wasting result from the severe weight loss characteristic of anorexia nervosa.

31.3 **C.** Laboratory abnormalities found in individuals with bulimia nervosa demonstrate hypochloremic-hypokalemic alkalosis resulting from repetitive emesis. Hyperamylasemia and hypomagnesemia are also not uncommonly seen in such patients. Various electrolyte imbalances can occur because of frequent laxative abuse. Thyroid abnormalities are not common in individuals with bulimia nervosa.

31.4 **E.** There is no clinical evidence for the use of atypical antipsychotics in a patient with bulimia, and they may only serve to increase the patient's appetite and binging.

CLINICAL PEARLS

▶ A diagnosis of bulimia nervosa requires both recurrent binging and purging or other compensatory behaviors to prevent weight gain. This behavior cannot occur exclusively during an episode of anorexia nervosa.

▶ Individuals with bulimia can be underweight, of normal weight, or overweight.

▶ Physical findings include dental caries, enlarged parotid or salivary glands, and esophageal tears.

▶ Abnormalities revealed in laboratory studies can include hypochloremic-hypokalemic alkalosis, hyperamylasemia, hypomagnesemia, and various electrolyte imbalances.

▶ Selective serotonin reuptake inhibitors are helpful in reducing both binging and purging behavior, but should be offered in association with cognitive behavioral psychotherapy or other evidence-based psychotherapies.

REFERENCES

American Psychiatric Association. *Practice Guideline for the Treatment of Patients with Eating Disorders.* 3rd ed. *Am J Psychiatry.* 2006;163(suppl 7):1-54.

Bulik CM, Marcus MD, Zerwas S, Levine MD, Via ML. The changing "weightscape" of bulimia nervosa. *Am J Psychiatry.* 2012:169(10);1031-1036.

Grange DL, Crosby RD, Lock J. Predictors and moderators of outcome in family-based treatment for adolescent bulimia nervosa. *J Am Acad Child Adolesc Psychiatry.* 2008;47(4):464-470.

Sadock BJ, Sadock VA, Ruiz P. *Kaplan and Sadock's Synopsis of Psychiatry: Behavioral Sciences/Clinical Psychiatry.* 11th ed. Baltimore, MD: Lippincott Williams & Wilkins; 2014.

A 17-year-old adolescent girl is brought to see a psychiatrist because her parents have become increasingly alarmed about her weight loss. The patient claims that her parents are "worrying about nothing" and that she has come to the office just to appease them. She states that she feels fine, although her mood is slightly depressed. She denies having problems with sleeping or appetite and denies any kind of drug or alcohol abuse. She says that she thinks she looks "fat," but that if she could lose another couple of pounds, she would be "just right." She notes that her only problem is that she stopped having her period 3 months ago; she is not sexually active and therefore cannot be pregnant.

When questioned separately, the parents report that the patient has been steadily losing weight over the past 8 months. They say that she started dieting after one of her friends commented that she "looked a little plump." At that point, they noted that their daughter weighed approximately 120 lb. The patient lost 5 lb and, according to the parents, felt good about the comments made by her friends. Since that time, she has eaten less and less. She now dresses in baggy clothes and does not discuss with her parents how much she weighs. Despite this, she helps her mother cook elaborate meals for party guests when the family entertains. She exercises throughout the day, and her parents say they can often hear her doing jumping jacks and sit-ups in her room in the evening. On physical examination, the patient is found to be 5 ft 2 in tall; she weighs 70 lb and appears cachectic.

▶ What is the most likely diagnosis?
▶ What are the next therapeutic steps?

ANSWERS TO CASE 32:

Anorexia Nervosa

Summary: A 17-year-old girl appears in a psychiatrist's office grossly underweight. Despite this, she denies having any problems other than being mildly depressed, and she has not come to the office willingly. She views herself as overweight despite obvious appearances to the contrary. Her parents note that she has increasingly restricted her intake of calories and exercises excessively. She has been amenorrheic for the past several months.

- **Most likely diagnosis:** Anorexia nervosa.

- **Next steps:** The patient might benefit from **hospitalization** or day treatment, but it is unlikely that she will agree. However, because she is 17 years old, her parents can sign her into a hospital without her consent. Her initial treatment should be aimed at restoring her nutritional status, as she is grossly malnourished. Dehydration, starvation, and electrolyte imbalances must be corrected. The patient should be weighed daily, and her daily fluid intake and output should be monitored. Therapy (behavioral management, individual psychotherapy, family education, and group therapy) should also be started, but her unstable nutritional status needs to be addressed first.

ANALYSIS

Objectives

1. Recognize anorexia nervosa in a patient.

2. Make recommendations about the treatment plan, initial and longer-term treatment of a patient with anorexia nervosa.

Considerations

This patient meets all three major criteria for anorexia nervosa: First, she has a refusal to maintain her body weight above a minimally normal level for her age. Her weight (70 lb) or a body mass index (BMI) of approximately 12 is 64% of the normally expected weight for her height (110 lb). Second, she has disturbance in the way her shape and body weight are perceived and a denial of the seriousness of her current low body weight. Her dieting began after she heard a derogatory comment about her weight, and it has accelerated over the past 8 months. The patient, **despite being quite cachectic, believes herself to be fat** and wants to lose still more weight. Third, her intense fear of gaining weight is consistent with anorexia nervosa. She has another symptom that had been part of the *DSM-IV* criteria, which is amenorrhea. However, in the *DSM-5*, this has been removed because of confusion in postmenopausal women, premenarcheal girls, or males. She is not interested in psychiatric treatment and denies that there is anything wrong with her other than a mildly depressed mood; this is commonly seen in patients with anorexia. Despite severely restricting her caloric intake, she seems very much interested in food and its preparation. She **exercises excessively** as well. Individuals with this disorder are often difficult to treat; they **deny** their behavior and try to mislead their parents or physicians. **This patient has the restricting type of the disorder. Anorexia nervosa can also present with a pattern in which the patient binge eats and then uses vomiting, laxatives, diuretics, and enemas to lose weight.**

Although not part of the official *Diagnostic and Statistical Manual of Mental Disorders, 5th edition (DSM-5)* criteria, these patients tend to be perfectionistic high achievers, who are socially withdrawn and have a poor self-concept. The anorexia is often an attempt to gain a sense of control over their lives as they are going through the physical and emotional changes of adolescence.

APPROACH TO:
Anorexia Nervosa

DEFINITIONS

AMENORRHEA: Absence of at least three consecutive menstrual cycles.

ANORECTIC ABNORMAL BODY WEIGHT: Body weight that is less than 85% of normal for age and produced by conscious weight loss efforts.

LANUGO: Fine body hair present on prepubertal children and commonly seen in patients with anorexia.

BODY MASS INDEX (BMI): A standardized measure of body fat based on a ratio calculation including height, weight, and age (in those younger than 18 years).

CLINICAL APPROACH

There is a strong female predominance of individuals with eating disorders. Anorexia nervosa is observed as either a food-restricting or a binge-eating/purging subtype. **A strong distortion of body image is present, and even at an extremely low weight, patients believe they are overweight. In addition, there is a great deal of evidence that family functioning may play an important role in the development of this disorder. A good family assessment is essential to treatment.** Table 32–1 lists the diagnostic criteria. Anorexia nervosa is rare in non-Western societies, and immigrants who move from these societies to Western cultures (and adopt Western concepts of female thinness as being desirable) have much higher incidences of anorexia.

Table 32–1 • DIAGNOSTIC CRITERIA FOR ANOREXIA NERVOSA
Refusal to maintain weight at or above the normal weight for one's age and height (85% of expected weight caused either by weight loss or by lack of expected weight gain).
Intense fear of gaining weight or becoming fat despite being underweight.
Disturbance in the way one's body weight or shape is experienced, undue influence of body weight or shape on self-evaluation, or denial of the severity of the current low body weight.

DIFFERENTIAL DIAGNOSIS

Weight loss caused by a general medical condition should be listed first on the differential diagnosis. Many medical conditions cause weight loss and must be ruled out prior to the initiation of treatment for anorexia nervosa. Major depressive disorder can be associated with weight loss caused by a decreased appetite; however, patients with this disorder are not concerned about their body image and readily admit that they have not put any effort into achieving the weight loss. If the decreased food intake is caused by odd or paranoid thoughts, then schizophrenia and obsessive-compulsive disorder must be considered. Patients with body dysmorphic disorder typically fixate on one particular part of their body which they consider imperfect rather than having the more global desire for thinness expressed by patients with anorexia.

Patients with bulimia nervosa have sudden urges to overeat and during one of these binges have a sense of lack of control over the ability to stop, resulting in their consuming large quantities of food followed by purging via laxatives, self-induced vomiting, diuretics, enemas, fasting, or exercise. These behaviors occur at least twice a week for 3 months. The self-concept of these patients is unduly influenced by their body shape, but not to the extent of individuals with anorexia nervosa. The extreme degree of cachexia that can be seen in anorexics is usually not present in bulimics, who may even remain at a normal body weight.

Diagnosing anorexia nervosa can sometimes be quite difficult. **Adolescents can be experienced at hiding the symptoms.** In addition, the onset of the illness is gradual, and changes may go unnoticed. Patients should be weighed regularly in a physician's office, and any significant weight loss should be evaluated with anorexia nervosa in the differential diagnosis. **Abnormalities in blood chemistries and electrocardiogram (ECG) changes** can be detected and considered evidence of anorexia if they are detected. Common laboratory abnormalities include hypokalemia, hypochloremic metabolic acidosis, low albumin levels (common in starvation), elevated liver enzymes and serum leptin levels, or leukopenia and a relative lymphocytosis. Recent imaging studies have also demonstrated region-specific gray matter loss in the anterior cingulate cortex, directly related to the severity of the disease. **This is a disease that by its nature tends to be hidden.** Clues should not be ignored by clinicians and, when found, should be addressed in a respectful but assertive manner.

The changes in *DSM-5* are minor. The most significant change is the removal of a criterion regarding amenorrhea to better reflect the presentation of patients with restricting eating disorders.

TREATMENT

The treatment of anorexia nervosa can be quite complicated and difficult. It is best accomplished in a series of steps. First, it is critical to engage in nutritional rehabilitation. This is often best done in a special inpatient psychiatric unit for eating disorders. This is because these patients are often able to subvert initial outpatient attempts to structure their eating to encourage weight gain, and even inpatient units must be alert for patient nonadherence. Patients are placed in structured regimens to restore weight, normalize eating patterns, achieve normal perceptions of hunger and satiety, and correct the biological and psychological effects of starvation. Given the cognitive impairment that goes along with starvation, **psychotherapy alone is not enough to treat severely malnourished patients with anorexia nervosa.** As nutritional status improves, psychotherapy becomes a critical component of the treatment. Psychiatric medications may have some role in the treatment of anorexia nervosa itself. A controlled study using olanzapine showed that adolescents achieved better weight gain and less obsessive symptoms as compared to controls. However, other studies examining neuroleptic use have shown no change. If the patient has other significant symptoms (depression, obsessions, anxiety), then use of medications for treating these symptoms is indicated as well. In general, use of psychiatric medications is delayed until metabolic abnormalities are corrected, and the patient's starvation status is significantly improved. There have been a few small studies showing that transcranial magnetic stimulation (TMS) may be of some benefit in reducing core symptoms of anorexia nervosa. After restoration of acute nutritional status problems, it is important to begin psychosocial interventions to treat anorexia. Treatments with the best evidence of effectiveness include both cognitive behavioral therapy (CBT), psychodynamic psychotherapy, exposure response prevention therapy, and family therapy.

A growing and consistent body of evidence shows that both short- and long-term family treatments have been found to be effective, depending on the severity of the eating disorder. These family interventions include a process for the parents to gain control of the adolescent's eating, a plan to gradually turn this control back over to the adolescent with improvement, and working on individual adolescent issues after weight stabilization to develop a healthy identity. Recent studies have shown some negative and positive patient factors associated with recovery. Negative factors include self-induced vomiting and high-trait anxiety. A factor positively influencing recovery is increased impulsivity.

CASE CORRELATION

- See also Case 19 and Case 31 for patients who may restrict their eating in public places. Social anxiety disorder patients may be embarrassed to be seen eating in public, but otherwise have normal eating habits. Bulimic patients may binge/purge in private and restrict their eating behavior in public; they also have a normal range of body weight as opposed to anorexics.

COMPREHENSION QUESTIONS

32.1 A 16-year-old girl is brought to a physician by her mother, who states that her daughter has been losing weight steadily. The adolescent denies there is a problem and states that she is in no way underweight. The physician determines that the girl is 5 ft 6 in tall and weighs 90 lb. Which of the following would be the next best step to work this patient up?

A. Complete blood count and differential white blood cell count

B. Thyroid function studies

C. Serum potassium level

D. Calculation and assessment of patient BMI

E. Liver function studies

32.2 Despite her protestations, the adolescent in the vignette above is diagnosed with anorexia. After stabilization of her nutritional status on a specialized inpatient unit, she is discharged home, with plans for follow-up therapy as an outpatient. Which of the following treatments have been shown to be effective in treating anorexia nervosa as an outpatient?

A. Neuroleptic therapy

B. Family therapy

C. Brief supportive therapy

D. Group therapy

E. Insight-oriented psychotherapy

32.3 The described patient has engaged in treatment. Which patient factor has been demonstrated to predict a positive outcome for recovery?

A. Higher trait anxiety

B. Self-induced vomiting

C. Greater impulsivity

D. Lower BMI at beginning of treatment

E. Age

ANSWERS

32.1 **D.** The BMI of a patient is calculated using the patient weight, height, and age (in those younger than 18) to create a ratio. BMIs of less than 19 may be the first indication of anorexia nervosa. It is an easy, noninvasive calculation that is done in the office quickly so should be done prior to more invasive, expensive, and time-consuming laboratory studies.

32.2 **B.** Family therapy, both short-term and long-term, has been demonstrated to improve outcomes in adolescent patients with anorexia nervosa. Many of these family treatments are completed in stages, generally beginning with developing parental control over the eating and gradually turning this control back over to the adolescent with improvement in nutritional status. Some cognitive behavioral therapies have been shown to be effective but there is little evidence for the others listed.

32.3 **C.** Greater impulsivity has been shown to be a positive prognostic characteristic in recent studies. Self-induced vomiting and trait anxiety have been shown to be negative prognostic factors.

CLINICAL PEARLS

▶ Anorexia nervosa is a serious, life-threatening disorder that can require inpatient medical and psychiatric hospitalization.

▶ Patients with anorexia nervosa rarely (at least at the beginning of their treatment) comply with refeeding and other treatment regimens willingly.

▶ Patients with anorexia nervosa can exhibit symptoms such as obsessions, performing rituals, and depression as a part of their clinical presentation.

REFERENCES

Fisher CA, Hetrick SE, Rushford N. Family therapy for anorexia nervosa. *Cochrane Database Syst Rev.* Apr 14, 2010;4:CD004780.

Föcker M, Timmesfeld N, Scherag S, et al. Screening for anorexia nervosa via measurement of serum leptin levels. *Neural Transm.* Apr 2011;118(4):571-578. Epub Jan 22, 2011.

Herpertz-Dahlmann B, Schwarte R, Krei M, et al. Day-patient treatment after short inpatient care versus continued inpatient treatment in adolescents with anorexia nervosa (ANDI): a multicentre, randomised, open-label, non-inferiority trial. *Lancet.* Apr 5, 2014;383(9924):1222-1229. Epub Jan 17, 2014.

Ornstein RM, Rosen DS, Mammel KA, et al. Distribution of eating disorders in children and adolescents using the proposed DSM-5 criteria for feeding and eating disorders. *J Adolesc Health.* Aug 2013;53(2):303-305. Epub May 15, 2013.

Steinglass JE, Albano AM, Simpson HB, et al. Confronting fear using exposure and response prevention for anorexia nervosa: a randomized controlled pilot study. *Int J Eat Disord.* Mar 2014;47(2):174-80. Epub Nov 8, 2013.

Van den Eynde F, Guillaume S, Broadbent H, Campbell IC, Schmidt U. Repetitive transcranial magnetic stimulation in anorexia nervosa: a pilot study. *Eur Psychiatry.* Feb 2013;28(2):98-101. Epub Aug 30, 2011.

Zerwas S, Lund BC, Von Holle A, et al. Factors associated with recovery from anorexia nervosa. *J Psychiatr Res.* Jul 2013;47(7):972-979. Epub Mar 25, 2013.

Zipfel S, Wild B, Groß G, et al; ANTOP study group. Focal psychodynamic therapy, cognitive behaviour therapy, and optimised treatment as usual in outpatients with anorexia nervosa (ANTOP study): randomised controlled trial. *Lancet.* Jan 11, 2014;383(9912):127-137. Epub Oct 14, 2013.

A 9-year-old boy is brought to the pediatrician by his mother with a chief complaint of wetting the bed at night. His mother states that the bedwetting began 3 months ago. Prior to this, the patient had "accidents" about once a month since completion of potty training at age 4. There are no other signs of regression and no other genitourinary complaints. Review of systems likewise reveals no recent issues. The boy has no past psychiatric or medical history. His parents separated 1 year ago and have divorced over the past 6 months. Three months ago, the mother's best friend moved into the home. She helps care for the patient, especially when his mother travels for work. The boy has visitation with his father every other weekend. The boy's mother disclosed his recent incontinence with the paternal grandmother; she revealed that the patient's father had the "same problem" around age 10.

When asked about bedwetting, the patient is quiet and appears uncomfortable. While his mother is interviewed, the boy promptly transitions into play appropriate for his age and seems generally at ease for the remainder of the encounter. On physical examination, the child appears healthy and well developed. There are no signs concerning for neglect or abuse. No abnormalities are noted.

▶ What is the most likely diagnosis for this patient?
▶ What is the best treatment?
▶ What is the most likely prognosis?

ANSWERS TO CASE 33:
Enuresis, Nocturnal Type

Summary: A 9-year-old boy presents with bedwetting in the context of psychosocial stressors, after a period of successful toilet training. There had been a chronic pattern of bedwetting, too infrequent to be deemed enuresis but indicative of persistent nighttime urinary incontinence. There are no other signs or symptoms indicative of an underlying medical condition. There are no signs of abuse or neglect. There is a paternal family history of enuresis.

- **Most likely diagnosis:** Enuresis (diagnostic criteria in Table 33–1).

- **Best treatment:** Psychoeducation, supportive psychotherapy, and behavioral modification with the alarm method are the mainstays of therapy. Desmopressin acetate (DDAVP) is the preferred pharmacologic agent, but should be reserved for patients 7 years of age and older. It may be advisable to delay treatment until the child has the motivation and capability to adhere to a treatment program. Treatment is often unnecessary if the behavior does not cause distress or impairment. In most cases, enuresis will spontaneously resolve without treatment.

- **Prognosis:** Spontaneous remission of enuresis, especially the nocturnal type, commonly occurs. Most children with **delay in establishing continence of urine (primary enuresis)** or **regression in control over micturition (secondary enuresis)** are successful at extinguishing the behavior though relapses are often interspersed with improvement. In fact, the majority of children will "grow out of it" even without direct management. If actively treated, the time course for resolution of atypical voiding patterns varies. Improvement depends on consistent adherence to the methods of behavioral modification. Patience is key to successful treatment.

ANALYSIS

Objectives

1. Recognize enuresis.
2. Understand the treatment recommendations for this disorder.
3. Be aware of the prognosis for this disorder.

Table 33–1 • DIAGNOSTIC CRITERIA FOR ENURESIS
Inappropriate elimination of urine into bed or clothes
Either frequency = 2× per week ≥ 3 months OR clinically significant distress/impairment
Chronological age or developmental age ≥ 5 years old
Not caused by a substance or medical condition
Specify if nocturnal, diurnal, or both

Considerations

This vignette presents a 9-year-old boy with secondary enuresis, nocturnal type with onset of incontinence in the context of significant environmental stressors. Over the last few years, he had periodic nighttime incontinence without the frequency or impairment to warrant a diagnosis of enuresis. At his age, monosymptomatic nocturnal enuresis is not uncommon, especially among boys. Previously, it was believed that the primary driver of enuresis was psychological. Psychosocial stress plays a role in enuresis, especially secondary enuresis. However, the predominant view today more heavily links biological features and cultural-familial-personal factors with the etiology of enuresis. Variability in toilet training adherence is an implicated cultural-familial-personal factor. This patient has a genetic propensity toward development of enuresis; the risk increases in a child whose father experienced enuresis. Other biological features include delayed maturation of neuroendocrine pathways leading to nocturnal polyuria and detrusor instability triggering bladder hyperreactivity.

APPROACH TO:

Enuresis

DEFINITIONS

NOCTURNAL ENURESIS: Inappropriate urinary voiding at night, that is, bedwetting.

DIURNAL ENURESIS: Abnormal daytime micturition.

PRIMARY ENURESIS: Failure to establish bladder control by 5 years of age.

SECONDARY ENURESIS: Loss of continence after previously achieved. Reemergence of a "wet period" after a relatively "dry period." Typically between 5 to 8 years of age, but may occur at any time.

CLINICAL APPROACH

Enuresis is defined by **repeated urinary voiding into inappropriate places** such as the clothes or bed. Although typically involuntary, enuresis may be intentional. To be considered diagnostic, the behavior must either occur twice weekly for 3 months or cause significant impairment. The development of normal bladder control typically occurs by age 4, thus enuresis can be first diagnosed by age 5 or the equivalent developmental age. Nocturnal enuresis represents the majority of cases. Daytime urinary incontinence may be because of social anxiety surrounding public toilet usage or engrossment in the task at hand. Primary enuresis exists when the child reaches age 5 without having sustained a period of appropriate toilet training. Secondary enuresis develops after a sufficient period during which the child has achieved continence. Secondary enuresis is often attributed

to a period of stress (eg, birth of a sibling, parental separation, geographic reloca-
tion). Established secondary enuresis should elicit a more thorough investigation
of psychosocial stressors. Screen carefully for trauma and neglect which may delay
the developmental process.

Determine the course of onset and the daily timing of urinary incontinence.
Asking the patient or parent to track symptoms in a voiding diary may be helpful.
Inquire about major life changes and other potential sources of stress. As inappropriate urinary voiding can be the result of a substance or another medical condition,
the patient and family should be asked about use of diuretics and antipsychotics
as well as medical conditions such as seizure disorders, diabetes, and spina bifida.
Clues to the presence of a nonenuretic cause of the abnormal micturition pattern include *the presence of other symptoms* such as increased/decreased frequency,
urgency, straining, a weak stream, and genital or lower urinary tract pain. In the
vast majority of enuresis cases, bedwetting is the only symptom. However, the presence of other symptoms does not rule out enuresis.

Changes from *DSM-IV-TR* to *DSM-5*: None

DIFFERENTIAL DIAGNOSIS

The differential for enuresis includes **substance-induced (eg, diuretics, neuroleptics)**
urinary incontinence and **medical conditions that may cause polyuria or urgency.**
Examples include neurogenic bladder, seizure disorder, diabetes, and spina bifida. If
the aberrant urinary voiding is attributable to any of these causes, enuresis should
not be diagnosed. However, if the symptoms presented **prior to** the medical condition or substance use or **continue after cessation/treatment**, then enuresis may still
be diagnosed.

In addition to a complete history, the evaluation of urinary incontinence should
include a comprehensive physical examination and **urinalysis.** The urinalysis screens
for diabetic ketoacidosis, diabetes insipidus, urinary tract infection (UTI), and
dilutional hyponatremia. Unless there is suspicion for a neurologic or urologic condition, urologic imaging (renal ultrasound) and urodynamic studies (eg, voiding
cystourethrogram) may be reserved for recurrent pediatric UTIs, multiple urinary
complaints, or other features suggestive of structural abnormality. For patients
reporting constipation, order an abdominal x-ray to determine the severity of stool
retention. As constipation can cause urinary incontinence, its treatment may correlate with resolution of enuresis. Constipation in children is often associated with
encopresis (the repeated inappropriate passage of feces), the other main elimination disorder.

TREATMENT

Psychoeducation is the most important element of treatment for patients and their
caretakers. The child's caretakers should be educated regarding the prevalence of
enuresis and its high rate of spontaneous resolution. Patients in the vast majority of cases "grow out of it." Parents should be helped to understand that for most
patients, the behavior is **not** voluntary. Children should not be punished or shamed

because this only exacerbates embarrassment and stress, potentially aggravating the condition. The disruptive behaviors often associated with enuresis are frequently in relation to the negative response by parents, siblings, and peers. The parents should also be educated about the impact of significant life changes; enuresis may be a manifestation of a stressor. Facilitate a nonjudgmental environment to help elicit important information and help the family feel at ease. The caretakers also require support; screen for caregiver burnout. Family therapy and parent management training may ease the strain of the family dynamic. Supportive psychotherapy emphasizing normalization and empowerment will help the patient adapt a healthy approach. It is advisable to initiate treatment only if the symptoms cause distress/ impairment to the child. The patient needs to be a willing, active participant in the treatment plan.

The most common strategy for behavioral modification involves **bell and pad training** for a course of 6 to 16 weeks. This method relies on a **sensor-equipped alarm** that detects fluid in the underwear or on the mattress pad. Other behavioral techniques, effective when used *in conjunction with* the alarm method, include positive reinforcement (rewarding alarm responsiveness or dry nights), dry-bed training, and overlearning. Dry-bed training refers to awakening the patient to use the bathroom at specified intervals by setting multiple alarms throughout the night. Overlearning involves a short-term treatment strategy of increasing fluid intake at night to improve bladder capacity. In the long-term, patients are encouraged to limit consumption of fluid and caffeine prior to bedtime. Acquiring a waterproof mattress can be vital for patients and families. Pharmacotherapy is reserved for short-term usage in the case of failed response to behavioral modifications. First-line treatment for enuresis is **DDAVP**. Patients with nocturnal polyuria and normal bladder capacity will show the most improvement on DDAVP. Imipramine, oxybutynin chloride, and tolterodine may reduce bedwetting but have less tolerable side-effect profiles. When the medications are stopped, patients typically relapse. The child and caretaker should be aware that relapse is common and does not necessarily indicate treatment failure. If relapse occurs, restart the management regimen.

CASE CORRELATION

- Neurogenic bladder or another medical condition such as diabetes mellitus can cause polyuria and urgency; this should not be diagnosed as enuresis. Likewise, medication side effects (antipsychotics, diuretics, etc) may cause incontinence and should be considered before a diagnosis of enuresis is made.

COMPREHENSION QUESTIONS

33.1 A 12-year-old boy is brought to the pediatrician by his father for recent night-time bedwetting over the last several months. The father appears frustrated and shows obvious signs of fatigue. On further questioning, he admits that his "stress levels have shot through the roof" because of layoffs in his department. The boy's father recently remarried and his new wife has been complaining about his son's "messes." The father has starting drinking more and feels easily irritated. The pediatrician evaluates the boy alone. The patient denies any physical abuse, but states that he does not feel welcome at home since his stepmother moved in. He feels ashamed about the bedwetting, but wishes "they wouldn't be so mean about it." What is the next step in management?

A. Bell and pad training

B. Biofeedback

C. DDAVP

D. Hypnosis

E. Psychoeducation

33.2 A 4-year-old boy without any known medical problems is brought in to the pediatrician by his mother because of recurrent bedwetting. His mother voices concern because the boy's four siblings were all toilet trained by age 3. The mother states her youngest is "almost 5 years old and cannot seem to learn to use the potty. I am really worried there is something wrong." He is meeting other developmental milestones. The boy does not show any signs of distress but does not engage in questions regarding incontinence. There are no abnormalities on physical examination. What is the most likely diagnosis?

A. Enuresis due to medication side effects

B. Normal development

C. Primary enuresis

D. Secondary enuresis

E. Urinary incontinence due to another medical condition

33.3 An 11-year-old girl is accompanied by her mother to establish care with her new pediatrician. The mother reports that since the family moved several weeks ago, the patient has been having episodes of incontinence. She also recalls that this problem occurred on three prior occasions over the last 4 years. Each time, the patient's former pediatrician treated her with antibiotics and the incontinence resolved. Today, the patient complains of suprapubic pain, urgency, and burning on urination. She reports enjoying her new school and feeling at home. She denies medical problems, drug use, sexual activity, or trauma. What is the most likely diagnosis?

A. Primary enuresis

B. Secondary enuresis

C. Substance-induced incontinence

D. Urinary incontinence resulting from structural anomaly

E. Urinary incontinence secondary to seizure disorder

ANSWERS

33.1 **E.** Psychoeducation is the next step prior to beginning any intervention. In this case, the child's father and stepmother would benefit from education about enuresis and how to manage the symptoms. The family unit needs to provide a supportive environment without further worsening the situation. Psychoeducation helps to put into perspective recent life stressors which may have contributed to the child's presentation. As the patient finds the symptoms clinically distressing, initiating behavioral modifications, such as the bell and pad training, could follow psychoeducation. Allowing the child to have autonomy over the treatment is essential. Short-term pharmacotherapy with DDAVP could be considered if the patient has not responded to behavioral modifications. Biofeedback and hypnosis are alternative treatment strategies, although not first line.

33.2 **B.** At 4 years old, the patient's symptoms should be considered within the scope of normal development. At the chronologic or developmental age of 5, continence is expected. Reassurance is the most appropriate next step in management.

33.3 **D.** Suspect a structural anomaly whenever there are recurrent urinary tract infections. In addition to the standard workup of enuresis, urological imaging and urodynamic studies should also be undertaken. Primary enuresis should not be diagnosed as the patient has previously established bladder control. Secondary enuresis may fit with the stress of moving, but she seems well adjusted. Also this would not explain the prior periods of incontinence. There is no evidence for seizure disorder nor substance-induced incontinence.

CLINICAL PEARLS

▶ Nocturnal enuresis is more common than diurnal enuresis especially among younger children (5 to 8 year olds).

▶ **Urinalysis** can reveal commonly associated conditions—diabetic ketoacidosis, diabetes insipidus, dilutional hyponatremia, urinary tract infection.

▶ Symptoms typically **resolve spontaneously**. Reassurance is critical.

▶ The behavioral modification technique of **bell and pad training** is first-line treatment.

▶ **DDAVP** is the first-line pharmacological agent.

REFERENCES

American Psychiatric Association. *Diagnostic and Statistical Manual of Mental Disorders*. 5th ed. Washington, DC: American Psychiatric Association; 2013.

Behrman RE, Jenson HB, Stanton BF. *Nelson Textbook of Pediatrics*. 19th ed. Philadelphia, PA: Elsevier/ Saunders; 2012.

Nevéus T, von Gontard A, Hoebeke P, et al. The standardization of terminology of lower urinary tract function in children and adolescents: report from the Standardisation Committee of the International Children's Continence Society. *J Urol*. 2006;176(1):314-324.

Sadock BJ, Sadock VA, Ruiz, P. *Kaplan & Sadock's Synopsis of Psychiatry* 11th ed. Baltimore, MD: Lippincott Williams & Wilkins; 2014.

A 28-year-old woman comes to her primary care physician with a chief complaint of not getting enough sleep and feeling fatigued for the past 3 months. She says that she has an almost daily problem falling asleep and often wakes up numerous times during the night as well. She claims that her sleep problems began after she had an argument on the telephone with her boyfriend. She noted that after that she was "all keyed up" and could not go to sleep that night. Subsequently, she faces every evening with dread because she is preoccupied with getting enough sleep. She becomes very frustrated with her inability to sleep, which just makes the problem worse. She has no other signs or symptoms other than the fatigue caused by failure to get her usual 8 hours of sleep each night. She states that her mood is "okay, except for this sleep thing." She is still seeing her boyfriend, and their relationship has been stable. She has no medical problems, she denies the use of drugs, and she drinks alcohol only very rarely—not at all since she began having problems sleeping. The results of her physical examination are entirely normal.

▶ What is the most likely diagnosis for this patient?
▶ What treatment recommendations should be made to this patient?

ANSWERS TO CASE 34:

Insomnia Disorder

Summary: A 28-year-old woman has had sleeping problems for the past 3 months that were precipitated by an argument with her boyfriend. Since that time, she is preoccupied with getting enough sleep and is worried and frustrated. She has problems falling and staying asleep. She reports no other medical or psychiatric problems, and the results of her physical examination are normal. She denies the use of drugs or alcohol.

- **Most likely diagnosis:** Insomnia disorder.

- **Recommended treatment:** Sleep hygiene education, stimulus control therapy, relaxation training, and cognitive behavioral therapy should be offered. Helpful medications include ramelteon, trazodone, and benzodiazepine receptor agonists such as zolpidem, zaleplon, and triazolam, although benzodiazepine receptor agonists should in general not be used for more than 2 weeks because tolerance and withdrawal can result.

ANALYSIS

Objectives

1. Recognize primary insomnia in a patient.

2. Understand the recommended treatment approaches for patients with this disorder.

Considerations

This patient experienced a psychological upset that interfered with her ability to sleep. Subsequently, she developed a vicious cycle of worrying about whether or not she will be able to sleep, which is invariably followed by a poor night's sleep. She has no signs or symptoms of a mood or other psychiatric disorder and no evidence of a physical disease or a substance abuse/dependence problem.

APPROACH TO:

Insomnia Disorder

CLINICAL APPROACH

Diagnostic Criteria

Insomnia disorder is diagnosed when problems sleeping have occurred for at least 3 months and cause significant distress or impairment. These problems include nonrestorative sleep or an inability to initiate or maintain sleep, often presenting as complaints of difficulty falling asleep and multiple awakenings during the night.

Patients are often quite preoccupied with getting enough sleep and the fact that they are not doing so, which further increases their frustration and inability to sleep. Psychological and physiologic arousal at night and negative conditioning for sleep are often evident. The sleep disorder cannot be caused by the effects of a substance or general medical condition or occur exclusively during an episode of another psychiatric disorder. Narcolepsy, breathing-related sleep disorder, circadian rhythm sleep disorder, or parasomnias (eg, sleepwalking, sleep terrors) must first be ruled out, which makes the diagnosis of insomnia disorder basically one of exclusion.

DIFFERENTIAL DIAGNOSIS

As noted earlier, **the diagnosis of insomnia disorder is one of exclusion**, and so physical factors (sleep apnea, sleep-related epilepsy, sleep-related asthma, sleep-related gastroesophageal reflux disease, etc) must all be ruled out before such a diagnosis can be made. In addition, mental disorders that cause disturbances in sleep, such as psychosis, major depression, alcoholism, anxiety disorders, and mania should also be excluded. Sleep-related disorders such as narcolepsy and circadian rhythm sleep disorder (in which the individual's sleep-wake pattern is out of synchrony with the desired schedule) must also be ruled out. Some individuals need a shorter amount of time to sleep. This should not be characterized as an insomnia disorder unless the patient has difficulty initiating or maintaining sleep, or has daytime symptoms such as fatigue, concentration problems, or irritability. Acute or situational insomnia occurs for a few days or weeks after disruptive life events or changes in sleep schedules. This insomnia does not last long enough to be diagnosed as an insomnia disorder, which must be present for at least 3 months.

TREATMENT

Insomnia disorder can be very difficult to treat. Initially sleep hygiene education (Table 34–1) should occur, with the clinician carefully going over each item to ensure the patient is not engaging in practices that will disrupt sleep. This should be combined with stimulus control therapy, where the association patients have made between their bedroom and not sleeping is broken. Patients are instructed to use their beds only for sleeping (and sex). They should go to bed only if sleepy. If they cannot fall asleep after 15 minutes, they should get up, do something else relaxing in another room, and return to bed only if sleepy. Relaxation training such as meditation, progressive relaxation, and guided imagery are helpful. Patients should maintain a regular wake-up time regardless of how they slept and avoid naps. Finally, cognitive behavioral therapy for insomnia (CBT-I) is useful to correct dysfunctional beliefs about sleep.

Ramelteon, an FDA-approved melatonin receptor agonist, appears to impact sleep onset latency with little effect on wakefulness during the middle of the night. The other FDA-approved agents for insomnia are benzodiazepine receptor agonists that impact both sleep onset latency and total sleep time. However, these drugs should not be used consecutively for more than 2 weeks because physiological and psychological dependence can occur with significant rebound insomnia and withdrawal when they are discontinued. Trazodone, while not FDA approved, is commonly used in psychiatry as a sleep aid that does not produce dependence. Melatonin is available as a nutritional supplement and may give some patients benefit.

Table 34–1 • SLEEP HYGIENE MEASURES
Eat at regular times during the day and not late at night.
Make sure that the sleeping room is dark and quiet, consider using "white" noise (running fan) to block out background noise.
Take a long, hot bath near bedtime.
Drink a glass of warm milk near bedtime.
Avoid daytime naps.
Get up at the same time every day.
Go to sleep at the same time every night.
Do not use substances that impair sleep, such as caffeine, alcohol, nicotine, or stimulants.
Begin a physical fitness program.
Avoid late evening stimulation with screens— turn off TVs, computers, smartphones. Listen to soft music or read a book instead.
Use the bed for sleep and sexual activity only, get out of bed and do something relaxing if not asleep within 15 minutes.

The herbal sleep aid valerian is available as a nutritional supplement but its overall efficacy is marginal. While some patients may utilize over-the-counter diphenhydramine as an occasional off-label sleep aid, tolerance to its side effect of drowsiness has been noted as quickly as after 4 days of regular use and so should not be used to treat chronic insomnia.

Telling patients that their health will not be endangered if they get fewer than 6 hours of sleep per night for a short time can reduce frustration and anxiety about their sleeplessness, which often contributes to their insomnia.

COMPREHENSION QUESTIONS

34.1 A 33-year-old married physician presents to your primary care practice with complaints of "depression." On interview, he denies pervasive feelings of sadness or anhedonia, and he has not had any change in appetite or weight, or any problems concentrating. He has felt tired much of the time for the past 6 weeks, with ongoing, multiple awakenings during the night. On further questioning, he reveals that these difficulties began when he was involved in a malpractice suit after the death of a patient. He was "up obsessing about it" prior to the trial when his sleep disturbance began. Although the suit was dropped, he continues to wake up frequently, worrying about not being able to fall back asleep. He denies medical problems, alcohol, or drug use. Which of the following is the most likely diagnosis for this patient?

A. Breathing-related sleep disorder

B. Circadian rhythm sleep disorder

C. Major depressive disorder

D. Insomnia disorder

E. Narcolepsy

34.2 You offer the patient in Question 34.1 a short course of lorazepam, but he declines. Which of the following should you next recommend to help his sleep?

A. Eat a late evening meal.

B. Exercise prior to bedtime.

C. Sleep later on the weekends.

D. Take a hot bath in the evening.

E. Take naps during the day.

34.3 A patient comes to her physician stating that for the last 6 months, since she started a new job, she has difficulty getting up in time for work. She notes that she is not tired around bedtime, and so she stays up for several hours playing computer games. When she finally does go to sleep, she has time to sleep for only 4 to 5 hours before she has to get up to go to work. She then finds herself groggy in the morning and fatigued throughout the day. This problem is interfering with her work at her job and thus is causing her distress. Prior to starting her new office job, the patient worked evening hours as a bartender and did not have a problem with sleeping. She takes no medications and uses no substances that could explain her sleep problems. The results of her physical examination are normal. Which of the following is the most likely diagnosis for this patient?

A. Breathing-related sleep disorder

B. Circadian rhythm sleep disorder

C. Primary hypersomnia

D. Insomnia disorder

E. Narcolepsy

ANSWERS

34.1 **D.** The patient likely suffers from insomnia disorder. There is no evidence of sleep apnea or a disconnect between the environment and the circadian rhythm of the patient. Despite the insomnia and fatigue, there is no pervasive depressed mood, anhedonia, or other neuro-vegetative symptoms suggestive of a major depression.

34.2 **D.** Taking a hot bath near bedtime is an effective technique for inducing sleep in some patients. The other options listed do not help and are actually likely to *worsen* insomnia.

34.3 **B.** This patient is suffering from a delayed-sleep-phase type of circadian rhythm sleep disorder. Circadian rhythm sleep disorder is characterized by a recurrent pattern of sleep disruption leading to excessive sleepiness and/or insomnia because of the mismatch between the sleep-wake schedule required in a person's environment (in this case, the demands of the patient's new job) and her circadian sleep-wake pattern. The sleep disorder must cause distress and must not be caused by a substance, a physical condition, or another mental disorder.

CLINICAL PEARLS

▶ Primary insomnia is characterized by trouble falling asleep and multiple awakenings throughout the night. Individuals with this disorder are often preoccupied with getting enough sleep and become more and more frustrated every night, which further inhibits their ability to sleep.

▶ Primary insomnia is a diagnosis of exclusion because interfering physical and mental disorders must all be ruled out before the diagnosis can be made.

▶ Primary insomnia can be treated to break the cycle of insomnia and worry with ramelteon, trazodone, or short-term use of benzodiazepine receptor agonists.

▶ Stimulus control therapy, relaxation training, and sleep hygiene training can be useful in helping patients with primary insomnia sleep.

REFERENCES

Buysse DJ. Chronic insomnia. *Am J Psychiatry*. 2008;165(6):678-686.

Kratochivil CJ, Owens JA. Pharmacotherapy of pediatric insomnia. *J Am Acad Child Adolesc Psychiatry*. 2009;48(2):99-107.

Pigeon WR, Bishop TM, Marcus JA. Advances in the management of insomnia. *F1000Prime Reports*. Jun 2, 2014;6:48. doi: 10.12703/P6-48. eCollection.

A 2½-year-old first-born son of married parents is brought to a pediatrician's office by his father. Before this visit, the patient visited the pediatrician only for regular well-child checks and for treatment of one episode of otitis media. The father is concerned about the behavioral problems his son has developed. He reports that for the past month, after the patient goes to bed and to sleep, the parents hear him get up in the middle of the night. This behavior occurs perhaps once or twice a week. On these occasions, the child is found standing somewhere in the house, crying and seemingly disoriented, with rapid breathing and profuse sweating. When the parents attempt to comfort him or return him to his room, he becomes quite upset, striking out at them and screaming loudly. He continues to scream and fight for several minutes but then stops spontaneously. Once he is awakened, he continues to act frightened and cannot share any dream content. Once the child is calmed, the parents put him back in his bed, and he sleeps through the rest of the night without incident. In the morning, he wakes up in his usual happy mood and does not remember what occurred the previous evening. The parents are worried that he might be having seizures or developing a severe behavioral problem.

▶ What is the most likely diagnosis for this child?
▶ What treatments would you recommend for this child?

ANSWERS TO CASE 35:
Nonrapid Eye Movement Sleep Arousal Disorder, Sleep Terror Type

Summary: The patient is a 2½-year-old boy with new-onset sleep problems who has no significant other history. He wakes at night, screaming and has autonomic hyperarousal, and his parents are unable to soothe him. These episodes last a few minutes, after which he goes back to normal sleep. The child has no memory of the events in the morning.

- **Most likely diagnosis:** Nonrapid eye movement sleep arousal disorder, sleep terror type.

- **Recommended treatments:** Protect the child from injury and do nothing. The disorder is usually time limited.

ANALYSIS

Objectives

1. Recognize nonrapid eye movement sleep arousal disorder, sleep terror type in a patient (Table 35–1).

2. Offer treatment suggestions to the parents.

Considerations

This patient's presentation is typical for nonrapid eye movement sleep arousal disorder, sleep terror type, a disorder that is found in 3% of all children and less than 1% of adults. It typically manifests itself as emotional and behavioral disturbances at night. These events usually occur early in the nightly sleep cycle during **delta (slow-wave) sleep.** In nonrapid eye movement sleep arousal disorder, sleep terror type, the affected **child does not remember the episodes in the morning. Fever, sleep deprivation, and central nervous system depressants may increase frequency of sleep terror episodes. Typically, these children have no other psychopathology.** The episodes are usually self-limiting without treatment, and the prognosis is very good. Reassuring the parents is the usual indicated intervention. Nightmares occur during rapid eye movement (REM) sleep and are typically associated with the report

Table 35–1 • DIAGNOSTIC CRITERIA FOR SLEEP TERROR DISORDER
Episodes of apparent abrupt awakening from sleep usually occurring in the early part of the sleep cycle.
Behavioral exhibition of intense emotion, often with extreme autonomic responses seen.
Patient is often unresponsive to efforts to soothe or calm.
Little memory of episode in the morning after a normal awakening.

of a "bad dream." If the child is awakened, he or she can typically recall the dream, even the next morning. Some recent studies have demonstrated a strong correlation of night terrors and other parasomnias with the presence of additional sleep disorders, such as sleep-disordered breathing and restless leg syndrome. In virtually all the children studied, the parasomnia, primarily sleep terrors and sleepwalking, was eliminated when appropriate interventions for the additional sleep disorder were implemented. It has been suggested that the sleep disorder may **trigger** the parasomnia, and when the trigger is eliminated, the parasomnia resolves. In addition, studies have also indicated a very strong correlation of sleep terrors with a family history of other parasomnias. A recent Canadian study looked at the correlation of sleep terrors among monozygotic and dizygotic twins and showed a considerable heritable component of this disorder.

APPROACH TO:
Nonrapid Eye Movement Sleep Arousal Disorder, Sleep Terror Type

DEFINITIONS

DELTA SLEEP: Sleep stage characterized by low-frequency (0.5-2 waves/s), high-voltage (amplitudes >75 µV) waves in at least 20% of the waves.

DYSSOMNIAS: Sleep difficulties associated with the duration and type of sleep.

PARASOMNIAS: Sleep disorders associated with problems during the stages of sleep.

RAPID EYE MOVEMENT (REM): A sleep stage characterized by fast eye movements and a wakeful pattern of electrical activity in the brain.

SLEEP CYCLE: The brain-wave activity associated with varying stages of sleep from light to deep.

SOMNAMBULISM: Sleepwalking.

SLEEP-DISORDERED BREATHING (SDB): Describes a group of disorders characterized by abnormalities of respiratory pattern (pauses in breathing) or the quantity of ventilation during sleep. Obstructive sleep apnea (OSA), the most common of this type of disorder, is characterized by the repetitive collapse of the pharyngeal airway during sleep and the need to arouse to resume ventilation.

CLINICAL APPROACH

Normal Sleep

The human sleep cycle is divided into several different stages defined by brain wave patterns that can be measured during a sleep study. Parameters measured include an electroencephalogram (EEG), which measures and records electrical activity on

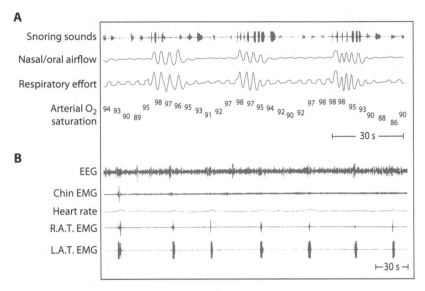

Figure 35-1. The parameters measured during a sleep study.

the surface of the brain, an electro-oculogram (EOG), which records eye movements during sleep, and an electromyogram (EMG), which records the electrical activity emanating from active muscles in the body (Figure 35–1). The stages of sleep defined by the sleep study include:

Stage 1: The EEG may show theta waves, muscle tone may be relaxed, and eye movements may be slow and rolling, typically the "nodding off" period.

Stage 2: The EEG shows K complexes and sleep spindles, no eye movements, and little muscle activity.

Delta sleep: The EEG shows low-frequency, high-voltage waves. Delta sleep has been divided into Stages 3 and 4 by some, depending on the number of delta waves seen.

Rapid eye movement: Low, fast voltage on the EEG, no muscle tone (cataplexy), and very rapid eye movements.

The sleep cycle is a dynamic presentation of the stages in a typical night's sleep. Sleep disorders are classified and defined based on their occurrence and manifestation in the context of the sleep cycle. Dyssomnias are disorders characterized by excessive sleepiness or difficulty initiating or maintaining sleep. They include such intrinsic sleep disorders as narcolepsy and OSA, and such extrinsic sleep disorders such as poor sleep hygiene, allergies, and insufficient sleep. Parasomnias are sleep disorders that occur during sleep or on arousal. They include such disorders as sleep terrors, sleepwalking (somnambulism), rhythmic movement disorder, sleep talking, nightmares, sleep paralysis, bruxism, and enuresis.

DIFFERENTIAL DIAGNOSIS

Non-REM sleep terrors are a fairly common disorder. A recent study showed a 10.4% lifetime prevalence and a 2.7% current prevalence. Night terrors and somnambulism tend to occur during periods of arousal from delta sleep. As a result, these disorders are more common in children (who have more delta sleep) and they often occur during the first half of the night when there is more delta sleep occurring. It is not uncommon for both disorders to occur in the same person. Patients with both disorders are difficult to awaken, confused if they are awakened during a parasomnia, and typically do not remember the incident. Sleepwalking (somnambulism) is characterized by repeated episodes of rising from bed and walking during sleep. Often patients have a blank look on their faces and seem indifferent to what is around them. They typically are not very reactive and thus do not show the behavior (such as screaming and violent thrashing), seen in sleep terror disorder. Patients who sleepwalk often show amnesia to the event on awakening as well. They are not dreaming but typically show an arousal pattern during delta sleep. The potential for harm to self or others from a sleepwalker (falls, walking into streets, starting a fire) means that families must take steps to protect these children. In serious cases, children may require pharmacologic intervention.

Individuals with nightmare disorders have dreams of a very frightening nature characterized by limited verbalization and movement. These dreams occur during REM sleep, and the patient can often recall them in detail on awakening. The absence of screaming and thrashing, plus the detailed memory of the dream, differentiates this disorder from sleep terror disorder. Patients with posttraumatic stress disorder may have frightening dreams or dissociative experiences, because this disorder is one of autonomic reactivity and an exaggerated startle response following exposure to a traumatic experience. However, these patients typically remember the frightening dreams and/or flashbacks and these do not occur exclusively at night. Temporal lobe epilepsy is a type of seizure disorder that includes active, often violent, motor responses, but these typically occur during waking hours.

Perhaps one of the most common disorders of sleep in childhood is **enuresis.** The treatment of enuresis in childhood is best approached by **diagnosing the core problem correctly and advising the parents to be supportive of and not punish the child. Primary enuresis is** defined as **nighttime urination** in a child **with no previous significant period of dryness. Secondary enuresis is nighttime urination following a period of dryness (usually at least several months).** Secondary enuresis is often because of a physical problem, such as a urinary tract infection, or a psychological stressor, such as regression associated with the arrival of a newborn sibling.

TREATMENT

The treatment of nonrapid eye movement sleep arousal disorder, sleep terror type usually consists of reassuring the parents that, with time, the child will outgrow these harmless events. They should be instructed to take measures to maintain the patient's safety during these episodes, as unrestrained thrashing can result in injury. Relief of the symptoms of sleep terror disorder is also shown in patients who have a demonstrated coexisting sleep disorder which is successfully treated.

In somnambulism, special care must be taken to ensure that the patient cannot wander out of windows or the house or access dangerous materials. There have been case reports using drugs such as diazepam or imipramine to treat this disorder, but no controlled studies.

Primary enuresis can be treated in a number of ways, although the developmental level of the child should be considered. It often remits spontaneously as the child becomes older. Generally, pharmacologic or extensive behavioral treatment should not be considered prior to **age 7.** The behavioral treatment for enuresis primarily involves the use of **an enuresis alarm, alternatively known as a "bell and pad."** This device consists of a moisture-sensitive sensor attached to the child's underwear and an alarm linked to the sensor close by. When the sensor is activated, the alarm goes off, waking the child as well as the caretaker. The child should then be quickly and directly taken to the bathroom to urinate. This method of enuresis control has a 75% success rate, as well as a low rate of recidivism after the alarm is removed. Buzzer ulcers sometimes can develop and should be discussed as a potential adverse effect.

Desmopressin (DDAVP) is a synthetic analog of a natural antidiuretic hormone that has been found effective in 18 randomized, controlled trials. A study comparing bell-and-pad method to DDAVP found comparable efficacy: bell-and-pad, 86% and desmopressin, 70%. It was used successfully in both tablet and nasal form to control enuresis in children. Again, it is an effective short-term treatment for enuresis, but there is a high rate of recidivism once the medication is discontinued.

Another common treatment for enuresis involves medication. **Imipramine** was an effective treatment in more than 40 double-blind studies. Given in relatively low doses, it is very effective in controlling nighttime wetting. However, there is a high rate of recidivism after the medication is discontinued. **Electrocardiogram (ECG) monitoring is recommended in doses above 3.5 mg/kg/d, and the danger of imipramine in overdose should be stressed to parents and children.**

CASE CORRELATION

- See Case 16 for patients who may also present with fearfulness upon awakening. Panic disorder patients may awaken abruptly from a deep sleep with fearfulness, but these episodes produce rapid and complete awakening, without confusion, amnesia, or the motor activity typical of nonrapid eye movement sleep arousal disorders.

COMPREHENSION QUESTIONS

35.1 Which of the following, in addition to sleep terrors, is considered a nonrapid eye movement sleep arousal disorder?

A. Nightmare disorder

B. Restless leg syndrome

C. Narcolepsy

D. Sleep apnea

E. Sleepwalking

35.2 A parent brings his child to the pediatrician's office because of concerns regarding sleep. The child is 3 years old and often wakes up at night screaming loudly, appearing very frightened, striking out when touched, and inconsolable. She remembers none of this when she wakes the next morning. Which of the following best describes this disorder?

A. Posttraumatic stress disorder

B. Non-REM sleep terror disorder

C. Rapid eye movement disorder

D. Nightmare disorder

E. Restless leg syndrome

35.3 The pediatrician orders a sleep study on this patient which documents the presence of sleep-disordered breathing, a commonly concurrent phenomenon with sleep terrors. What treatment for the sleep terror might best be considered at this point?

A. A selective serotonin reuptake inhibitor

B. A benzodiazepine sleeping agent

C. Adenoidectomy or tonsillectomy

D. Reassuring the parents that the patient will not harm herself

E. Restraining the patient in bed

ANSWERS

35.1 **E.** Sleepwalking is also categorized as a nonrapid eye movement sleep arousal disorder which is characterized by a mixture of both wakefulness and non-REM sleep.

35.2 **B.** This case is typical for sleep terrors. Sleep terrors often occur in the presence of another sleep disorder—in particular, restless leg syndrome and sleep-disordered breathing. However, this particular disorder is categorized as a nonrapid eye movement sleep arousal disorder. These disorders represent a mixture of both wakeful activity and non-REM behaviors.

35.3 **C.** The best treatment for night terrors with the documented presence of another sleep disorder is definitive treatment of that sleep disorder. In this case, an adenoidectomy or tonsillectomy should be considered in consultation with an ear, nose, and throat specialist. Nearly all cases of sleep terrors resolve if the primary sleep disorder is addressed appropriately.

CLINICAL PEARLS

▶ Patients with sleep terror disorder need to be protected from injuring themselves during these episodes, but otherwise do not require pharmacologic intervention.

▶ Sleep terror disorder occurs almost exclusively during delta sleep.

▶ Enuresis may be effectively treated with the bell-and-pad method, desmopressin, and imipramine.

REFERENCES

American Psychiatric Association. *Diagnostic and Statistical Manual of Mental Disorders*. 5th ed. Washington, DC: American Psychiatric Publishing; 2013.

Bjorvatn B, Grønli J, Pallesen S. Prevalence of different parasomnias in the general population. *Sleep Med*. Dec 2010;11(10):1031-1034. doi: 10.1016/j.sleep.2010.07.011. Epub Nov 18, 2010.

Sadock BJ, Sadock VA, Ruiz P. *Kaplan and Sadock's Synopsis of Psychiatry: Behavioral Sciences/Clinical Psychiatry*. 11th ed. Baltimore, MD: Lippincott Williams & Wilkins; 2014.

A 26-year-old chromosomal man dressed as a woman comes to see a psychiatrist as part of the workup required before he is allowed to have the sex change operation that he desires. He tells the psychiatrist that he has always felt he is a girl. He says, "When I was born, there must have been some mistake. I should have had the body of a woman." He notes that as a child he enjoyed playing with dolls and female playmates; he never seemed to fit in with those of his own male gender. He claims that he has adopted all the mannerisms of a woman, including dressing like one, since leaving home at age 16. He states that he always would have dressed this way but was forbidden to do so by his parents, from whom he is now estranged. He admits that he has had no sexual experiences with women. His first sexual encounter with a man occurred when he was 18 years old, and he is currently in a relationship with another man lasting for the past 4 years. He considers himself a "straight woman" and has never seen himself as a gay man.

On his mental status examination, the patient appears alert and oriented to person, place, and time. He is dressed in a blouse, skirt, jacket, nylons, and high heels and purports himself to be a woman. His grooming is good, and he cooperates fully during the examination. No abnormalities were found on his mental status examination.

▶ What is the most likely diagnosis?
▶ What options are open to the patient other than sex reassignment surgery?

ANSWERS TO CASE 36:
Gender Dysphoria

Summary: A 26-year-old man is referred to a psychiatrist as part of the workup for a sex change operation. He has a strong, persistent desire to be female and has dressed as a woman since age 16. His sexual experiences have been exclusively with men. The results of his mental status examination are normal.

- **Most likely diagnosis:** Gender dysphoria

- **Options other than sex reassignment surgery:** Patients can take estrogen to create breasts and other feminine contours and undergo electrolysis to remove their male hair.

ANALYSIS

Objectives

1. Recognize gender dysphoria in a patient (Table 36–1 for diagnostic criteria).
2. Understand treatment options open to patients with this disorder.

Considerations

This patient has had a persistent desire to be female and has always been uncomfortable with his male body. As soon as he could, he adopted female dress and mannerisms, although this resulted in estrangement from his family. He has requested surgery in order to fulfill his desire to be a woman. His sexual preference is for men because he sees himself as a woman. He does not consider himself a homosexual. True gender dysphoria will present with a history of having the cross-gender identity from a very young age.

Table 36–1 • DIAGNOSTIC CRITERIA FOR GENDER DYSPHORIA
A strong, persistent, cross-gender identification.

In children, this desire is manifested by:
  • Repeatedly stating that one is a member of the other sex
  • Dressing in the attire of the other sex
  • A preference for cross-sex roles in make-believe play and preferred toys
  • A strong preference for playmates of the other sex

In adults, this desire is manifested by stated wishes to live and be treated as a member of the other sex.
A persistent discomfort with the patient's own sex and a sense of inappropriateness in this gender role; in adults, this is often accompanied by a preoccupation with getting rid of the sex characteristics with which one was born.
The disturbance is not concurrent with a physical intersex condition.
The disturbance is distressing to or impairs the functioning of the individual.

APPROACH TO:
Gender Dysphoria

DEFINITIONS

ANATOMICAL SEX: Sex based on appearance of genitals. In ambiguous cases, see intersex and sexual assignment definitions.

ANDROGEN INSENSITIVITY SYNDROME: A type of intersex presentation where the patient is chromosomally a male, but does not respond developmentally to androgen, and therefore develops externally female genitalia.

CHROMOSOMAL SEX: The sex of the individual based on karyotyping. It is also necessary to detect individuals who are genetic mosaics (eg, 45X/46 XY with 60% the latter).

GENDER IDENTITY: How the patient perceives oneself as male or female.

INTERSEX: Intersex states are conditions where a newborn's sex organs (genitals) appear unusual, making it impossible to identify the sex of the baby from its outward appearance.

SEXUAL ASSIGNMENT: Assignment by parents and physicians as to whether an infant is male or female in cases of ambiguous genitalia. The decision is made based on presence and adequacy of what genital structures are present, expected sexual functionality of these structures, and parental preference with completion of surgical reconstruction by age 3. Female sex is more commonly assigned (constructing a functional vagina more likely than functional penis) and most children adopt assigned sex.

SEXUAL PREFERENCE: Whether the individual prefers male or female sexual partners or has no preference (bisexual).

CLINICAL APPROACH

There are no epidemiologic data on the prevalence of gender dysphoria in children, adolescents, or adults. Males seem to be more affected than females. These individuals often suffer internal and external conflict and ridicule and need to be approached with sensitivity. They often face barriers to getting help in the health care system ranging from stigmatization by health care providers to insurance not covering needed procedures to providers who are sensitive to their situation but lack the expertise to effectively help.

In order to fully assess the origins of the patient's gender identity, a thorough medical history and physical examination, a detailed psychiatric evaluation with psychological testing, karyotyping in the cases of individuals who had ambiguous genitalia at birth, and an endocrine evaluation of sexual hormones are required prior to any hormonal therapies or surgery. Patients may not always be aware of their medical history of ambiguous genitalia if sexual assignment surgery was performed as an infant.

It is especially important to assess whether the patient's cross-gender identification is because of the presence of other psychiatric disorders. Approximately 45% of patients presenting with cross-gender identification are eventually found to have this as part of another psychiatric disorder, most commonly personality disorders, mood disorders, dissociative disorders, and psychotic disorders.

According to the minimum standards of the Harry Benjamin International Gender Dysphoria Association, the real-life experience of living in the community in the desired sex role for at least 3 months before hormonal reassignment, and 12 months before surgical reassignment, is recommended. When participation in a real-life experience is successful, there is a much higher probability of a positive outcome for sex reassignment. Following protocols of this type, 85% to 97% of individuals report being satisfied with their rehabilitation.

The most common issue in the differential diagnosis for gender dysphoria is recognizing simple nonconformity with stereotypic sex role behavior. For example, this includes being a "tomboy" as a girl or a "sissy" as a boy. Gender dysphoria goes far beyond this type of behavior. There is a profound disturbance in the patient's sense of identity regarding being a male or a female.

Homosexuality is not seen as a psychiatric disorder.

Transvestic fetishism, cross-dressing in the clothes of the other sex, serves to create sexual excitement. Patients displaying these behaviors generally do not have other symptoms of gender identity disorder such as childhood cross-gender behaviors and their gender identity matches their assigned sex.

In schizophrenia, delusions can occur in which patients believe that they are members of the other sex. However, these individuals actually believe that they *are* members of the other sex. Patients with gender identity disorder usually say that they *feel* as if they are members of the other sex but do not actually believe that they *are*.

CASE CORRELATION

- See Case 6 for patients who might (although rarely) present with delusions of belonging to some other gender. These patients have other psychotic symptoms (other delusions, hallucinations, or thought disorders) as well, distinguishing them from patients with gender dysphoria. In the absence of other psychotic symptoms, the belief that one is misassigned to the wrong gender is not considered a delusion.

COMPREHENSION QUESTIONS

36.1 A 35-year-old man being seen for major depression shares that he enjoys dressing as a woman and masturbating in private. He finds cross-dressing very arousing sexually but is married and his wife has become aware of this. She is very upset and there have been marital problems over his behavior. At work and in other settings he functions in typical male roles and activities. He had two sexual experiences with men before he got married. He feels very committed to his marriage and finds his wife sexually attractive. The best diagnosis for this patient would be which of the following?

A. Mixed personality disorder with schizotypal and borderline features

B. Gender dysphoria

C. Transsexual fetishism

D. No diagnosis

E. Body dysmorphic disorder

36.2 Gender dysphoria with a sexual attraction to males has been diagnosed in a 15-year-old boy sent to a psychiatrist. His parents are extremely unhappy with the boy's insistence on wearing women's clothes and want the psychiatrist to provide therapy "so that he won't think like this anymore." The boy is willing to talk to the psychiatrist but only if he can discuss the problems caused by the social ostracism he endures because of his wish to be a woman. Which of the following actions should the psychiatrist take?

A. Inform the patient that his gender dysphoria will likely remit in time with psychotherapy alone.

B. Inform the patient that psychotherapy has been found to be helpful but that sexual reassignment surgery is also an option once he is an adult.

C. Inform the parents that their child will likely only experiment with homosexual behavior and will turn to heterosexuality once he is an adult.

D. Inform the parents that they should forbid their son to wear women's clothes.

E. Inform the patient's school that mechanisms must be put in place to reduce his social ostracism.

36.3 A 29-year-old man with a diagnosis of gender dysphoria wishes to undergo sex reassignment surgery. Which of the following treatment steps is strongly related to a positive outcome of sex reassignment?

A. Screening the patient for psychopathology

B. Treating the patient with an antidepressant before surgery

C. Treating the patient with hormones

D. Real-life experience in the community

E. Ongoing supportive psychotherapy

36.4 Patients with schizophrenia or other psychotic disorders may present with delusional claims of cross-gender issues. Which of the following pieces of history would suggest a male patient's claim of cross-gender identity is due to delusions?

A. The patient says he feels as if he is a member of the other sex but does not actually believe that he is a member of the other sex.

B. He has felt that he was the wrong gender from a young age.

C. He dresses in the attire of the other sex.

D. He actually believes he is a member of the other sex.

ANSWERS

36.1 **C.** This individual has transvestic fetishism. He has a male gender identity and is comfortable with male role function. He cross-dresses for sexual excitement but it has a negative impact on his marriage. There is nothing present to support a diagnosis of personality disorder, that is, he does not seem to have problems functioning at home or at work in his life in general. He also does not seem to have symptoms supportive of body dysmorphic disorder—he does not seem displeased or disgusted with his body shape or presence/appearance of sexual organs per se. While it is true that bisexuality and homosexuality are not psychiatric diagnoses, transvestic fetishism is characterized as such.

36.2 **B.** Gender dysphoria can be treated with psychotherapy and sex reassignment rehabilitation. Psychotherapy alone has not been found to be effective in relieving gender dysphoria and does not stop patients from continuing to be preoccupied with altering their sexual characteristics.

36.3 **D.** According to the minimum standards of the Harry Benjamin International Gender Dysphoria Association, the real-life experience of living in the community in the desired sex role for at least 3 months before hormonal reassignment, and 12 months before surgical reassignment, is recommended, because these experiences are correlated with a positive outcome.

36.4 **D.** Gender dysphoria begins at a young age and individuals with this disorder frequently cross-dress. They realize what their physical assigned sex is but feel that they should be a member of the opposite sex. Individuals with delusions actually believe they are a member of the opposite sex even without sex change surgery (a male who believes he is physically a female even with male anatomy).

CLINICAL PEARLS

► Patients with gender dysphoria feel as if they should have been born a member of the other sex.

► In the diagnosis of gender dysphoria, specifiers are used that identify the sexual attraction of the patient to others: sexually attracted to males, females, both, or neither.

► Psychotherapy should address, primarily, the problems these patients have with social ostracism and conflict.

► Patients with gender identity issues should be asked how they prefer to be referred to.

► Sexual reassignment surgery is an option for such patients.

REFERENCES

Menvielle E, Gomez-Lobo V. Management of children and adolescents with gender dysphoria. *J Pediatr Adolesc Gynecol.* 2011;24(4):183-188.

Roberts TK, Fantz CR. Barriers to quality health care for the transgender population. *Clin Biochem.* 2014;47(10-11):983-987.

Sadock BJ, Sadock VA, Ruiz P. *Kaplan and Sadock's Synopsis of Psychiatry: Behavioral Sciences/Clinical Psychiatry.* 11th ed. Baltimore, MD: Lippincott Williams & Wilkins; 2014.

A 15-year-old girl is brought to a psychiatrist by her parents because they are concerned that she might be depressed. The parents had no complaints until 2 or 3 years ago. The patient's grades have fallen because she cuts classes. She gets into fights, and her parents claim that she hangs out with the "wrong crowd"; some nights she does not come home until well past her curfew.

The patient says that there is "nothing wrong" with her and that she wants her parents to "butt out of her life." She claims that she is sleeping and eating well. She says she skips school to hang out with her friends and admits that they frequently steal food from a convenience store and spend time watching movies at one of their homes. She claims that she fights only to prove that she is as tough as her friends but admits that she often picks on younger students. She shows limited guilt or remorse about this. She seems cold and uncaring about how her behavior might affect others. She is not concerned about her grades and just wants her parents to "lay off" and let her enjoy her youth. She denies the use of drugs or alcohol other than occasionally at parties. Her blood alcohol level is zero, and the results of a urinalysis are negative for drugs of abuse.

▶ What is the most likely diagnosis?
▶ What treatment should be started?

ANSWERS TO CASE 37:
Conduct Disorder

Summary: A 15-year-old girl gets into fights, intimidates others, steals, skips school (resulting in falling grades), and breaks her curfew regularly. She does not exhibit any remorse over her behavior. She denies having any depressive symptoms such as sleep or appetite disturbances and says she feels pretty good about herself. She does not report any suicidal or homicidal thoughts.

- **Most likely diagnosis:** Conduct disorder (CD).

- **Best treatment:** A multisystemic treatment (MST) approach with involvement of parents and teachers. The treatment of CD can be difficult. There are only a few studies that look at the treatment of CD systematically. Over the last few years, a number of new studies have begun to look at how to treat CD. In terms of behavioral interventions, multisystemic therapeutic approaches are quite helpful. These approaches combine a well-coordinated plan to help parents develop new skills at home, such as parent–child interaction training, to help the relationship between parents/caregivers and the child. In addition, it is helpful to teach classroom social skills, institute playground behavior programs, and facilitate and encourage communication between teachers and parents. Psychopharmacologic interventions also show some promise. Many children with CD have a comorbid diagnosis of attention deficit hyperactivity disorder (ADHD). This needs to be identified and treated. Even if a child does not meet full diagnostic criteria for ADHD, there is evidence that CD is amenable to treatment with stimulants—often leading to less aggression and impulsiveness. Although no medication has yet to be approved for use in children with conduct disorder, there is a growing body of evidence that atypical neuroleptics may be useful in helping to control the aggression associated with this diagnosis. In particular, risperidone seems to be helpful, but olanzapine, quetiapine, and aripiprazole may also be useful. Behavioral and cognitive behavioral group-based parenting interventions are effective and cost effective for improving child conduct problems, parental mental health, and parenting skills in the short term.

ANALYSIS

Objectives

1. Understand the diagnostic criteria for CD.

2. Understand when medications should be used in CD.

Considerations

This patient presents with a pattern of aggression, truancy, deceitfulness, theft, and serious violations of the rules of expected behavior for her age that fits the

Table 37–1 • DIAGNOSTIC CRITERIA FOR CONDUCT DISORDER

Persistent, repetitive pattern of behavior that infringes on the basic rights of others or violates major age-appropriate societal norms. This pattern is manifested by the presence of at least three of the following symptoms in the last 12 months with at least one occurring in the last 6 months. The symptom categories are:
  • Aggression toward people or animals (7 symptoms in category)
  • Destruction of property (2 symptoms in category)
  • Deceitfulness or theft (3 symptoms in category)
  • A serious rule violation (3 symptoms in category)

The person can have more than one symptom in a category.
The disturbance causes clinically significant impairment.
If the patient is older than age 18, the criteria for antisocial personality disorder are not met.

criteria for CD (Table 37–1). This behavior has been ongoing for 2 or 3 years and appears to be at least in part peer-mediated. Although her parents are concerned that she might be depressed, she appears engaged and nonchalant. It is important to collect information about substance use or abuse as well. Girls with CD have lower general intelligence and poorer performance on visuospatial, executive function, and academic achievement domains. School performance and programming should always be assessed. This often requires gathering information from sources outside of the child, such as teachers, parents, siblings, and so on. It is important to remember that CD is a mental illness that is amenable to treatment. Some studies have demonstrated that boys with CD and comorbid ADHD show brain abnormalities in frontolimbic areas which are typically observed in adults with antisocial behavior. Psychopathic traits consist of a callous-unemotional component and an impulsive-antisocial component, which are associated with two core impairments. The first is a reduced empathic response to the distress of other individuals, which primarily reflects reduced amygdala responsiveness to distress cues; the second is deficits in decision making and in reinforcement learning, which reflects dysfunction in the ventromedial prefrontal cortex and striatum. Without treatment, a large percentage of these children will go on to develop antisocial personality disorder and possible imprisonment. Treatment as children reduces the likelihood of this.

APPROACH TO:
Conduct Disorder

DEFINITIONS

ANTISOCIAL PERSONALITY DISORDER: Pervasive disregard for and violation of rights of others starting by age 15.

WRAPAROUND: A framework for organizing services in high-needs, mentally ill children involving a number of core values including cultural sensitivity, strengths focus, creativity, natural supports, and team approaches.

CLINICAL APPROACH

Differential Diagnosis

Oppositional defiant disorder (ODD) is also characterized by a negative behavior pattern; however, the offences **do not typically cause significant harm to others** or involve violations of major societal norms. The behavior cannot occur exclusively in the context of an episode of mania or as a reaction to some stressor (in which case, adjustment disorder with disturbance of conduct is diagnosed instead). Finally, **antisocial personality disorder** is diagnosed if the symptoms appear **after the age of 18. Many clinicians pragmatically see ODD as a precursor to CD, which is a precursor to antisocial personality disorder.**

WORKING WITH CHILDREN AND THEIR FAMILIES

Conduct disorder is a very difficult disorder to treat, requiring participation from a number of systems involved with the child. The recommended interventions require considerable effort and change on the part of the parents who are often frustrated and feel hopeless. By the time the family comes in for evaluation, many years of maladaptive behavior and parental responses to this behavior have already passed. **The parents have lost control of their home and their child, and a great effort will be required to make an impact on the situation.** The child has also learned that even if the parents change for a while, the change is not likely to last. He or she **can simply outlast the latest parental efforts** or "up the ante" on the problematic behavior. However, it is important to note that with appropriate community interventions and support, such as with wraparound programs or MST, the outcome of this disorder can be hopeful. More than just about any other psychiatric illness in children, the prognosis is related to the degree in which one can organize a community-oriented intervention.

> ## CASE CORRELATION
>
> - See Case 3 and Case 12 for patients that might also present with conduct problems. ADHD patients are often hyperactive and impulsive, though this behavior does not violate social norms or the rights of others. Patients with major depressive disorder may be irritable or have conduct problems (especially in childhood and adolescence) but the course of their illness is also marked by mood symptoms, while conduct disordered patients exhibit the behavior problems in the absence of these.

COMPREHENSION QUESTIONS

37.1 For a patient with conduct disorder, which neuroleptic medication has been found the most useful?

 A. Haldol

 B. Lithium

 C. Methylphenidate

 D. Risperidone

 E. Latuda

37.2 Which evidence-based treatment is likely most cost effective for treatment of conduct disorder?

 A. Parent training

 B. Intensive outpatient (IOP)

 C. Incarceration

 D. Military school

 E. Corporal punishment

37.3 Which of the following treatments is best employed to treat comorbid depressive symptoms of an adolescent with CD?

 A. Multisystemic therapy

 B. Attendance in group therapy

 C. An antidepressant medication

 D. Treatment of the family to address the underlying reasons for the depression

 E. Helping the adolescent change schools

ANSWERS

37.1 **D.** Risperidone. The other medications are either not neuroleptics or are a neuroleptic with little or no evidence of effectiveness with conduct disorder.

37.2 **A.** Parent training. Group-based behavioral and cognitive behavioral treatment has demonstrated effectiveness as well as cost effectiveness.

37.3 **C.** If the criteria for a comorbid condition are met, this disorder should be the first target of psychopharmacologic intervention.

> ## CLINICAL PEARLS

▶ Conduct disorder can be a predecessor of antisocial personality disorder.

▶ Oppositional defiant disorder can be a predecessor of conduct disorder.

▶ Treatment of CD is very difficult and typically involves a community-oriented and highly organized treatment approach.

▶ When there are comorbid psychiatric conditions, they should be the target of psychopharmacologic interventions.

▶ Conduct disorder can be diagnosed prior to age 18, whereas antisocial disorder cannot be diagnosed until after age 18.

REFERENCES

Blair RJ. The neurobiology of psychopathic traits in youths. *Nat Rev Neurosci.* Nov 2013;14(11): 786-799. doi: 10.1038/nrn3577. Epub Oct 9, 2013.

Furlong M, McGilloway S, Bywater T, Hutchings J, Smith SM, Donnelly M. Cochrane review: behavioural and cognitive-behavioural group-based parenting programmes for early-onset conduct problems in children aged 3 to 12 years (Review). *Evid Based Child Health.* Mar 7, 2013;8(2):318-692. doi: 10.1002/ebch.1905.

Loy JH, Merry SN, Hetrick SE, Stasiak K. Atypical antipsychotics for disruptive behaviour disorders in children and youths. *Cochrane Database Syst Rev.* Sep 12, 2012;9:CD008559. doi: 10.1002/14651858.CD008559.pub2.

Sadock BJ, Sadock VA, Ruiz P. *Kaplan and Sadock's Synopsis of Psychiatry: Behavioral Sciences/Clinical Psychiatry.* 11th ed. Baltimore, MD: Lippincott Williams & Wilkins; 2014.

A 45-year-old married man presents to his primary care physician with a chief complaint of fatigue lasting for the past 9 months. He states that he goes to sleep easily enough but then wakes up repeatedly throughout the night. He has had this problem since he was injured on the job 9 months ago. On further questioning, he reports low mood, especially regarding not being able to do his job. He states that his alcohol consumption is 6 to 12 beers a day, as well as several ounces of hard liquor to "take the edge off the pain." He discloses that it takes more alcohol than it used to in order to "get me relaxed." The patient states he has experienced several blackouts caused by drinking during the past 2 months and admits that he often has a drink of alcohol first thing in the morning to keep him from feeling shaky. Despite receiving several reprimands at work for tardiness and poor performance and his wife threatening to leave him, he has been unable to stop drinking.

On his mental status examination, the patient is alert and oriented to person, place, and time. He appears rather haggard, but his hygiene is good. His speech is of normal rate and tone, and he is cooperative with the physician. His mood is noted to be depressed, and his affect is congruent, although full range. Otherwise, no abnormalities are noted.

▶ What is the most likely diagnosis for this patient?
▶ What are some of the medical complications resulting from this disorder?

ANSWERS TO CASE 38:
Alcohol Use Disorder

Summary: A 45-year-old man comes to see his physician with a chief complaint of fatigue. Because of his heavy drinking, he has received several reprimands at work and his wife has threatened to leave him. He drinks 6 to 12 beers a day plus several ounces of hard liquor. He reports blackouts, an inability to quit drinking, tolerance for alcohol, and likely withdrawal symptoms. He has tried to quit on several occasions but has been unable to do so.

- **Most likely diagnosis:** Alcohol use disorder.

- **Commonly associated medical complications:** Withdrawal seizures, delirium tremens, Wernicke-Korsakoff syndrome (encephalopathy, anterograde amnesia), cerebellar degeneration, peripheral neuropathy, fetal alcohol syndrome (low birth weight, mental retardation, facial and cardiac abnormalities), hepatic encephalopathy, malabsorption syndromes, pancreatitis, cardiomyopathy, macrocytic anemia (increased MCV), and an increased incidence of trauma (all types).

ANALYSIS

Objectives

1. Recognize alcohol use disorder in a patient.

2. Be familiar with the many medical complications that are caused by the excessive use of alcohol.

Considerations

A 45-year-old man comes to see his physician with a chief complaint of fatigue. He has not been sleeping well for the past several months, and the pattern he describes is characteristic of alcohol use disorder. His wife has threatened to leave him, and his job is in jeopardy, but despite this, he is unable to quit drinking. He drinks 6 to 12 beers plus several ounces of hard liquor per day. He reports blackouts, an inability to quit drinking, tolerance (it takes more alcohol to "make him relaxed"), and withdrawal symptoms (shakes).

> APPROACH TO:
> ## Alcohol Use Disorder

DEFINITIONS

DELIRIUM TREMENS: A delirium characterized by disorientation, fluctuation in the level of consciousness, elevated vital signs, and tremors because of an abrupt reduction in or cessation of heavy alcohol use that has lasted for a prolonged period of time.

WERNICKE ENCEPHALOPATHY: An acute, usually **reversible,** encephalopathy resulting from a **thiamine deficiency** and characterized by the **triad of delirium, ophthalmoplegia (typically sixth nerve palsy), and ataxia.**

KORSAKOFF SYNDROME: May be referred to as Korsakoff psychosis, although not a psychotic disorder. It is an alcohol-induced, persisting amnestic disorder (alcohol-induced neurocognitive disorder according to the *DSM-5*) characterized by an anterograde amnesia, classically with confabulation. It is usually **irreversible** and is also caused by a **thiamine deficiency.**

CLINICAL APPROACH

Alcohol-related disorders are the most common substance-related disorders. Alcohol is associated with damage to almost every organ system in the body, particularly with increased rates of cancer (esophagus, stomach, and other parts of the gastrointestinal tract), cardiovascular disease (hypertension, cardiomyopathy), and hepatic disease (liver cirrhosis, pancreatitis). In the United States, 40% of individuals have experienced an alcohol-related adverse event (eg, a blackout, driving while intoxicated [DWI], missing work, automobile accident). The 12-month prevalence for alcohol use disorder is approximately 4.9% for women and 12.4% for men. Adoption and twin studies indicate a genetic basis; the risk of alcohol use disorder is three to four times higher in close relatives of people with alcohol use disorder.

Alcoholics have a much higher prevalence of comorbid psychiatric disorders. Major depressive disorder is comorbid in approximately 20% of individuals with alcohol use disorder, and therefore should be evaluated carefully. **Alcohol is associated with up to 50% of all homicides and more than 25% of suicides.** Four percent of all deaths worldwide are due to alcohol use. Alcohol use is also strongly associated with illicit drug use.

Alcohol use disorder can be characterized by a variety of drinking patterns. For example, some individuals require a large amount of alcohol each day, others drink heavily only on weekends, and some binge heavily for days followed by days of no alcoholic intake at all. Alcohol use disorder is also associated with behaviors such as an inability to cut down or stop drinking, repeated attempts to curb drinking (going on the wagon), binging (intoxication throughout the day for a minimum of 2 days), episodes of amnesia (blackouts), and drinking despite a known medical disorder that is exacerbated by the intake of alcohol (Table 38–1). Individuals with alcohol use disorder show impairment in social and occupational functioning.

Table 38–1 • DIAGNOSTIC CRITERIA FOR ALCOHOL USE DISORDER[a]
Two or more of the following are present within a 12-month period:
• Alcohol taken in larger amounts or over a longer period of time than was intended
• Persistent desire or unsuccessful efforts to cut down or control alcohol use
• A great deal of time spent obtaining alcohol, using alcohol, or recovering from the effects of alcohol
• Craving or a strong desire to use alcohol
• Recurrent alcohol use resulting in a failure to fulfill major obligations at work, home, or school
• Continued alcohol use despite having persistent or recurrent social or interpersonal problems caused by alcohol
• Important social, occupational, or recreational activities given up or reduced because of alcohol use
• Alcohol use continued despite the knowledge that it causes or worsens physical or psychological problems (eg, ulcer disease, depression)
• Tolerance for alcohol
• Withdrawal symptoms (eg, elevated vital signs, tremors, delirium tremens, seizures)

[a]*It is important to note that these are the same general criteria for all substances of abuse.*

This behavior can be manifested by violence toward others, absence from work, legal difficulties (DWI, intoxicated behavior), and finally, strained relationships with friends and family.

TREATMENT

The essential treatment of alcohol use disorder rests with the patient controlling his or her alcohol use, which is usually best achieved through total abstinence and relapse prevention. Twelve-step programs such as the one sponsored by Alcoholics Anonymous (AA) are extremely helpful, as they address important issues necessary for recovery. These issues include denial that one has an addiction (prevalent in all addictive disorders), feelings of responsibility and blame, discouraging the enabling behavior of loved ones, establishing social support systems (through a sponsor), and a sense of hope within a community. Membership in these groups is free; they often meet daily and are located throughout the United States.

The first-line pharmacologic treatment option is naltrexone, an opioid antagonist believed to reduce craving for alcohol through blocking the dopaminergic (rewarding) pathways in the brain. Naltrexone can be given orally or via a long-acting injectable. Meta-analyses have found it to be more effective than placebos in reducing craving, maintaining abstinence, and reducing heavy drinking.

Another medication option is acamprosate (Campral). The precise mechanism is unknown, but it is believed to stabilize glutaminergic functioning. Although the studies are more mixed than with naltrexone, acamprosate has shown to help promote abstinence, as well.

Disulfiram (Antabuse) is a medication that blocks the enzyme acetaldehyde dehydrogenase. The purpose of taking this drug is to deter a patient from consuming alcohol, as concurrent use with alcohol (or alcohol-containing products such as foods and aftershave) causes extremely uncomfortable (and in high doses potentially fatal) physical symptoms. For this reason, the patient needs to be motivated, responsible, and without significant cognitive deficits, so that adherence with treatment instructions can be ensured.

Chronic alcohol use results in the depletion of many vitamins, most notably **thiamine.** This occurs because of both decreased absorption and poor nutrition often seen in individuals with alcohol dependence. It is therefore important for any individual with a pattern of heavy, chronic alcohol consumption to receive vitamin supplements. **Acute thiamine depletion causes Wernicke encephalopathy, and chronic thiamine depletion causes Korsakoff syndrome.** Wernicke encephalopathy is not an uncommon presentation in the emergency department setting. If suspected, intravenous administration of thiamine should be given to all patients *prior* to intravenous glucose administration, as administering glucose in a thiamine-deficient state will exacerbate the process of cell death and worsen the condition.

CASE CORRELATION

- See also Case 49 for patients who, in the majority of cases, have a coexisting alcohol use disorder. For individuals with antisocial personality disorder, it is important to diagnose the coexisting alcohol use disorder if it is present, because the personality disorder is associated with a worse prognosis for the alcohol use disorder.

COMPREHENSION QUESTIONS

38.1 A 58-year-old man with hypertension and hyperlipidemia is admitted to the medicine unit for intravenous antibiotics for treatment of pneumonia. After 2 days he becomes increasingly anxious, with complaints of "shaking" and sweating. His vitals demonstrate a temperature of 100.4 F, blood pressure of 170/97 mm Hg, pulse of 110 beats per min, and respirations of 16 breaths/min. On examination he appears diaphoretic and flushed, with a coarse tremor of his upper extremities bilaterally. Laboratory test results are significant for slightly elevated AST, ALT, and GGT. Review of his chart reveals a long history of daily, heavy alcohol use. When confronted with this information, the patient reluctantly admits to drinking "one fifth" of vodka plus several beers daily, with little sobriety. His last drink was the day prior to admission. Administration of which of the following medications would be the most appropriate for this patient?

A. Acamprosate

B. Disulfiram

C. Lorazepam

D. Naltrexone

E. Thiamine

38.2 The above patient in Question 38.1 is treated appropriately, with normalization of his vitals and laboratory test results, and he is released from the hospital after 8 days. He immediately enrolls in an outpatient rehabilitation program, for which he is required to attend 3 times per week, as well as AA meetings daily. He is quite hopeful about his recovery and denies significant depression, although he is greatly concerned about a possible relapse. While he is interested in medication to minimize his risk, he admits to being "very forgetful" with medications. Which of the following medications would be most appropriate to initiate in this patient?

A. Acamprosate

B. Disulfiram

C. Lorazepam

D. Naltrexone

E. Sertraline

38.3 A 48-year-old woman is brought to the emergency department. She is unresponsive to questions, stumbles around the room, and is agitated. On physical examination, you notice that she smells of alcohol, and she is not cooperative during the remainder of the examination. Administration of what medicine would be the most appropriate initial treatment?

A. Antipsychotic

B. Benzodiazepine

C. Disulfiram

D. Glucose

E. Thiamine

38.4 A 60-year-old man is brought to the emergency room by his wife for "confusion." She reluctantly confides to the staff that he is a "heavy drinker," and that he has drunk up to a case of beer almost every day for the past 30 years. Although he has not changed his alcohol intake significantly, over the past year he has eaten less, preferring alcohol to large meals. She has noticed a gradual weight loss as a result. His last drink was earlier this day. Which of the following would be the most likely finding on the mental status examination of this patient?

A. Confabulation

B. Delusions

C. Elevated affect

D. Fluctuating consciousness

E. Loose associations

ANSWERS

38.1 **C.** This patient is most likely experiencing acute alcohol withdrawal, characterized by signs of sympathetic nervous system stimulation, such as elevated vital signs, diaphoresis, flushing, tremor, as well as insomnia and anxiety. It can occur anywhere between 1 and 4 days after cessation or significant reduction in alcohol intake. This patient's history, clinical presentation, and laboratory results are consistent with a history of regular, heavy alcohol use. Other complications of alcohol withdrawal include withdrawal seizures (12-48 hours after the last drink) and delirium tremens (24-96 hours after the last drink). The mainstay of treatment for alcohol withdrawal is with benzodiazepines (eg, lorazepam, oxazepam), either tapering the dose over several days, or (in mild-to-moderate withdrawal), with a symptom-triggered approach, utilizing the Clinical Institute Withdrawal Assessment (CIWA) scale. Acamprosate and naltrexone are not appropriate for treating alcohol withdrawal, rather they are used in some cases to reduce craving and promote abstinence. Disulfiram is also not used to manage alcohol withdrawal, instead it is used as a deterrent to prevent a patient from consuming alcohol. Thiamine, while often depleted in alcoholics and necessary in the treatment of Wernicke-Korsakoff syndrome, also does not address the pathophysiology of alcohol withdrawal.

38.2 **D.** Naltrexone, an opioid antagonist, has been shown to help reduce craving, maintain abstinence, and reduce heavy drinking. Another advantage is that it can be given in a long-acting injectable form, beneficial in patients (like this one) who demonstrate poor adherence with medications. While acamprosate has also demonstrated benefit in promoting abstinence, the evidence is not as strong as for naltrexone, and adherence would likely be an issue in this individual. Disulfiram can be useful as a deterrent in patients, but should be reserved for motivated patients who are reliable with taking medications. Benzodiazepines such as lorazepam are used for treatment of alcohol withdrawal and are not indicated (and even contraindicated) in patients with alcohol use disorder for maintenance therapy. Selective serotonin reuptalce inhibitors like sertraline have not demonstrated efficacy in patients with alcohol use disorder in the absence of an additional mood disorder (such as major depressive disorder).

38.3 **E.** The most appropriate treatment is the immediate administration of thiamine. This patient presents with Wernicke encephalopathy, characterized by the triad of delirium, ataxia, and ophthalmoplegia. Thiamine must be given *prior to* glucose in patients suspected of having this disorder.

38.4 **A.** This patient has a long history of heavy, regular alcohol use and likely malnutrition. A common sequelae of this is chronic thiamine deficiency, resulting in Korsakoff syndrome. Korsakoff syndrome is characterized by an anterograde amnesia; this memory impairment is often (poorly) compensated for by the patient's confabulation, or filling in the missing memories with false information.

CLINICAL PEARLS

▶ Alcohol use disorder is characterized by the recurrent use of alcohol, craving, tolerance, withdrawal, as well as resulting occupational, academic, or interpersonal problems, or use in potentially dangerous situations.

▶ Alcohol withdrawal occurs between 1 and 4 days after cessation or reduction in alcohol use: withdrawal symptoms/elevated vitals—12 to 48 hours; seizures—24 to 48 hours; delirium tremens—24 to 96 hours.

▶ The mainstay of treatment for alcohol withdrawal is benzodiazepines.

▶ Both Wernicke and Korsakoff syndromes are caused by a thiamine deficiency. The classic triad of Wernicke syndrome is encephalopathy, ataxia, and ophthalmoplegia. The hallmark of Korsakoff syndrome is amnesia, especially anterograde amnesia.

▶ In a patient with suspected Wernicke encephalopathy, thiamine should be administered intravenously *prior* to glucose.

REFERENCES

American Psychiatric Association. *Diagnostic and Statistical Manual of Mental Disorders.* 5th ed. Arlington, VA: American Psychiatric Publishing; 2013.

Brière FN, Rohde P, Seeley JR, Klein D, Lewinsohn PM. Comorbidity between major depression and alcohol use disorder from adolescence to adulthood. *Compr Psychiatry.* 2014;55:526-533.

Kaplan MS, Huguet N, McFarland BH, Caetano R. Use of alcohol before suicide in the United States. *Ann Epidemiol.* 2014;24:588-592.

Kuhns JB, Exum ML, Clodfelter TA, Bottia MC. The prevalence of alcohol-involved homicide offending: a meta-analytic review. *Homicide Studies.* Aug 2014;18(3):251-270.

Maisel NC, Blodgett JC, Wilbourne PL, Humphreys K, Finney JW. Meta-analysis of naltrexone and acamprosate for treating alcohol use disorders: when are these medications most helpful? *Addiction.* 2013;108:275-293.

Nelson DE, Jarman DW, Rehm J, et al. Alcohol-attributable cancer deaths and years of potential life lost in the United States. *Am J Public Health.* April 2013:103(4):641–648.

Sullivan JT, Sykora K, Schneiderman J, Naranjo CA, Sellers EM. Assessment of alcohol withdrawal: the revised clinical institute withdrawal assessment for alcohol scale (CIWA-Ar). *Br J Addict.* 1989;84(11):1353.

A 29-year-old single woman is brought to the emergency department by the police after they picked her up attempting to break into a grocery store. When they apprehended her, they noticed that she "seemed high" and that she was sweating with dilated pupils. The patient admits to "doping" daily for the majority of the past year and losing 30 lb in the past 6 months. She claims that her habit now costs more than $100 per day, although she used to get the "same high" for $20. When intoxicated, she describes her mood as "really good" and that she has "loads" of energy. When she does not use, she craves for the drug, becomes very sleepy, feels depressed, and has a large appetite. She has tried to quit on numerous occasions, even entering an inpatient treatment program at one point, but she always quickly begins using again. The patient used to work part-time as a secretary, but she lost her job as she was chronically late and, in fact, stole money in order to pay her dealer. She freely admits that she was trying to rob the grocery store to "pay off my debts."

► What is/are the most likely diagnosis/diagnoses?

ANSWER TO CASE 39:

Stimulant (Cocaine) Intoxication and Stimulant (Cocaine) Use Disorder

Summary: A 29-year-old woman was arrested while attempting to rob a grocery store. She lost her job because she was always late and stole from her employer to support her habit. The patient needed increased amounts of her drug of choice to get high, and she suffers from cravings, hypersomnia, depression, and hyperphagia when she is unable to obtain it. When intoxicated, the patient notes a feeling of euphoria and heightened energy. She has tried to stop using but has been unsuccessful. Upon presentation, she displays mydriasis, diaphoresis, and has lost 30 lb in a short period of time.

- **Most likely diagnoses:** Stimulant (cocaine) intoxication and stimulant (cocaine) use disorder.

ANALYSIS

Objectives

1. Recognize substance use disorder in a patient.

2. Identify the likely drug based on a patient's history and physical examination.

Considerations

This patient exhibits the classic signs of substance use disorder—she has a tolerance for the drug (requires more to achieve the same effect) and withdrawal symptoms when lacking it. She also demonstrates unsuccessful attempts to cut down, a strong desire to use, and continued use of cocaine despite the negative effects it has had on her life. During intoxication, she feels euphoric and energetic, with mydriasis, diaphoresis, and decreased appetite. During withdrawal, she feels depressed, hungry, and sleepy.

APPROACH TO:
Cocaine Use Disorder

CLINICAL APPROACH

The criteria for stimulant (cocaine) use disorder are the same as for all substance use disorders (see Table 38–1). Cocaine intoxication can produce numerous behavioral and physiologic changes (Table 39–1). Note that these are also seen in amphetamine and other stimulant use and intoxication. Individuals can also develop hallucinations (both auditory and visual), paranoia, delusions, and risk-taking behavior (including promiscuity and violence). There can be serious physical health risks associated with cocaine use, including cerebral infarctions, transient ischemic attacks, seizures (including status epilepticus), myocardial infarctions, and cardiomyopathies.

Stimulant (cocaine) withdrawal typically lasts 2 to 4 days, although can be longer in heavy users. The **"crash"** is commonly accompanied by **dysphoria**, irritability, fatigue, increased appetite, psychomotor agitation or retardation, vivid/unpleasant dreams, and insomnia or hypersomnia. Patients can develop marked depressive symptoms with suicidal ideation and can require hospitalization. They frequently experience strong cravings for the drug during the withdrawal period.

DIFFERENTIAL DIAGNOSIS

There are many psychiatric conditions which may be comorbid with stimulant (cocaine) use disorder. Some disorders, including anxiety disorders, antisocial personality disorder, and attention deficit hyperactivity disorder, can predate the development of stimulant (cocaine) use disorder. Patients with stimulant (cocaine) use disorder can also have major depressive disorder, bipolar disorder, cyclothymic

---

Table 39–1 • COCAINE (AND OTHER STIMULANT)-ASSOCIATED BEHAVIORAL AND PHYSICAL CHANGES

Behavioral changes include:
- Euphoria or blunting of feelings
- Hypervigilance or hypersensitivity
- Heightened anxiety or irritability/anger
- Stereotyped behaviors
- Impaired judgment

Physical changes include:
- Dilated pupils
- Autonomic instability such as elevated (or lowered) blood pressure, tachycardia, or bradycardia
- Chills or sweating
- Nausea/vomiting
- Psychomotor agitation or retardation
- Muscle weakness
- Chest pain/arrhythmias
- Confusion, seizures, stupor, dystonias, or coma
- Weight loss

disorder, or various anxiety disorders. Because cocaine also creates depression (in withdrawal), euphoria, aggression, irritability, mood lability, anxiety, and even psychotic symptoms, the diagnosis of a primary mood or psychotic disorder can be difficult if an individual is actively using cocaine. Therefore, a period of abstinence lasting up to several months may be required before an accurate diagnosis of other disorders can be made. In addition, stimulant (cocaine) use disorder is often accompanied by other substance use disorders, especially those associated with opiates and alcohol—these drugs are often used to temper the irritability and hypervigilance that can follow cocaine intoxication and withdrawal.

TREATMENT

Cocaine is a very addictive substance, with studies showing that up to one in six persons who use cocaine will develop a cocaine use disorder. Because cocaine delivers a particularly positive and reinforcing high, most users do not seek treatment voluntarily until the behavioral patterns have resulted in significant impairment in functioning (job and relationship losses, legal consequences) or health problems. Craving for cocaine is often so intense that a patient may need to be initially entered into residential treatment in order to establish abstinence from the drug.

Treatment must be multimodal, including medical, psychological, and social strategies to help the patient establish and maintain abstinence. Frequent unscheduled urine toxicology screenings are essential in both short- and long-term treatment of stimulant (cocaine) use disorder, as denial is a prominent aspect of *all* addictions. Individual and group therapies can focus on support, education, and reduction of denial, as well as on building skills to avoid further drug use. Various behavioral therapies (clinical management, coping skills approaches, motivational interviewing) have been shown to help reduce cocaine use. Narcotics Anonymous sponsors a well-known, widely available, and free group therapy that offers all of the previously mentioned components. Family therapy can also be helpful in confronting both the patient, with the effects of his or her drug-related behavior, and the family, with ways they enable or reinforce the addictive behavior. Social interventions can include abstinence-focused housing programs and vocational training. Unlike in alcohol and opiate addictions, somatic treatments (eg, antidepressants, mood stabilizers, dopamine agonists, and acupuncture) have not been consistently shown to reduce cocaine craving; research in this area continues to be pursued. However, psychotropic medications such as antidepressants, anxiolytics, or mood stabilizers are indicated for treating any comorbid psychiatric illnesses in patients with stimulant (cocaine) use disorder.

CASE CORRELATION

- See also Case 6 and Case 8 for patients who might present with the same symptoms of euphoria and/or hypervigilance which may be present in individuals with stimulant intoxication. Schizophrenia and bipolar disorder, however, are longer lasting than the half-life of a stimulant, and do not present with the signs and symptoms of stimulant intoxication that are described in category C of the diagnostic criteria (tachycardia, pupillary dilation, perspiration or chills, etc).

COMPREHENSION QUESTIONS

39.1 A 50-year-old homeless male veteran is brought to the emergency department by the police for disruptive behavior. On mental status examination, he has an elevated affect, but also has psychomotor agitation and paranoia; he says he "feels fantastic" but is wary of answering any questions, quickly becoming irritated. On physical examination, the patient exhibits a moderately elevated blood pressure and pulse rate. He is most likely intoxicated with which of the following substances?

   A. Alcohol

   B. Barbiturates

   C. Benzodiazepines

   D. Cocaine

   E. Opiates

39.2 Which of the following physical complications would be most likely to occur in the above patient in Question 39.1?

   A. Bradycardia

   B. Chest pain

   C. Delirium

   D. Hypothermia

   E. Respiratory depression

39.3 The above patient in Questions 39.1 and 39.2 is subsequently admitted to a detoxification unit in the hospital. After his euphoria and paranoia resolve, he is able to give a more complete history. He describes a 5-year history of almost daily crack cocaine use, with no periods of sobriety lasting for more than 7 to 10 days. During these periods of sobriety, he feels "depressed," with an increased appetite, disrupted sleep, difficulty concentrating, and fatigue. He describes rare alcohol use and denies other drug use, and his psychiatric review of systems is otherwise negative. Which of the following would be the most appropriate treatment for this patient?

   A. Antidepressant

   B. Dopamine antagonist

   C. Dopamine agonist

   D. Mood stabilizer

   E. Narcotics Anonymous

ANSWERS

39.1 **D.** Cocaine (or other stimulants such as amphetamine) intoxication can present with euphoria, irritability, anxiety, and psychotic symptoms such as paranoia, as well as with elevated vital signs. Conversely, intoxication with alcohol, barbiturates, benzodiazepines, and opiates generally causes depression, somnolence, and depressed vital signs.

39.2 **B.** Cocaine (or other stimulant) intoxication causes numerous physical complications, including chest pain (believed to be from coronary vasospasm), tachycardia, diaphoresis, hypertension, and mydriasis. In severe overdose or when combined with other substances, it may cause seizures; however, delirium or respiratory depression is not commonly seen in intoxication with stimulants such as cocaine.

39.3 **E.** The most beneficial approach to cocaine addiction without additional psychopathology is to stress abstinence and relapse prevention. Narcotics Anonymous meetings are free, easily accessible, approachable, and provide ongoing group and individual support. No medications have been consistently proven to prevent cocaine cravings or relapse. While the patient admits to depressive symptoms when abstinent from cocaine, these symptoms are quite common (and self-limiting) during withdrawal. In addition, the time period (< 2 weeks) is not typical of a major depressive disorder. After 4 to 6 weeks of sobriety, if depressive symptoms are still present, he should be reevaluated with consideration to begin an antidepressant.

CLINICAL PEARLS

▶ Cocaine acts like a stimulant, causing euphoria, anxiety, increased energy/activity, and psychotic symptoms, as well as elevated vital signs, dilated pupils, weight loss, chest pain, and seizures.

▶ Denial is more the rule than the exception regarding a patient's awareness and acknowledgment of cocaine use.

▶ On average, cocaine is cleared from the body within 72 hours, and so a 3-day period following its use is necessary for a patient to yield negative results on urine toxicology screening.

REFERENCES

American Psychiatric Association. *Diagnostic and Statistical Manual of Mental Disorders*. 5th ed. Washington, DC: American Psychiatric Publishing; 2013.

National Survey on Drug Use and Health, 2006, Report no. SMA 07-4293, Office of Applied Studies, Substance Abuse and Mental Health Services Administration. National Survey or Drug Use and Health www.icpsr.umicedu/icpsrweb/SAMHDA/studies/21240. Accessed August 15 2014. Rockville, MD; 2005.

Anthony, JC, Warner, LA, Kessler, RC. Comparative epidemiology of dependence on tobacco, alcohol, controlled substances, and inhalants: basic findings from the National Comorbidity Survey Experimental and Clinical Psychopharmacology. 1994;23:244.

A 56-year-old divorced, unemployed man with a long-standing history of substance abuse presents to the emergency department with abdominal pain, sweats, diarrhea, and body aches. On initial evaluation, the patient is noted to have a watery nose and eyes, a slightly elevated temperature of 100°F (37.8°C), and dilated pupils. His mood is dysphoric, and his affect is irritable and labile. His abdominal examination is benign. Laboratory examinations including electrolytes, complete blood count, liver function tests, amylase, and lipase are all normal. A plain abdominal x-ray showed no clear cause for his abdominal pain.

▶ What is the most likely diagnosis for this patient?
▶ What medications are the most appropriate for alleviating this patient's symptoms?

ANSWERS TO CASE 40:

Opioid Withdrawal

Summary: A 54-year-old man presents with abdominal pain, sweats, diarrhea, and body aches. A physical examination shows pupillary dilation, lacrimation, rhinorrhea, and a mild fever of 100°F (37.8°C). His mood is dysphoric, and he is irritable.

- **Most likely diagnosis:** Opioid withdrawal.

- **Medication to help alleviate symptoms**: Methadone or clonidine.

ANALYSIS

Objectives

1. Recognize opioid withdrawal in a patient.

2. Understand the use of methadone, clonidine, and buprenorphine in ameliorating opioid withdrawal symptoms.

Considerations

Shortly after he ceased using his drug of choice after years of heavy use, this patient began to experience classic signs and symptoms of opioid withdrawal. Whereas opiate intoxication causes apathy, psychomotor retardation, constricted pupils, and drowsiness, opiate withdrawal results in nausea and vomiting, muscle aches, lacrimation, rhinorrhea, diarrhea, diaphoresis, chills, fever, and dilated pupils. These symptoms can develop within hours or days of the last opiate dose, depending on the half-life of the agent used and the individual's tolerance. In general, agents with a short half-life (eg, heroin) tend to induce a rapid, severe withdrawal, whereas opiates with a long half-life (eg, methadone) tend to be associated with a less severe, more gradual (but prolonged) withdrawal course. The introduction of clonidine (an alpha 2-adrenergic agonist) to treat many of the withdrawal symptoms, along with the short-term administration and gradual tapering of methadone (a long-acting opiate) or buprenorphine (a long-acting partial agonist), is effective.

APPROACH TO:
Opioid Withdrawal

CLINICAL APPROACH

Opioid withdrawal is just one of many recognized substance withdrawal syndromes. All these syndromes have in common the development of a substance-specific pattern of symptoms following cessation of use of the drug in question. The drug use is generally heavy and prolonged, and a physiologic dependence develops; thus a withdrawal syndrome occurs on its cessation or with a reduction in use. The symptoms of **opioid withdrawal** specifically include **a depressed or anxious mood, gastrointestinal distress (nausea or vomiting), muscle aches, lacrimation/rhinorrhea, pupillary dilation/piloerection/sweating, diarrhea, yawning, autonomic hyperactivity (including fever), and insomnia.** An intense craving for the drug is also commonly present. Although very uncomfortable, opiate withdrawal is not life threatening unless complicated by a severe preexisting physical condition. For the diagnosis of opioid withdrawal, these symptoms must cause significant distress or impairment in functioning, and they cannot be caused by either another medical condition or mental disorder.

DIFFERENTIAL DIAGNOSIS

The differential diagnosis for opioid withdrawal is generally straightforward because patients experiencing withdrawal are conscious, usually able to give their history, and know when the last dose of their drug was taken. Other withdrawal syndromes do not present in the same way as opioid withdrawal. For example, while patients undergoing alcohol and/or benzodiazepine withdrawal can also demonstrate autonomic hyperactivity, they also typically present with anxiety, restlessness, irritability, and insomnia, as well as hyperreflexia and tremor. As withdrawal progresses, hallucinations or illusions can be seen. In severe cases, seizures, delirium, and death can occur. Withdrawal from stimulants, including cocaine, includes a "crash," as well as fatigue, vivid or unpleasant dreams, insomnia or hypersomnia, hyperphagia, psychomotor agitation or retardation, and depressed mood. Withdrawal from tobacco produces anxiety, depression, irritability, poor concentration, increased appetite, restlessness, and sleep disturbances. Opioid withdrawal generally does not cause tremors, confusion, delirium, or seizures. Patients are seldom lethargic or tired. If any of these former symptoms are present, the concurrent or separate use of other drugs of abuse should be considered.

TREATMENT

A rule of thumb regarding opioid withdrawal symptoms is that the **shorter the duration of action of the drug ingested, the more acute and intense the withdrawal symptoms. The longer the duration of action of the drug being used, the more prolonged, but mild, the symptoms are.** An exception to this rule occurs when an opioid antagonist (eg, naltrexone) is given to a person who is dependent on a long-acting opioid. In this case, the withdrawal symptoms can be severe. **Clonidine can been**

used to decrease the autonomic as well as other symptoms of opioid withdrawal, such as hypertension, tachycardia, sweating, nausea, cramps, diarrhea, lacrimation, and rhinorrhea. It does not, however, remove the cravings for the drug. Blood pressure levels must be monitored carefully if clonidine is used. Its mechanism of action involves binding to alpha 2-adrenergic receptors in the locus ceruleus that share potassium channels with opioids, thereby blunting symptoms of withdrawal. **Methadone** can be used instead of, or in addition to, clonidine. It is given orally, in one daily dose, and is very effective in ameliorating opioid withdrawal syndromes. Unless the patient will subsequently be placed on methadone maintenance, the dose will need to be slowly tapered over several days. **Buprenorphine** (a mixed opioid agonist-antagonist) can also be used in lieu of methadone. It is also administered once daily but in a sublingual form, and should be gradually tapered as well.

> ### CASE CORRELATION
> - See also Case 44 for patients who might also present with anxiety and restlessness. However, opioid withdrawal patients present with rhinorrhea, lacrimation, and pupillary dilation, which do not occur in sedative, hypnotic, or anxiolytic withdrawals.

COMPREHENSION QUESTIONS

40.1 A 25-year-old man arrives to the emergency room with symptoms of gastrointestinal distress, muscle aches, rhinorrhea, lacrimation, and an anxious mood. He states that he "wants to kick this thing once and for all." Which of the following medications would be most helpful in ameliorating his symptoms?

   A. Antabuse

   B. Clonidine

   C. Haloperidol

   D. Lorazepam

   E. Naloxone

40.2 A 30-year-old homeless woman with an 18-year history of daily intravenous heroin use comes into the community rehabilitation clinic asking to be "detoxed" in order to "kick my heroin habit" once and for all. While she is motivated for treatment, she currently is shivering, with rhinorrhea, tearing, gagging, and grabbing her abdomen in pain due to cramps. When questioned about her last use, she claims she used shortly before arriving, but that a peer gave her "something different to shoot up." Which of the following substances would be most likely to cause her current symptoms?

A. Alprazolam

B. Buprenorphine

C. Cocaine

D. Methadone

E. Morphine

40.3 A 32-year-old man with a long-standing heroin addiction has recently started maintenance treatment with methadone. Three days since starting the methadone regimen, he is now experiencing some craving, diarrhea, and mild sweating. His urine toxicology screen is negative for any opiates besides methadone. Which of the following is the most appropriate course of action?

A. Increase the dose of methadone.

B. Decrease the dose of methadone.

C. Keep the dose of methadone the same and assure the patient that the symptoms will subside.

D. Begin clonidine to be taken in addition to the methadone.

E. Put the patient on a 1-week methadone taper program and refer him to Narcotics Anonymous.

ANSWERS

40.1 **B.** Clonidine can be used to help ease the symptoms of opioid withdrawal. It is not an opioid and does not have any addictive properties. However, the withdrawal may not be as painless or rapid as it would be if methadone were used. Blood pressure levels should be monitored when clonidine is used. Antabuse or disulfiram is a treatment option for alcoholics. It is not used to treat acute opioid withdrawal. Haloperidol, an antipsychotic, has no use in treating withdrawal. Lorazepam, a benzodiazepine, is commonly used in the treatment of alcohol withdrawal. Naloxone is used to counter the effects of life-threatening depression of the central nervous respiratory systems from opioid (eg, heroin or methadone) overdose; it would worsen this patient's withdrawal symptoms.

40.2 **B.** This patient is suffering from classic symptoms of opioid withdrawal. Buprenorphine is a partial agonist which, when given to a patient actively using another opiate, will precipitate withdrawal. Alprazolam and cocaine would not present with this clinical picture. Methadone and morphine are opioids which would cause further intoxication, not withdrawal.

40.3 **A.** Clinical signs of withdrawal appearing very early in methadone maintenance treatment of heroin use disorder are an indication that the methadone dose is not sufficient to ameliorate all the withdrawal symptoms. Because the patient is at great risk of returning to the use of heroin at this point in the process, a dose increase (in order to minimize craving and withdrawal) would be appropriate.

CLINICAL PEARLS

▶ The history of a current use of other substances of abuse should always be obtained in the presence of opioid addiction.

▶ A mnemonic that is helpful in remembering the signs and symptoms of opioid withdrawal is SLUDGE—salivation, lacrimation, urination, defecation, gastrointestinal distress, and emesis.

▶ Opioid withdrawal is extremely uncomfortable but is rarely life threatening.

▶ Clonidine, methadone (a long-acting opioid), and buprenorphine (a long-acting mixed opiate agonist-antagonist) are the most beneficial treatments for the relief of opioid withdrawal symptoms.

▶ Loperamide (for loose stools), promethazine (for nausea and vomiting), and ibuprofen (for muscle/joint aches) are useful *adjunctive* treatments for the symptoms of opioid withdrawal.

▶ The presence of dilated pupils, sweating, and anxiety are often the first signs of opioid withdrawal which can be noticed by a physician.

▶ Methadone maintenance programs substitute one opioid for another, but the social and physical advantages gained make it one of the best choices for treatment of opiate addiction.

REFERENCES

Amato L, Davoli M, Minozzi S, Ferroni E, Ali R, Ferri M. Methadone at tapered doses for the management of opioid withdrawal (Review). *The Cochrane Collaboration*. Published by John Wiley & Sons, Ltd; 2013.

American Psychiatric Association. *Diagnostic and Statistical Manual of Mental Disorders*. 5th ed. Washington, DC: American Psychiatric Publishing; 2013.

Gowing L, Farrell MF, Ali R, White JM. Alpha$_2$-adrenergic agonists for the management of opioid withdrawal. *Cochrane Database of Syst Rev*. 2014;3:CD002024.

Sigmon SC, Dunn KE, Saulsgiver K, et al. A randomized, double-blind evaluation of buprenorphine taper duration in primary prescription opioid abusers. *JAMA Psychiatry*. 2013;70(12):1347-1354.

A 50-year-old married man shows up for a new appointment with his internist. He has not seen a physician for many years, and he doesn't take medications except for occasional multivitamins. He describes chronic insomnia and being "easily irritated," although he denies pervasive depression. He also complains of difficulty walking long distances without becoming fatigued and short of breath. He has smoked 1½ packs of cigarettes per day for the last 32 years, smoking a cigarette immediately after waking up and directly before going to sleep; he reluctantly admits to getting up in the middle of the night in order to smoke. He spends most of his work breaks and lunch smoking. He was recently laid off from his job and complains "a pack is too expensive" but "I can't wait for my next cigarette." This has resulted in arguments with his wife. He has attempted to quit smoking "dozens" of times over the last 15 years "but it never lasts more than one-to-two weeks." He drinks several six packs of beer on the weekends and denies drug use, although he smoked marijuana daily for several months in high school.

On physical examination, his vitals are within normal limits except for an elevated blood pressure of 158/92 mm Hg. He has decreased breath sounds bilaterally, with occasional wheezes. The rest of his physical is unremarkable. His laboratory values are normal, as well, with the exception of slightly elevated liver function tests.

▶ What are some of the medical complications resulting from this disorder?
▶ What is the most appropriate approach to promote abstinence?

ANSWERS TO CASE 41:

Tobacco Use Disorder

Summary: A 50-year-old man comes to see his physician for a health maintenance appointment. He complains of insomnia, irritability, and dyspnea on exertion. He gives a 48-pack-year history of cigarette smoking, spending a lot of time smoking, craving, spending too much money despite unemployment, arguments with his spouse because of his ongoing tobacco use, and multiple, unsuccessful attempts to quit smoking. His physical examination demonstrates likely hypertension, as well as evidence of chronic obstructive pulmonary disease and elevated liver function tests, likely from alcohol use.

- **Commonly associated medical complications:** Cardiovascular diseases (eg, heart disease, stroke), chronic obstructive pulmonary disease, cancers, diabetes (as well as perinatal problems such as low birth weight and miscarriage in women).

- **Most appropriate approach:** Interventions which combine behavioral and pharmacologic approaches have shown the greatest success in promoting smoking cessation.

ANALYSIS

Objectives

1. List the many medical complications that are caused by tobacco use.

2. Be familiar with various treatments for promoting abstinence in patients with tobacco use disorder.

Considerations

A 50-year-old man comes to see his new physician with complaints of easily becoming short of breath. He also has had ongoing insomnia and is easily irritated. He has a long history of heavy tobacco use, with an inability to cut down, which has led to marital conflict. His physical examination is consistent with high blood pressure and obstructive pulmonary disease.

APPROACH TO:
Tobacco Use Disorder

CLINICAL APPROACH

Tobacco use, while decreasing in the United States, is increasing in developing countries. The 12-month prevalence for nicotine dependence (according to *DSM-5*) is approximately 13% for adults in the United States. Most, although not all, tobacco users use daily, and many use to relieve withdrawal symptoms (Table 41–1). A majority of adolescents try smoking, although rarely begin after age 21. The diagnostic criteria for tobacco use disorder are the same as that of all substance use disorders.

Tobacco is the leading cause of preventable deaths worldwide. It kills over 5 million people per year (an average of one person every 6 seconds) and kills up to half of all users. Tobacco use is a risk factor for six of the eight leading causes of deaths in the world. Tobacco has been associated with causing multiple medical complications, including numerous cancers (eg, neck, larynx, throat, lung, kidney, liver, bladder, cervix), stroke, aneurysm, coronary artery disease, peripheral vascular disease, cataracts, chronic obstructive pulmonary disease, ectopic pregnancy, infertility, and erectile dysfunction.

Because of its addictive nature, legal status, ease of access, and significant withdrawal syndrome, abstaining from tobacco is extremely difficult for individuals with tobacco use disorder. Most (80%) attempt to quit, but most of those (60%) relapse within 1 week and only 5% remain abstinent. While the majority of patients make multiple attempts, one-half eventually abstain for life.

TREATMENT

Interventions which combine behavioral and pharmacologic approaches have shown the greatest success in promoting smoking cessation. All tobacco users should be encouraged to quit and offered treatment. Both counseling (eg, clinician, group therapy, skills training) and social support (from friends and family) are helpful in treatment.

Nicotine replacement therapy (NRT) includes a nicotine patch, gum, lozenge, inhaler, or spray. There is often benefit with combining the nicotine patch

Table 41–1 • SYMPTOMS COMMONLY SEEN DURING TOBACCO WITHDRAWAL
-Irritability, anger
-Anxiety
-Difficulty concentrating
-Increased appetite
-Restlessness
-Depressed mood
-Insomnia

(a long-acting replacement) and a short-acting formulation (eg, nicotine patch daily with nicotine gum or lozenge as needed for acute cravings).

Treatment with NRT may be combined with other pharmacologic interventions, including bupropion or varenicline. Bupropion is an antidepressant believed to increase the central nervous system levels of both norepinephrine and dopamine. Varenicline is a partial agonist at the alpha-4 beta-2 subunit of the nicotinic acetylcholine receptor. Both have demonstrated efficacy in promoting abstinence. Patients on either of these need to be closely monitored, however, as varenicline and bupropion may cause increased suicidality. Evidence for clear benefit of one medication over the other is lacking.

> ## CASE CORRELATION
> - None

COMPREHENSION QUESTIONS

41.1 A 30-year-old married man presents to your office wanting to "quit smoking cold turkey." He gives a 14-year history of tobacco use, smoking 1 to 1½ packs per day. He has attempted to cut back or stop on his own on numerous occasions, but without lasting success. He feels more motivated now given that his wife is 15 weeks pregnant. Despite education, he is reluctant to try medications and decides to stop suddenly. He sheepishly returns several days later complaining about his inability to stop smoking due to withdrawal symptoms. Which of the following symptoms would be most likely to occur in this patient?

A. Anxiety

B. Decreased appetite

C. Hypersomnia

D. Nausea

E. Tremors

41.2 The patient in Question 41.1 subsequently agrees to a more formal treatment regimen in order to promote cessation. Which of the following would be the most efficacious approach to maintain abstinence?

A. Education

B. Social support

C. Education plus social support

D. Nicotine replacement therapy (NRT)

E. NRT plus social support

41.3 The patient in Question 41.2 is referred to a smoking cessation group and also begun on a nicotine patch daily. After 1 month he returns for follow-up and has decreased his smoking to ½ pack per day. While he denies withdrawal, he occasionally has intense cravings for cigarettes during the day. He is started on bupropion, which is quickly increased to a therapeutic dose. Which of the following side effects would be the most important to monitor for?

A. Activation

B. Decreased appetite

C. Headache

D. Insomnia

E. Suicidality

ANSWERS

41.1 **A.** Withdrawal from tobacco products (nicotine) can be severe and a significant impediment to abstaining from use. Psychological symptoms, such as anxiety, anger, depression, and irritability, as well as physical symptoms, such as increased appetite, insomnia, restlessness, and decreased concentration may occur. Nausea and tremor are not commonly seen with tobacco withdrawal.

41.2 **E.** While education, social support, and NRT are all beneficial in promoting abstinence from tobacco products, the most efficacious approach has been shown to be a combination of behavioral (such as social support) and pharmacologic (such as NRT).

41.3 **E.** Both bupropion and varenicline have demonstrated efficacy in promoting abstinence from tobacco. However, they also have been associated with an increase in suicidal thoughts. While activation, anorexia, headache, and insomnia can occur with bupropion, the emergence of suicidal ideation would be the most concerning side effect.

CLINICAL PEARLS

▶ Tobacco is the leading cause of preventable deaths worldwide.

▶ Tobacco is associated with multiple medical complications, including cancer, stroke, cardiovascular disease, and chronic obstructive pulmonary disease.

▶ Most individuals make multiple attempts to quit, however only one-half eventually abstain.

▶ All tobacco users should be encouraged to quit, and the greatest chance of success is in utilizing both behavioral and pharmacologic treatments.

REFERENCES

American Psychiatric Association. *Diagnostic and Statistical Manual of Mental Disorders.* 5th ed. Arlington, VA: American Psychiatric Publishing; 2013.

Fiore MC, Jaen CR, Baker TB, et al. Treating tobacco use and dependence: 2008 update. US Department of Health and Human Services; 2008.

Stead LF, Lancaster T. Combined pharmacotherapy and behavioural interventions for smoking cessation. *Cochrane Database Syst Rev.* 2012;10:CD008286. doi: 10.1002/14651858.CD008286.pub2.

A clinical practice guideline for treating tobacco use and dependence: a US Public Health Service report. The Tobacco Use and Dependence Clinical Practice Guideline Panel, Staff, and Consortium Representatives. *JAMA.* 2000;283(24):3244.

An 18-year-old man is brought to the emergency department after he became belligerent at a party, screaming, throwing punches at other guests, and ripping a flat screen television off the wall and throwing it through a window. In the emergency department, the patient is unable to provide any kind of history and is so agitated, paranoid, and hostile that he requires placement in four-point leather restraints. One of the patient's friends claims that the patient is normally "a really nice guy" and that his current behavior is completely out of character.

The mental status examination is limited because of the patient's extreme hostility and lack of cooperation. He struggles fiercely against the restraints, his speech is mildly slurred, and he appears to have vertical nystagmus. The patient is unable or unwilling to give any meaningful history, although is clearly extremely angry and agitated. It is impossible to assess his thought process or thought content.

▶ What is most likely diagnosis for this patient?
▶ What is the best treatment?

ANSWERS TO CASE 42:

Phencyclidine Intoxication

Summary: An 18-year-old man is brought to the emergency department after possibly ingesting an unknown substance at a party. He is belligerent, paranoid, hostile, and violent and requires leather restraints. The patient's speech is slurred, and he has vertical nystagmus.

- **Most likely diagnosis:** Phencyclidine (PCP) intoxication.

- **Best treatment:** A PCP urine screen should be ordered to confirm the diagnosis. Medical monitoring in a hospital setting is required for severe intoxication, as well as to provide a safe environment. Antipsychotics can worsen the symptoms because of their anticholinergic side effects but may be necessary nonetheless to control violent behavior. Benzodiazepines are generally considered to be a safer, first option in cases where psychosis is not as prominent.

ANALYSIS

Objectives

1. Recognize PCP intoxication in a patient.

2. Understand the emergency treatment for this disorder.

Considerations

This patient became hostile, paranoid, and violent after ingesting an unknown substance at a party. This behavior is not characteristic of the patient. The **dysarthria** and **nystagmus** observed are typical of **PCP intoxication.**

APPROACH TO:

Phencyclidine Intoxication

DEFINITIONS

ATAXIA: A disturbance in gait; the patient cannot remain steady on his feet.

DYSARTHRIA: A disturbance in speech, which appears slurred, garbled, or unclear.

HYPERACUSIS: Hearing that is especially sensitive.

NYSTAGMUS: Rhythmic, oscillating motion of the eyes. This to-and-fro motion is generally involuntary and can occur in the vertical or horizontal plane.

PHENCYCLIDINE: Phencycline may be referred to by various street names, including angel dust, horse tranquilizer, supergrass, boat, tic tac, hog, ozone, rocket fuel, zoom, Sherman, wack, crystal, and embalming fluid. Marijuana laced with PCP may be referred to as killer joints, supergrass, fry, lovelies, wets, and waters. PCP is a piperidine similar to ketamine that was originally developed as an anesthetic agent. It is very potent, long acting, and causes marked behavioral, physiologic, and neurologic toxic effects in humans, including agitation, disorientation, hallucinations, and delirium. Its effects are similar to those of lysergic acid diethylamide (LSD), and it is often used in conjunction with other drugs of abuse such as marijuana, heroin, and cocaine. PCP can be smoked or injected intravenously and is easily synthesized and distributed.

CLINICAL APPROACH

Diagnostic Criteria

Phencyclidine intoxication is considered a psychiatric emergency because of the potential for psychosis and destructive behavior. The short-term effects last up to 6 hours, but the full effect of the drug can last for several days. Behavioral manifestations are very unpredictable; the individual can be sociable and cooperative 1 minute, becoming hostile and extremely violent the next. Auditory and visual hallucinations are common, as are confused and disorganized thoughts. Common findings on a physical examination include hypertension, hyperthermia, and nystagmus, as well as muscle rigidity. The criteria for PCP intoxication are listed in Table 42–1.

DIFFERENTIAL DIAGNOSIS AND TREATMENT

Laboratory evidence (a PCP assay) can confirm the diagnosis, but in the meantime other possible diagnoses must be considered. A manic episode of bipolar disorder, a psychotic decompensation in schizophrenia, or a brief episode of psychosis must be considered. Intoxication caused by other sedatives, stimulants, or narcotics should also be included, particularly those produced by hallucinogens, amphetamines, and ketamine.

The treatment of PCP intoxication must address the numerous aspects of the effects of PCP. Gastric lavage is controversial in light of the risk of electrolyte

Table 42–1 • CRITERIA FOR PHENCYCLIDINE INTOXICATION
Recent use of phencyclidine (PCP) or a similar substance
Disturbed behavior such as hostility and violence, impulsivity, and psychomotor agitation after ingestion of PCP.
Two or more of the following signs within an hour of ingestion: • Nystagmus • Hypertension or tachycardia • Numbness • Ataxia • Dysarthria • Muscle rigidity • Seizures or coma • Hyperacusis
The symptoms are not secondary to a medical condition or to another mental illness.

imbalance, emesis, and aspiration. The patient should be kept in a room with minimal stimulation, that is, in the dark and away from the confusion of the usual emergency department setting. Physical restraints should be avoided if possible because of the risk of muscle breakdown but are often necessary in the early stages of treatment.

Benzodiazepines are preferred as first-line treatment in nonpsychotic patients to treat muscle spasms, seizures, and sedation. If agitation and psychosis are marked, antipsychotic medication may be indicated, but can prove problematic given the potential risk of increasing PCP-induced hyperthermia, dystonia, anticholinergic reactions, and lowering the seizure threshold. As such, typical low-potency antipsychotics should be avoided. Haloperidol remains frequently used, although atypical antipsychotics are gaining in popularity.

Hypertension can be treated with intravenous antihypertensive medications. Acidification of the urine (eg, with cranberry juice, ascorbic acid, or ammonium chloride) to promote excretion of PCP is no longer recommended. Most importantly, the patient may need to be hospitalized for several days to allow the danger of violence or central nervous system complications to pass.

CASE CORRELATION

- See Case 39 and Case 45 for presentations of other patients with intoxication diagnoses and how they differ from that of PCP intoxication.

COMPREHENSION QUESTIONS

42.1 A 39-year-old man presents to the emergency room at the behest of his girlfriend, who reports that he has barely slept in the past week. The patient speaks extremely rapidly and switches topic so frequently as to be incomprehensible. His affect is happy and elevated, but he quickly snaps and becomes belligerent when he is accidentally bumped by a nurse. Which of the following symptoms would most likely distinguish this patient's presentation from PCP intoxication?

A. Disorganized thoughts

B. Hostile or violent behavior

C. The absence of nystagmus

D. Hallucinations

E. Pressured speech

42.2 A 15-year-old boy is brought to the emergency department by the police due to violent, psychotic behavior. Phencyclidine intoxication is confirmed via urine toxicology. Which of the following treatment interventions is associated with the lowest risk of adverse complications?

A. Low-potency, traditional antipsychotic agents to treat hallucinations

B. Ammonium chloride to acidify the urine and increase clearance of the drug

C. Benzodiazepines for agitation

D. Gastric lavage to remove unabsorbed, excess drug

E. Full-leather restraints to prevent harm to self or others

42.3 An obtunded young woman is discovered by the police sitting in the middle of the street and is subsequently brought to the emergency department. She is unable to verbalize any history. Which of the following sets of findings is most indicative of PCP intoxication?

A. Nystagmus, muscle rigidity, cannabinoids present on urine toxicology

B. Dilated pupils, bradycardia, runny nose

C. Pinpoint pupils, tachycardia, orthostatic hypotension

D. Ocular nerve palsy, cardiac arrhythmias, pseudobulbar palsy

E. Hallucinations, heart block, lower limb weakness

ANSWERS

42.1 **C.** Individuals with mania and PCP intoxication can have hallucinations, display hostility, and have disordered thoughts and pressured speech; nystagmus is commonly associated with PCP use but not with mania.

42.2 **C.** Low-potency traditional antipsychotics may worsen the intoxication syndrome via anticholinergic side effects. Acidification of the urine has been found to be ineffective and increases the risk of acute tubular necrosis due to myoglobinuria from rhabdomyolysis. Gastric lavage is contraindicated due to risk of emesis and aspiration, while restraints may lead to muscle breakdown (though they may still be necessary).

42.3 **A.** The triad of nystagmus, muscle rigidity, and numbness points strongly to PCP intoxication. Other symptoms that can occur include hypertension, tachycardia, ataxia, dysarthria, seizures or coma, and hyperacusis. PCP is very commonly smoked upon application to marijuana. B would be consistent with opioid withdrawal.

CLINICAL PEARLS

▶ Phencyclidine intoxication is an emergency; if it is suspected, the clinician must take precautions to protect both patient and staff from potential violent behavior.

▶ The patient can ingest PCP without knowing; it is a substance that is sometimes added to marijuana cigarettes.

▶ Nystagmus is commonly associated with PCP intoxication.

▶ Individuals with PCP intoxication often exhibit extraordinary physical strength.

REFERENCES

American Psychiatric Association. *Diagnostic and Statistical Manual of Mental Disorders*. 5th ed. Washington, DC: American Psychiatric Publishing; 2013.

Black BW, Andreasen NC. *Introductory Textbook of Psychiatry*. 6th ed. Washington, DC: American Psychiatric Publishing; 2014:164-170, 551-570.

Phencyclidine. Drug Enforcement Administration, Office of Diversion Control, Drug & Chemical Evaluation Section. www.deadiversion.usdoj.gov/drug_chem_info/pcp.pdf.

Sadock BJ, Sadock VA, Ruiz P. *Kaplan and Sadock's Synopsis of Psychiatry: Behavioral Sciences/Clinical Psychiatry*. 11th ed. Baltimore, MD: Lippincott Williams & Wilkins; 2014.

Twelve hours after a surgical admission because of broken arm, a 42-year-old woman begins to complain of feeling jittery and shaky. Six hours later, she tells staff members that she is hearing the voice of a dead relative shouting at her, although on admission she denied ever having heard voices previously. She complains of an upset stomach, irritability, and sweatiness. Her vital signs are BP 150/95 mm Hg, pulse 120 beats/min (bpm), respirations 20 breaths/min, and temperature 100.0°F (37.8°C). The patient reports no prior significant medical problems and says that she takes no medications. She has not had prior complications due to general anesthesia.

▶ What is the most likely diagnosis?
▶ What is the next step in the treatment of this disorder?

ANSWERS TO CASE 43:

Alcohol Withdrawal

Summary: Twelve hours after admission to a hospital, a 42-year-old woman complains of feeling shaky. Six hours later, she is irritable, has gastrointestinal disturbances and hallucinations, and is diaphoretic. She is hypertensive, mildly febrile, and tachycardic. She reports no previous medical problems.

- **Most likely diagnosis:** Alcohol withdrawal.

- **Next step in treatment:** The patient should be treated with a benzodiazepine immediately, starting with high doses and tapering as she recovers.

ANALYSIS

Objectives

1. Recognize the symptoms of alcohol withdrawal in a patient (Table 43–1 for diagnostic criteria).

2. Be aware of the treatment recommendations that should be instituted immediately in a patient with this disorder.

Considerations

Because of her admission to the hospital, this patient was unable to continue her alcohol intake, and 12 hours after her last drink, she began to experience the signs and symptoms of alcohol withdrawal, which then worsened over the next 6 hours.

Table 43–1 • DIAGNOSTIC CRITERIA FOR ALCOHOL WITHDRAWAL
Cessation of or reduction in heavy, prolonged, alcohol use.
Two or more of the following develop within hours to days: • Autonomic hyperactivity • Hand tremor • Insomniagn • Nausea or vomiting • Transient hallucinations • Agitation • Anxietyn • Seizures
The symptoms cause distress or impairment in functioning.
The symptoms are not due to a general medical condition or to another mental disorder.

APPROACH TO:
Alcohol Withdrawal

DEFINITIONS

DIAPHORESIS: Excessive sweating.

SYMPATHOMIMETIC: A substance that mimics at least some adrenalin or catecholamine responses. Examples of sympathomimetic substances include caffeine, ephedrine, and amphetamines.

CLINICAL APPROACH

Alcohol functions as a depressant much like benzodiazepines and barbiturates. It has an effect on serotonin and gamma-aminobutyric acid type A (GABA-A) receptors, producing tolerance and habituation. Positron emission tomographic (PET) studies have suggested a globally low rate of metabolic activity, particularly in the left parietal and right frontal areas in otherwise healthy persons withdrawing from alcohol. Withdrawal symptoms usually, but not always, occur in stages: tremulousness or jitteriness (6-8 hours), psychosis and perceptual symptoms (8-12 hours), seizures (12-24 hours), and delirium tremens ([DTs], 24-72 hours, up to 1 week). Notably, **alcohol withdrawal, particularly DTs, can be fatal.**

DIFFERENTIAL DIAGNOSIS

Included in the differential diagnosis for alcohol withdrawal are other drug withdrawal states, especially sedative-hypnotic withdrawal. In fact, the criteria for withdrawal from substances such as benzodiazepines (most commonly short-acting, high-potency drugs) and barbiturates are identical to those for alcohol withdrawal. A carefully recorded history, a physical examination, and laboratory results indicative of long-term, heavy alcohol use (eg, evidence of cirrhosis or liver failure, macrocytic anemia, elevated liver transaminase levels—particularly gamma-glutamyl transpeptidase) will point to the correct diagnosis.

Medical conditions with similar signs and symptoms must be ruled out. Examples of such conditions include thyroid storm (thyrotoxicosis), pheochromocytoma, and inappropriate use of beta-agonist inhalers or sympathomimetics.

Although hallucinations are rare in alcohol withdrawal without delirium, if present they can be confused with those of schizophrenia. Several features distinguish the two conditions: In alcohol withdrawal, the perceptual disturbances are transient, there is not necessarily a history of a preexisting psychotic illness, the associated symptoms of schizophrenia are not present, and the patient's reality testing ability remains intact.

TREATMENT

Severe alcohol withdrawal with autonomic instability (delirium tremens or DTs) has a high mortality and requires stabilization in an acute medical facility. The most common treatment for alcohol withdrawal remains **benzodiazepines,** administered either orally or parenterally. If liver function is not impaired, a long-acting benzodiazepine such as chlordiazepoxide or diazepam is generally preferable given PO or IV. If there is concern about decreased liver function, lorazepam can be administered either orally or parenterally, as its metabolism is not as dependent on liver function, and, as such, is probably the most popular agent utilized. Similarly, oxazepam may be preferred in these instances. Whatever the specific drug used, it should be given as frequently as necessary in order to normalize the vital signs and sedate the patient. The medicine should then be gradually tapered over the next several days, and the patient's vital signs monitored. Use of the Clinical Institute Withdrawal Assessment for Alcohol Scale, Revised (CIWA-Ar) may be useful in standardizing the assessment of withdrawal severity and assist in guiding treatment. Anticonvulsants such as carbamazepine and valproic acid are also effective in treating alcohol withdrawal, although it is a much less popular option in the United States given familiarity with treatment with benzodiazepines. Antipsychotics should be avoided, because of their potential to lower the seizure threshold.

CASE CORRELATION

- See also Case 44 for another diagnosis that is very similar to alcohol withdrawal. Other medical conditions such as hypoglycemia and diabetic ketoacidosis may also cause symptoms similar to alcohol withdrawal.

COMPREHENSION QUESTIONS

43.1 A 47-year-old man is admitted to a psychiatric unit for depression with suicidal ideation and detoxification. He has a long history of dependence upon both alcohol and cocaine. Which of the following signs is most characteristic of early alcohol withdrawal?

  A. Decreased blood pressure

  B. Hypersomnia

  C. Persistent hallucinations

  D. Tremor

  E. Increased appetite

43.2 A 54-year-old man is admitted to the hospital for elective surgery. He has been through alcohol rehabilitation, but has continued to struggle with his drinking. He alerts the primary service taking care of him that he has continued to drink up to the time of his admission. In what time frame after cessation of all drinking is he at most risk for delirium tremens?

  A. 6 to 8 hours

  B. 8 to 12 hours

  C. 12 to 24 hours

  D. 48 to 96 hours

  E. Over 1 week

43.3 An elderly woman presents to the emergency department due to a hip frac-
ture. She reports that she "hasn't been feeling very well" recently, and is vague
and hard to pin down regarding details. You think that there might be the
odor of alcohol on her breath and suspect alcohol use disorder. Which of the
following findings would be most supportive of your concern?

    A. A healed scar from a previous fall several years ago

    B. Microcytic anemia

    C. Elevated gamma-glutamyl transpeptidase

    D. Slightly elevated aspartate aminotransferase (AST), with normal alanine
aminotransferase (ALT)

    E. Mini-mental state examination score of 28/30

43.4 A 63-year-old man presents to the emergency department with complaints
of anxiety. He describes a long history of daily heavy alcohol use and 2 days
ago "quit cold turkey." He appears visibly tremulous, flushed, and diaphoretic.
His temperature, blood pressure, and pulse rate are elevated. The results of
his physical examination are otherwise unremarkable, but his laboratory tests
demonstrate low serum albumin and low protein levels, as well as an elevated
prothrombin time/partial prothrombin time value. He is admitted to the
medical service for alcohol detoxification. Which of the following medications would be most appropriate in treating this patient?

    A. Alprazolam

    B. Chlordiazepoxide

    C. Diazepam

    D. Lorazepam

    E. Clonazepam

Match the timing of the following symptoms with the time frame that it usually
occurs, after the last alcoholic drink ingested:

43.5 Delirium tremens

43.6 Hallucinations with intact orientation

43.7 Withdrawal seizures

43.8 Tremulousness

43.9 Hallucinations with delirium

    A. Immediately

    B. 6 to 8 hours

    C. 8 to 12 hours

    D. 12 to 24 hours

    E. 24 to 72 hours

ANSWERS

43.1 **D.** Tremor is the most characteristic sign of alcohol withdrawal. Vital signs are elevated in alcohol withdrawal because of autonomic hyperactivity. Patients generally have insomnia as a result, not hypersomnia. Hallucinations associated with alcohol withdrawal usually resolve within a week, while those occurring in delirium tremens usually resolve with the delirium. Cocaine withdrawal more typically involves hypersomnia and hyperphagia.

43.2 **D.** Withdrawal symptoms usually, but not always, occur in stages: tremulousness or jitteriness (6-8 hours), psychosis and perceptual symptoms (8-12 hours), seizures (12-24 hours), and DTs (24-72 hours, up to 1 week).

43.3 **C.** Laboratory tests in alcoholics commonly show macrocytic anemia and elevated liver transaminase levels—particularly gamma-glutamyl transpeptidase.

43.4 **D.** Although all these medications are benzodiazepines, only lorazepam is metabolized solely by glucuronidation, which is not as dependent on liver functioning. The metabolism of the other benzodiazepines is much more dependent on liver function. In this patient (who has evidence of poor liver function), using high doses of medications that are dependent on liver function for their degradation could result in excessive drug levels in the blood of an overly sedated patient.

43.5 **E.** Withdrawal symptoms usually, but not always, occur in stages: tremulousness or jitteriness (6-8 hours), psychosis and perceptual symptoms (8-12 hours), seizures (12-24 hours), and DTs (24-72 hours, up to 1 week).

43.6 **C.** Withdrawal symptoms usually, but not always, occur in stages: tremulousness or jitteriness (6-8 hours), psychosis and perceptual symptoms (8-12 hours), seizures (12-24 hours), and DTs (24-72 hours, up to 1 week). Of note, alcoholic hallucinosis occurs earlier than hallucinations associated with delirium tremens, and are not usually associated with a clouded sensorium or abnormal vital signs.

43.7 **D.** Withdrawal symptoms usually, but not always, occur in stages: tremulousness or jitteriness (6-8 hours), psychosis and perceptual symptoms (8-12 hours), seizures (12-24 hours), and DTs (24-72 hours, up to 1 week).

43.8 **B.** Withdrawal symptoms usually, but not always, occur in stages: tremulousness or jitteriness (6-8 hours), psychosis and perceptual symptoms (8-12 hours), seizures (12-24 hours), and DTs (24-72 hours, up to 1 week).

43.9 **E.** Withdrawal symptoms usually, but not always, occur in stages: tremulousness or jitteriness (6-8 hours), psychosis and perceptual symptoms (8-12 hours), seizures (12-24 hours), and DTs (24-72 hours, up to 1 week).

CLINICAL PEARLS

▶ Alcohol withdrawal can occur within hours to days after heavy use and can include elevated vital signs, tremor, transient hallucinations, anxiety, and seizures.

▶ The criteria (and symptoms) of alcohol withdrawal are identical to those for sedative-hypnotic withdrawal.

▶ The treatment of choice for alcohol withdrawal is benzodiazepines. Anticonvulsants can also be used.

▶ Benzodiazepines are not dependent on liver function, such as lorazepam, but are often preferred in the treatment of alcohol withdrawal.

REFERENCES

Hoffman RS, Weinhouse GL. Management of moderate and severe alcohol withdrawal syndrome. UpToDate. www.uptodate.com. Accessed Sep 11, 2013.

Kosten TR, Newton TF, De La Garza R, Haile CN. Substance-related and addictive disorders. *Textbook of Psychiatry*. 6th ed. Washington, DC: American Psychiatric Publishing; 2014:735-814.

CASE 44

A physician is called to see a 42-year-old man who was jailed on a robbery charge 48 hours previously. Twelve hours before the physician arrived, the patient began to complain of feeling anxious. The correctional officers noted that he was nauseous, diaphoretic, and had muscle tics, so they alerted medical personnel. By the time the physician came to see the patient, the patient had a witnessed, generalized tonic-clonic seizure, 30 seconds in duration. He is now postictal. The results of a subsequent urine toxicology screening are positive for cocaine, opiates, and benzodiazepines.

▶ What is the most likely etiology of the patient's seizures?
▶ What treatment would you recommend for this patient?

ANSWERS TO CASE 44:
Benzodiazepine Withdrawal

Summary: A 42-year-old man whose urine toxicology screening showed positive results for cocaine, opiates, and benzodiazepines had a seizure 48 hours after he was arrested and put in jail. Twelve hours prior to the seizure, he noted feeling anxious and was observed to be nauseous, diaphoretic, and to have muscle tics.

- **Most likely diagnosis:** Benzodiazepine withdrawal. Additionally, stimulant use disorder, opioid use disorder, and sedative-, hypnotic- or anxiolytic use disorder should be considered and assessed.

- **Best treatment:** The patient should be transferred to an acute care medical facility and initially treated with a benzodiazepine which should then be slowly tapered so that the withdrawal symptoms do not reappear.

ANALYSIS

Objectives

1. Recognize benzodiazepine withdrawal in a patient (Table 44–1 for diagnostic criteria).
2. Understand the principles of treatment for patients in this state.

Considerations

Forty-eight hours after he was jailed, this patient began displaying signs and symptoms classic for benzodiazepine withdrawal, namely, anxiety, sweating, intolerance of loud noises or lights, muscle twitching, and ultimately seizures. The other drugs in his system are less likely to contribute to the etiology. Opiate withdrawal (see Case 40) is usually characterized by abdominal cramping, rhinorrhea, diarrhea, nausea, and vomiting. Cocaine withdrawal typically causes depressive symptoms, anxiety, irritability, hypersomnolence, and fatigue. In contrast to benzodiazepine withdrawal, opiate withdrawal and cocaine withdrawal are not life threatening. Because of the danger involved, the patient should be transferred to a hospital where he can be carefully monitored.

Table 44–1 • DIAGNOSTIC CRITERIA FOR ANXIOLYTIC WITHDRAWAL
Cessation or reduction in the use of an anxiolytic drug.
Two or more of the following symptoms occur following cessation of use of the drug: autonomic hyperactivity, hand tremor, insomnia, nausea or vomiting, hallucinations, psychomotor agitation, anxiety, and grand mal seizures.
Symptoms should not be due to a general medical condition.

APPROACH TO:

Sedative, Hypnotic, or Anxiolytic Withdrawal

DEFINITIONS

ANXIOLYTIC DRUGS: Medications used to treat anxiety. Most commonly, they include the class of drugs called benzodiazepines but can also include barbiturates as well as miscellaneous medications such as buspirone and chloral hydrate.

FLUMAZENIL: A benzodiazepine antagonist that is used in the emergency department to treat benzodiazepine overdose. Its principal danger is that it can precipitate severe withdrawal.

WITHDRAWAL: The pattern of symptoms exhibited by a person after repeated use of a drug and the physiologic effect that occurs on its discontinuation. Withdrawal is also called discontinuance syndrome.

CLINICAL APPROACH

A large number of Americans use benzodiazepines, either properly prescribed (as an anxiolytic or hypnotic) or recreationally. Like barbiturates, **benzodiazepines have their primary effect on the gamma-aminobutyric acid type A (GABA-A) receptor complex**, altering chloride ion influx (Figure 44–1). Withdrawal from both barbiturates and benzodiazepines can be life threatening. Seizures can result from

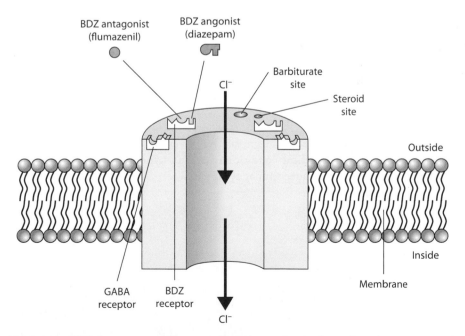

Figure 44-1. GABA-A receptor complex on a cell membrane, showing benzodiazepine receptors and chloride channel.

benzodiazepine withdrawal. The severity of benzodiazepine withdrawal varies according to duration of use, dose, and the half-life of the offending agent. Symptoms such as anxiety, photophobia, nausea, diaphoresis, muscle twitching, and seizures can occur.

DIFFERENTIAL DIAGNOSIS

Withdrawal from anxiolytics can be confused with withdrawal from other substances, but a carefully recorded history of the symptoms can usually differentiate the two. Opioid withdrawal typically induces abdominal pains, salivation, lacrimation, rhinorrhea, urination, and defecation. Cocaine withdrawal causes a "crash" in which the individual becomes hypersomnic and hyperphagic, in addition to having a strong craving for the drug. Alcohol withdrawal can be manifested by many symptoms similar to those of benzodiazepine withdrawal and can be life threatening as well, but a history of heavy, sustained use of alcohol is usually present. Panic disorder can cause acute anxiety, diaphoresis, and palpitations, but they typically occur "out of the blue," and a history of a recent cessation of benzodiazepine use is not present. However, because many patients with panic disorder are treated with benzodiazepines, the clinical picture is often confounded.

TREATMENT

To prevent seizures and other withdrawal symptoms, the clinician should, if possible, **slowly taper the dose of the benzodiazepine** rather than abruptly discontinuing it. Some reports have noted that the addition of carbamazepine can be useful in preventing withdrawal seizures in individuals prone to developing them.

Flumazenil, a benzodiazepine receptor antagonist, reverses the effects of benzodiazepines. Although it may have some future use as a disulfiram-like medication to help patients addicted to benzodiazepines refrain from using them, it is currently not used in this manner and is **restricted to use in the emergency department in instances of benzodiazepine overdose.**

> ## CASE CORRELATION
>
> - See also Case 38 for another diagnosis that is very similar to benzodiazepine withdrawal. Other medical conditions such as hypoglycemia and diabetic ketoacidosis may also cause similar symptoms.

COMPREHENSION QUESTIONS

44.1 A 55-year-old unresponsive woman is brought to the emergency department after an apparent suicide attempt. Earlier that day, she refilled her monthly prescription for a benzodiazepine, which she had been prescribed for panic disorder. The empty pill bottle was found on her nightstand by the paramedics. Concurrent ingestion of which of the following substances is most likely to worsen the prognosis of her overdose?

A. Cannabis

B. Cocaine

C. Citalopram

D. Alcohol

E. Lysergic acid diethylamide (LSD)

44.2 Treatment of the case in Question 44.1 would likely involve administration of which of the following?

A. Lorazepam

B. Flumazenil

C. Chlordiazepoxide

D. Disulfiram

E. Naltrexone

44.3 The acute crisis of the woman in Question 44.1 is averted. She is subsequently hospitalized for detoxification. Which of the following benzodiazepines is most likely to cause a withdrawal syndrome?

A. Chlordiazepoxide

B. Clonazepam

C. Alprazolam

D. Diazepam

E. Lorazepam

44.4 Which agent would be safest to employ in a patient with severe hepatic pathology?

A. Chlordiazepoxide

B. Clonazepam

C. Alprazolam

D. Diazepam

E. Lorazepam

44.5 Withdrawal from which of the following substances is potentially the most lethal?

A. Heroin

B. Cocaine

C. Cannabis

D. Valium

E. Ethanol

ANSWERS

44.1 **D.** Benzodiazepines are rarely lethal in overdose by themselves. However, when taken with other sedative-hypnotic drugs, especially alcohol, the effects of their potentiation can be lethal. None of the other listed drugs would potentiate the benzodiazepine overdose.

44.2 **B.** Flumazenil is a benzodiazepine receptor antagonist, which reverses the effects of benzodiazepines. Its use is restricted to use in the emergency department in instances of benzodiazepine overdose. Lorazepam and chlordiazepoxide are benzodiazepines, which would be contraindicated in benzodiazepine overdose. Disulfiram and naltrexone are used in the treatment of alcohol addiction, and opiate overdose (respectively) and have no use in benzodiazepine withdrawal.

44.3 **C.** Generally speaking, shorter-acting agents are more likely to cause a withdrawal syndrome. Alprazolam is the shortest acting of all the benzodiazepines listed.

44.4 **E.** Lorazepam is directly conjugated to an inactive glucuronide metabolite that is excreted by the kidneys. All the other benzodiazepines listed are excreted primarily by the liver.

44.5 **E.** Ethanol withdrawal can be lethal. Although valium is a benzodiazepine and benzodiazepine withdrawal can be lethal, valium has such a long half-life that it essentially tapers itself; the symptoms of benzodiazepine withdrawal are not often seen with this drug. Heroin, cocaine, and cannabis withdrawals are not lethal (except in some cases in those with preexisting medical conditions).

CLINICAL PEARLS

▶ Anxiolytic medications include several classes of medication, most commonly benzodiazepines.

▶ A withdrawal syndrome is most likely associated with the abuse of benzodiazepines with shorter half-lives and shorter onsets of action.

REFERENCES

American Psychiatric Association *Diagnostic and Statistical Manual of Mental Disorders*. 5th ed. Washington, DC: American Psychiatric Publishing; 2013.

Greller H, Gupta A. Benzodiazepine poisoning and withdrawal. UpToDate. www.uptodate.com. Accessed May 15, 2013.

A 26-year-old chemistry graduate student is brought to the emergency department after throwing a punch at his roommate. The patient insists that he must return home to study for his upcoming examinations, quickly becoming angry and belligerent with staff members when they refuse to let him leave. He claims that he has been studying "like a fiend" for the past 3 weeks. The patient's best friend reports that the patient has not slept in days, and he has lost at least 10 lb. The patient has no medical or psychiatric problems of which his friend is aware.

On a physical examination, the patient is found to have a BP of 140/94 mm Hg and a pulse rate of 100 beats/min. His pupils are dilated; he is sweaty and has a fine tremor in both hands. The results of the rest of the physical examination are normal, although the patient is uncooperative. On a mental status examination, the patient is seen to be alert and oriented to person, place, and time. He is belligerent and uncooperative, and his speech is rapid and loud. He describes his mood as "just great," but his affect is angry. He denies suicidal or homicidal ideation. He has had occasional worries recently that people are staring at him too much and might be trying to sabotage his laboratory projects.

▶ What is most likely diagnosis for this patient?
▶ What is the best diagnostic test?

ANSWERS TO CASE 45:

Amphetamine Intoxication

Summary: A 26-year-old man is brought to the emergency department after becoming physically aggressive with his best friend. He is belligerent, angry, and mildly paranoid. The patient has not been sleeping or eating well, resulting in a weight loss of approximately 10 lb. The patient has no medical or psychiatric history. In the emergency department, he is oriented but belligerent and uncooperative. He states that his mood is fine, although he appears angry. The patient's physical examination shows hypertension and tachycardia, as well as dilated pupils, diaphoresis, and a fine bilateral tremor in his hands.

- **Most likely diagnosis:** Amphetamine intoxication.

- **Diagnostic test:** A urine toxicology screening for amphetamines to verify the suspected diagnosis.

ANALYSIS

Objectives

1. Recognize amphetamine intoxication in a patient (see diagnostic criteria in Table 45–1).

2. Understand what laboratory tests can be used to confirm this diagnosis.

3. Be aware of the psychological and physical sequelae that can occur as a patient recovers from amphetamine intoxication.

Considerations

This patient has a history of taking pills to help him stay awake and study. After using these pills consistently for several weeks, he becomes belligerent and physically

Table 45–1 • DIAGNOSTIC CRITERIA FOR STIMULANT INTOXICATION
Recent use of a stimulant.
Clinically significant maladaptive behavioral or psychological changes that developed during or shortly after use of substance.

Two or more symptoms develop during or shortly after use of the amphetamine or related substance such as:
    A change in heart rate
    Dilation of pupils
    A change in blood pressure
    Perspiration or chills
    Nausea or vomiting
    Weight loss
    Muscular weakness, respiratory depression, chest pain, arrhythmias
    Confusion, seizures, dyskinesia, dystonia, or coma

The symptoms are not caused by another medical condition, including another mental disorder.

violent with a friend. The friend notes that the patient has not been sleeping or eating. His pulse rate and blood pressure are elevated, his pupils are dilated, he is sweaty, and he has a fine tremor in both hands. If the patient stops taking the pills, what will happen? He will probably "crash," with resulting dysphoria, fatigue, psychomotor slowing, increased appetite, and need for sleep. But, unlike schizophrenia, his paranoia will likely resolve after discontinuing the amphetamine.

APPROACH TO:
Amphetamine Intoxication

DEFINITIONS

DYSKINESIAS: Abnormal movements.

DYSTONIAS: Abnormal contracture of muscle or muscle groups; typically transient, but can be life threatening if the muscles used in breathing are involved.

CLINICAL APPROACH

Amphetamines were first synthesized to treat medical and mental disorders but have been widely abused. Currently, they are approved for use in attention deficit hyperactivity disorder, narcolepsy, and depressive disorders. The classic amphetamines, dextroamphetamine (Dexedrine), methamphetamine, "crystal meth" (Desoxyn), and methylphenidate (Ritalin), affect the dopamine system. Designer amphetamines have both dopaminergic and serotoninergic effects and can cause hallucinations. They include "ecstasy," "eve," and "serenity, tranquility, and peace" (STP). Amphetamines are quickly absorbed orally, although the illicit varieties can also be injected intravenously or smoked. The neurobiochemical response depends on the specific receptor activated; **adrenergic hyperactivity (dilated pupils, elevated blood pressure, weight loss, confusion, or seizures) with or without hallucinations** is common. Additionally, amphetamines have central-acting effects in several areas of the brain, including the orbitofrontal cortex, dorsolateral prefrontal cortex, and amygdala. Tolerance and habituation occur, although to a lesser degree than with cocaine. **Withdrawal symptoms** include **anxiety, tremors, lethargy, fatigue, nightmares, headache, and extreme hunger.**

In recent years, methamphetamine has grown to epidemic proportions, particularly in western, midwestern, southern, and rural areas of the United States. Methamphetamine ("meth," "crank," "chalk," "ice," "crystal," and "glass") can be smoked, snorted, injected, or ingested. Smoking has become the more common method, given its fast uptake to the brain by this route. Long-term effects may include paranoia, hallucinations, repetitive motor activity, memory loss, aggressive behavior, mood disturbance, severe dental problems ("meth mouth"), and weight loss. Recent legislation to control access to ephedrine and pseudoephedrine has led to decreased production in homegrown meth laboratories, but have shifted production to more industrial, criminal enterprises. Despite these interventions, methamphetamine remains widely available and a significant drug problem in this country, as well as other areas of the world.

DIFFERENTIAL DIAGNOSIS

Other psychoactive substances can cause behavioral abnormalities; therefore, amphetamine-induced psychotic disorder, cocaine intoxication, hallucinogen intoxication, and phencyclidine intoxication must be ruled out prior to making this diagnosis. Urine toxicology screening can establish the diagnosis if the patient is unable to give a coherent history of which substance has been used. Psychosis related to amphetamine intoxication can be distinguished from schizophrenia best by history, with no premorbid negative symptoms of schizophrenia such as anhedonia, and flat affect strengthening the diagnosis of amphetamine intoxication.

TREATMENT

The treatment of amphetamine intoxication is generally supportive, with the passing of time being the most useful element; symptoms of intoxication clear in 48 hours. The resulting "crash" of the patient, with dysphoria, excessive sleepiness, fatigue, and increased appetite, are also time limited and do not need treatment unless the depressed mood is severe. In this case, an antidepressant can be considered if the depressed mood does not clear within several weeks. Emergency treatment of amphetamine intoxication can include the use of antipsychotic agents and/or restraints if the psychosis is severe and violent behavior is present. Hospitalization can be necessary if delusions or paranoia are present, and/or patients are a danger to themselves or others.

CASE CORRELATION

- See also Case 39 for a stimulant intoxication presentation due to another chemical.

COMPREHENSION QUESTIONS

45.1 A 19-year-old girl is brought to the emergency department by her friends, who are worried that she is not behaving normally. They suspect that she was experimenting with some type of drug, but are unsure what. Which of the following syndromes would be most consistent with amphetamine intoxication?

   A. Flushed face, slurred speech, unsteady gait

   B. Anorexia, diaphoresis, pupillary dilation

   C. Prominent hallucinations, pupillary dilation, incoordination

   D. Miosis, slurred speech, drowsiness

   E. Hyperphagia, conjunctival injection, tachycardia

45.2 In the previous case, urine toxicology confirms intoxication with amphetamines. Which of the following withdrawal syndromes would be expected?

A. Diarrhea, piloerection, yawning

B. Delirium, autonomic hyperactivity, visual or tactile hallucinations

C. "Crash" of mood into depression, lethargy, increased appetite

D. Tremor, headache, hypertension

E. Postural hypotension, psychomotor agitation, insomnia

45.3 A 20-year-old man is brought to a mental health center by his parents, who
are at their wit's end because of their son's drug problem. The son is sul-
len and completely uncommunicative. The parents who are extremely naïve
about the world of street drugs can only guess by his behavior that he is
abusing "uppers." Which of the following findings might help differentiate
between the abuse of cocaine versus amphetamine?

A. Rhinorrhea

B. "Track marks" on his arms

C. Severe smoker's cough and respiratory problems

D. Extremely poor dentition

E. Weight loss

45.4 A 38-year-old white man is brought into the emergency department by the
police. Several officers are needed to control the patient, who is psychotic and
extremely agitated, requiring placement in full-leather restraints. The officers
had received a complaint that the patient attacked several individuals at a
biker party for no apparent reason, although witnesses on the scene indicate
that the patient had been smoking methamphetamine. Which of the following pharmacological interventions is the most appropriate?

A. Citalopram

B. Diazepam

C. Ascorbic acid

D. Haloperidol

E. Bupropion

ANSWERS

45.1 **B.** Symptoms of amphetamine intoxication include anorexia, tachycardia,
hypertension, pupillary dilation, and diaphoresis. A = alcohol intoxication,
C = hallucinogen intoxication, D = opioid intoxication, E = cannabis
intoxication.

45.2 **C.** The withdrawal symptoms from amphetamines include depressed mood,
lethargy, and increased appetite. A = opioid withdrawal, B = delirium
tremens, D = alcohol withdrawal, E = sedative-hypnotic withdrawal.

45.3 **D.** Cocaine, amphetamines, and other stimulant drugs are quite similar in their presentation. Both cocaine and amphetamine may be used via smoking, insufflation (potentially leading to nasal problems), or intravenously. However, "meth mouth" is commonly seen with prolonged abuse of methamphetamine, caused by lowered saliva production in conjunction with cravings for sugar.

45.4 **D.** Haloperidol and antipsychotic medications are best suited to target psychosis and agitation. Diazepam would be preferable to address agitation in the absence of psychosis. Antidepressants such as citalopram and bupropion would not be useful acutely. Bupropion may be preferable to treat depression after acute withdrawal. The use of ascorbic acid to acidify the urine in amphetamine intoxication is not recommended.

CLINICAL PEARLS

► Urine toxicology screening is the definitive test in making a diagnosis of amphetamine intoxication.

► The symptoms should resolve once the amphetamine has been eliminated from the body.

REFERENCES

American Psychiatric Association. *Diagnostic and Statistical Manual of Mental Disorders.* 5th ed. Washington, DC: American Psychiatric Publishing; 2013.

Sadock BJ, Sadock VA, Ruiz P. *Kaplan and Sadock's Synopsis of Psychiatry: Behavioral Sciences/Clinical Psychiatry.* 11th ed. Baltimore, MD: Lippincott Williams & Wilkins; 2014.

The night float psychiatry resident is paged to evaluate a 64-year-old man in the telemetry unit after he began screaming about strange men in his hospital room. The patient has a history of multivessel coronary artery disease (CAD) and underwent a coronary artery bypass graft (CABG) surgery three days ago. He claims that he saw several ominous-appearing men standing in his room, glaring at him threateningly. The patient denies ever having any unusual experiences like this before and has no prior psychiatric history. The nurses' notes from the last shift indicate that the patient has been agitated and restless, although at other times he appeared stuporous. On mental status examination, the patient is alert and oriented to person, place, and situation, but the date is off by several months. He denies any current hallucinations, and no delusions were elicited.

▶ What is the most likely diagnosis for this patient?
▶ What is the next step in the treatment of this patient?

ANSWERS TO CASE 46:

Delirium

Summary: The patient is a 64-year-old man with CAD and no prior psychiatric history who experienced visual hallucinations, paranoia, and fluctuation of attention and awareness on the evening of postoperative day number three following CABG. On examination later that night, the patient is oriented to person, place, and situation, but not to time. Otherwise, his mental status examination and physical examination are essentially unremarkable.

- **Most likely diagnosis:** Delirium.

- **Next step in treatment:** A cause of the delirium should be sought by reviewing the patient's medical record, performing a focused history and physical examination, and obtaining clinically guided laboratory and imaging studies.

ANALYSIS

Objectives

1. Recognize and diagnose delirium in a patient.

2. Be familiar with the steps to be followed in the case of new-onset delirium.

3. Understand that delirium represents a psychiatric emergency and carries a poor prognosis.

Considerations

This patient, with no history of psychosis, began having visual hallucinations and paranoia 3 days after undergoing a CABG. Intensive care settings and/or major surgical procedures are risk factors for delirium, especially for geriatric patients. He also experienced waxing and waning of consciousness and was disoriented. The short-term nature of the event and the fluctuations in attention and awareness observed are consistent with delirium (Table 46–1).

Table 46–1 • DIAGNOSTIC CRITERIA FOR DELIRIUM[a]
Disturbance in baseline attention and awareness.
The disturbance develops over a short period of time (hours to days) and fluctuates in severity over the course of the day.
A disturbance in cognition such as memory deficit, language, visuospatial ability, or perception is present.
The disturbances are not better explained by a neurocognitive disorder and do not occur in the context of a severely reduced level of arousal, such as coma.

[a]Note that the criteria are essentially the same regardless of the etiology.

APPROACH TO:
Delirium

DEFINITIONS

ATTENTION: Ability to maintain focus on a particular stimulus or activity.

AWARENESS: Orientation to situation and surroundings.

SUNDOWNING: A phenomenon characterized by worsening of neurocognitive symptoms during the late afternoon or evening hours, usually in elderly and/or cognitively impaired individuals.

CLINICAL APPROACH

The hallmark of delirium is a fluctuation in the level of attention and awareness. The Confusion Assessment Method (CAM) can be used to evaluate for delirium. Associated symptoms include memory deficits, visuospatial dysfunction, and perceptual disturbances, such as visual hallucinations. These can result in behavioral problems which interfere with management, such as agitation, wandering, and pulling out intravenous lines, catheters, etc.

Delirium is a medical and psychiatric emergency, often described as "acute brain failure." It should viewed as akin to failure of other organ systems (ie, heart failure, respiratory failure, or renal failure). Early recognition and treatment are essential to prevent progression to stupor, coma, or death. Delirium carries a poor prognosis. Mortality 1 year after diagnosis is estimated to be up to 40%.

Any disease process, illicit substance, toxin, or medication that affects the central nervous system can cause delirium. Risk factors include dementia, elderly age, medical illness, polypharmacy, and recent surgery. Several causes of delirium may be present simultaneously.

Table 46–2 lists many of the causes of delirium.

A mnemonic for common contributing factors to the development of delirium in those with preexisting cognitive impairment includes:

PInCH ME: **P**ain, **In**fection, **C**onstipation, **H**ydration status, **M**edications, **E**nvironment Evaluation of delirium should include an assessment of potential contributing factors. History and physical examination findings should guide further workup. Bedside testing, such as pulse-oximetry, electrocardiography, fingerstick glucose testing, arterial blood gas analysis, and bladder scan may reveal hypoxemia, hypercapnia, hypo/hyperglycemia, or urinary retention. Laboratory and radiographic studies to consider include a comprehensive metabolic panel with ammonia, complete blood count with leukocyte differential, B_{12} and folate levels, urinalysis, urine drug screen, blood and urine cultures, cerebrospinal fluid (CSF) analysis and culture, and chest radiography. Electroencephalography (EEG) has poor sensitivity and specificity for delirium, but may help in ruling out nonconvulsive epilepsy. EEG findings suggestive of delirium include increased generalized slow-wave activity, which may also be seen in dementia. Delirium associated with alcohol withdrawal is associated with increased fast waves on EEG.

Table 46–2 • PRECIPITANTS OF DELIRIUM
Acute intermittent porphyria
Cardiovascular diseases: Arrhythmias, congestive heart failure, myocardial infarction
Central nervous system disorders: Brain trauma, epilepsy, neoplasm, cerebral vascular accident, subdural hematoma, vasculitis
Drugs of abuse (in intoxication or withdrawal): Alcohol, barbiturates, benzodiazepines, narcotics
Electrolyte imbalances
Endocrine disorders: Adrenal insufficiency, hypoglycemia, parathyroid dysfunction
Hepatic encephalopathy
Infections: UTI, pneumonia, sepsis, meningitis, encephalitis
Medications: Anticholinergics, anticonvulsants, antihypertensive agents, antiparkinsonian agents, H_2 blockers, digitalis, corticosteroids, narcotics, benzodiazepines
Pulmonary disorders: Hypercarbia, hypoxemia
Sleep deprivation
Uremia
Vasculitis
Vitamin deficiencies: B_{12}, folic acid, thiamine

DIFFERENTIAL DIAGNOSIS

Major neurocognitive disorder, specifically dementia, increases the risk of developing delirium, but delirium cannot be diagnosed if the condition is better explained by dementia. This can be clinically challenging because both delirium and dementia can exhibit very similar symptoms (eg, memory impairment, cognitive disturbances, and behavioral problems). Several characteristics help distinguish between the two, which are compared in Table 46–3.

Other diseases in the differential diagnosis for delirium include psychotic disorders such as schizophrenia and acute mania. However, individuals with delirium display a fluctuating level of consciousness, and patients with schizophrenia and mania usually maintain an alert level of consciousness. Delirious patients often have visual hallucinations, but primary psychotic disorders more frequently manifest as auditory hallucinations and delusions.

Table 46–3 • CHARACTERISTICS OF DELIRIUM AND DEMENTIA		
Characteristic	Delirium	Dementia
Onset	Short	Long
Course	Fluctuating	Stable
Level of alertness	Hypoactive, hyperactive, mixed	Stable
Prognosis	Reversible	Irreversible

TREATMENT

The cornerstone of treatment for delirium is identification and correction of the underlying abnormality. This approach ideally results in reversal of the delirious state, typically over the course of 1 week. However, patients may show subtle signs of delirium for months afterwards.

The level of psychomotor activity exhibited by the patient helps to guide the treatment approach. Hyperactive delirium is characterized by a high level of psychomotor activity that may be accompanied by mood lability, agitation, and refusal to cooperate with care. Hypoactive delirium manifests as decreased psychomotor activity that may be associated with sluggishness, lethargy, or stupor. In mixed delirium, one may have a normal level of psychomotor activity, but have altered awareness and alertness. Alternatively, mixed delirium may present with rapid fluctuation of activity level, similar to the patient described in the case above. It is important to note that hypoactive delirium may go unnoticed due to its less disruptive nature.

Thoroughly review the medication list as a preventive measure. Common iatrogenic causes include sedative-hypnotics (ie, benzodiazepines), anticholinergics, H_2-receptor antagonists, corticosteroids, narcotics, and antibiotics (especially fluoroquinolones). Discontinue or switch medications if this is an option. If possible, use dexmedetomidine instead of a benzodiazepine for sedation of critically ill individuals.

Maintain adequate pain control to avoid precipitating delirium. The concept of the "ICU triad," which consists of pain, agitation, and delirium, emphasizes the interrelationship among these conditions. The treatment of one affects the others. Opiates are the medications of choice for treatment of non-neuropathic pain. However, opiates can worsen delirium if dosed too high. Meperidine and codeine should in particular be avoided.

Environmental modification is another significant aspect of the treatment approach. Hospitalization can be very distressing and disorienting. The presence of family members, items from home (ie, pictures), and reminders of location, date, and time help maintain patient orientation. Efforts should be made to reduce excess noise, dim the lights at night, and cluster care activities to minimize disruption to the patient's sleep-wake cycle. Minimize "tethers," such as IV lines, urinary catheters, telemetry wires, and restraints. Restraints may be indicated, however, if the patient poses a risk to himself or others.

If behavioral interventions do not adequately manage agitation, pharmacologic intervention may be necessary. Judicious use of antipsychotics can be implemented for delirium not caused by alcohol or benzodiazepine withdrawal. The decision to use antipsychotics should not be taken lightly, as these medications have been linked to an increased risk of mortality in the elderly. Special caution should be exercised when treating patients with known baseline QTc prolongation, patients receiving other QTc prolonging agents, and individuals with a history of torsade de pointes. Benzodiazepines should be avoided, unless treating alcohol or sedative-hypnotic withdrawal. The Revised Clinical Institute Withdrawal Assessment for Alcohol (CIWA-Ar) scale can be used in gauging the severity of alcohol withdrawal and determining the dose of benzodiazepines needed.

CASE CORRELATION

- See also Case 25 and Case 60 for patients that may present with similar symptoms. Delirium may be associated with fear, anxiety, and dissociative symptoms. This must be distinguished from acute stress disorder, which may present with these symptoms, but is precipitated by a severely traumatic event. Patients who are malingering may present with atypical symptoms of delirium, and there will be the absence of a medical condition or substance related to them.

COMPREHENSION QUESTIONS

46.1 A 32-year-old man with a 12-beer per day drinking history for the last year presents to the emergency department with headache, stomach upset, and tremulousness after deciding to quit drinking cold turkey earlier that day. On examination, he is afebrile with normal vital signs. He is alert and oriented to person, place, time, and situation. The man appears diaphoretic and anxious. If this patient were to progress to delirium tremens, how many hours would this be expected take?

  A. 6 to 12 hours after his last drink

  B. 12 to 24 hours after his last drink

  C. 24 to 48 hours after his last drink

  D. 48 to 96 hours after his last drink

46.2 In the previous case, what class of medication would be an appropriate first-line treatment for delirium tremens?

  A. First-generation antipsychotic

  B. Second-generation antipsychotic

  C. Benzodiazepine

  D. Barbiturate

46.3 A 71-year-old woman with a history of early Alzheimer disease is brought to the hospital by her family because "she is just not acting like her normal self" since waking up this morning. She takes no medications. On mental status examination, she is lethargic, easily distractible, and oriented only to person. At baseline, she is oriented to person and place, but has difficulty recalling the date and time. Physical examination and diagnostic workup are suggestive of an uncomplicated urinary tract infection (UTI). What is the most important component of treating this patient's delirium?

  A. Begin oral antipsychotic therapy.

  B. Treat her UTI with antibiotics.

  C. Start her on an oral benzodiazepine.

  D. Start maintenance intravenous fluids and place a Foley catheter.

46.4 In the previous case, which of the following features most distinguishes delirium from early dementia?

A. Decreased attention

B. Disorientation

C. Cognitive deficits

D. Behavioral disturbances

46.5 During morning pre-rounds, a medical student finds her 72-year-old male patient unresponsive to verbal stimuli. The patient groans to sternal rub but does not otherwise respond. What is the best descriptor for this patient's level of attention and awareness?

A. Mild delirium

B. Moderate delirium

C. Severe delirium

D. Coma

ANSWERS

46.1 **D.** This patient is experiencing early symptoms of alcohol withdrawal which typically begin within the first 6 to 12 hours following the last drink. Alcoholic hallucinosis, characterized by visual, tactile, and auditory hallucinations without disturbances in attention or awareness, occurs within 12 to 24 hours and lasts up to 48 hours. Delirium tremens rarely occurs before the 48-hour mark and may not appear until up to 96 hours from the last drink.

46.2 **C.** Delirium tremens (DTs) is one of the only forms of delirium for which benzodiazepines are useful. Oral benzodiazepines can be used early in alcohol withdrawal to reduce agitation and prevent progression to seizures or DT. Once a person has developed DT, medication must be given by intravenous route. Sedation with phenobarbital (a barbiturate) or propofol may be necessary for refractory DT and requires intubation. Antipsychotics are generally not used in DT, as they can lower the patient's seizure threshold.

46.3 **B.** The most important component of delirium treatment is to detect and treat the precipitating factor(s). In this case, the patient's dementia predisposes her to delirium, while the acute onset of the UTI precipitated her change in mental status. Of note, all antibiotics have the potential to contribute to the worsening of delirium, so a change in medication may be necessary if the patient needs a prolonged course. Use of antipsychotics has been associated with increased mortality in the elderly. Thus, these agents should be reserved for situations in which the patient's behaviors put herself or others at risk for harm. Benzodiazepines are not appropriate, as they may cause excessive sedation, disinhibition, or paradoxical excitation. While maintenance intravenous fluids or a Foley catheter may be necessary in certain cases, these items may restrict patient mobility, thereby exacerbating delirium and increasing risk of falls.

46.4 **A.** Both delirium and dementia can result in behavioral disturbances, cognitive deficits, and poor orientation. However, in all cases of delirium there is an alteration (reduction) in the level of attention. In early dementia, attention and concentration are typically maintained.

46.5 **D.** Coma is defined by unresponsiveness to verbal stimuli and precludes a diagnosis of delirium. Delirium can be conceptualized on a continuum, lying between normal attentiveness/awareness and coma.

CLINICAL PEARLS

▶ The hallmark of delirium is a fluctuation in the level of attention and awareness.

▶ Delirium carries a poor prognosis and constitutes a medical and psychiatric emergency requiring early detection and intervention.

▶ Medications are a common cause of delirium.

▶ The occurrence of symptoms during delirium is an exclusion criterion for many psychiatric disorders.

▶ The most important aspect of delirium treatment is detection and correction of the underlying condition.

▶ Antipsychotics may be used judiciously for agitation, but are associated with increased mortality in the elderly.

▶ Benzodiazepines are the treatment of choice for delirium associated with alcohol or sedative-hypnotic withdrawal.

REFERENCES

American College of Critical Care Medicine. Clinical practice guidelines for the management of pain, agitation, and delirium in adult patients in the intensive care unit. *Crit Care Med.* Jan 2013;41(1): 263-306.

American Psychiatric Association. *Diagnostic and Statistical Manual of Mental Disorders.* 5th ed. Washington, DC: American Psychiatric Association; 2013.

Kaufman D, Milstein M. *Clinical Neurology for Psychiatrists.* 7th ed. London, England: Elsevier; 2013.

Sadock BJ, Sadock VA, Ruiz P. *Kaplan & Sadock's Synopsis of Psychiatry.* 11th ed. Philadelphia, PA: Lippincott Williams & Wilkins; 2014.

A 69-year-old man is brought to the clinic by his wife due to her concern about his memory problems. Over the past several months, the patient has had increasing difficulty remembering the names of friends and family members. On two separate occasions, he has become lost while driving in his own neighborhood. As a retired engineer, he had always been meticulous about his work and appointments. Now, he needs constant reminders about every aspect of his daily affairs, including his medications. His only known medical problems are hypertension and hyperlipidemia.

On mental status examination, the patient is alert and oriented only to person and place. When asked questions, he looks to his wife for assistance in answering. He does not remember his physician's name, although he has been coming to the same office for several years. When he speaks, he seems to have difficulty finding the right words to express himself. On further cognitive testing, the patient is unable to draw a clock as directed and can only recall one of three objects after 3 minutes. The rest of his neurological and other physical examination findings are unchanged in comparison to prior evaluations.

▶ What is the most likely diagnosis for this patient?
▶ What is the next step?

ANSWERS TO CASE 47:

Major Vascular Neurocognitive Disorder (Vascular Dementia)

Summary: A 69-year-old retired engineer with a history of hypertension and hyperlipidemia has been suffering from memory problems over the last several months. Previously, he functioned at a much higher level. Mild aphasia, memory impairment, and executive dysfunction are evident on mental status examination.

- **Most likely diagnosis:** Major vascular neurocognitive disorder (NCD).

- **Next step:** Obtain laboratory tests to identify potentially reversible causes of cognitive impairment. Also consider brain imaging.

ANALYSIS

Objectives

1. Recognize and differentiate mild and major NCDs.

2. Identify the steps in the medical workup of a patient with cognitive impairment.

3. Become familiar with medications that are commonly used to treat NCDs.

Considerations

This patient has experienced worsening of memory and speech problems, which have recently become noticeable to his wife. His overall functional status has declined, and he has begun to require assistance with his daily activities. These findings are consistent with the diagnostic criteria for major NCD. His history of hypertension and hyperlipidemia are risk factors for vascular NCD. Additional evaluation is needed to determine the severity of impairment and identify the etiology.

APPROACH TO:

Major Vascular Neurocognitive Disorder (Vascular Dementia)

DEFINITIONS

AGNOSIA: Loss of ability to recognize or identify objects/people, despite intact sensory function.

APHASIA: Language impairment.

APRAXIA: Impaired ability to carry out motor activities despite intact motor function.

ACTIVITIES OF DAILY LIVING (ADLs): Essential self-care tasks (eg, feeding, bathing, dressing, grooming, toileting, and transfers).

EXECUTIVE FUNCTIONING: Ability to utilize and coordinate the various cognitive faculties (eg, planning, organizing, sequencing, and abstracting).

INSTRUMENTAL ACTIVITIES OF DAILY LIVING (IADLs): The set of skills that are necessary for independent functioning in society (eg, managing personal finances, buying groceries, meal preparation, telephone use, housekeeping, laundering clothes, medication self-administration, and driving/transportation).

SOCIAL COGNITION: Ability to recognize and consider the mental state of others.

SUNDOWNING: Phenomenon characterized by an increase in behavioral disturbances during the late afternoon or early evening hours in patients with major NCDs.

CLINICAL APPROACH

Mild and major NCDs are characterized by a decline in cognitive functioning that is **not attributable to delirium.** Especially in early stages, deficits may go unnoticed by the patient and his or her family and friends. Forgetfulness and difficulty making decisions may be attributed to normal aging. Thus, significant functional decline may occur before it is realized. An episode of delirium may be the first sign of an underlying mild NCD, or deficits may be discovered during a routine geriatric examination.

When a mild or major NCD is suspected, the physician should initiate a thorough workup to confirm the diagnosis, assess the severity, and determine the underlying etiology. History should be obtained from both the patient and collateral sources. The diagnostic criteria for mild and major NCDs are listed in Table 47–1. Severity

Table 47–1 • DIAGNOSTIC CRITERIA FOR MILD AND MAJOR NEUROCOGNITIVE DISORDERS[a]
Findings suggestive of functional decline[b] in **one or more** of the following cognitive domains based on observation/self-report and impaired cognitive performance: • Complex attention • Executive function • Learning and memory • Language • Perceptual motor • Social cognition
Occurrence of deficits outside of delirium.
Deficits not attributable to another psychiatric disorder.

[a]Note that the criteria for mild and major NCDs are essentially the same regardless of the different etiologies, with the exception of evidence from a history, a physical examination, or laboratory studies indicating a specific cause (eg, vascular disease, substance-induced, other medical condition).
[b]The difference between mild and major NCD is the degree of functional deficits, from modest to substantial. In major NCDs, cognitive deficits interfere with performing IADLs independently whereas these abilities are preserved in mild NCD.

Table 47–2 • ETIOLOGIES OF MILD AND MAJOR NEUROCOGNITIVE DISORDERS
Alzheimer disease
Vascular disease
Parkinson disease
Traumatic brain injury
Frontotemporal lobar degeneration (Pick disease)
Human immunodeficiency virus infection
Substance/medication use
Prion disease
Huntington disease
Other medical conditions

is defined in terms of ability to perform IADLs and ADLs. Patterns of cognitive and noncognitive symptoms, as well as time course, may suggest one or more of the etiological subtypes (Table 47–2). Identification of behavioral disturbances, such as agitation or depression, helps to guide treatment.

Evaluation of cognitive impairment requires a complete physical examination, including mental status and neurologic assessments. Formal neuropsychological testing is preferable for identification of specific deficits, but more readily available bedside tests may also be used. Two of the most commonly used bedside examinations are the Montreal Cognitive Assessment (MoCA) and the Mini-Mental State Examination (MMSE) (Table 47–3). The final score ranges from 0 to a perfect score of 30. A score of less than 25 is suggestive of *major* NCD, and a score of less than 20 indicates significant cognitive impairment. The MMSE is useful not only as a screening tool but also as a means of monitoring change. When scoring the MMSE, the patient's education level needs to be taken into account. Tests such as the Mini-Cog (clock drawing and three item recall at 3 minutes) is more useful for the detection and monitoring of *mild* NCDs.

Changes from *DSM-IV-TR* to *DSM-5*: *DSM-5* includes delirium, dementia, and amnestic disorders under the broad category of neurocognitive disorders (NCDs). The dementias and amnestic disorders now fall within the category of *major neurocognitive disorders*. The *DSM-5* also introduces the term *mild neurocognitive disorder*, which refers to cognitive impairments that lie on a spectrum between the deficits associated with normal aging and dementia. The mild and major NCDs are subcategorized by etiology. Cognitive domains in which deficits are noted include complex attention, executive function, language, perceptual-motor skills, learning, memory, and social cognition.

DIFFERENTIAL DIAGNOSIS

NCDs can be confused with delirium, as both can result in marked cognitive impairment. However, in NCD an alert level of consciousness is maintained, whereas **delirium manifests as a fluctuating level of consciousness.** The NCD course spans

Table 47–3 • MINI-MENTAL STATE EXAMINATION[a]

Orientation (10 points)
- Year, season, date, day of week, month
- State, county, town, or city
- Hospital or clinic, floor

Registration (3 points)
- Name three objects: apple, table, penny.
- Each must be spoken distinctly and with a brief pause.
- Patient repeats all three (1 point for each).
- Repeat process until all three objects have been learned.
- Record the number of trials needed to learn all three objects.

Attention and calculation (5 points)
- Spell WORLD backward: DLROW.
- Points are given up to the first misplaced letter.
  Example: DLORW scores as only 2 points

Recall (3 points)
- Recite the three objects memorized earlier.

Language (9 points)
- Patient names two objects when they are displayed, for example, pencil and watch (1 point each).
- Repeat a sentence: "No ifs, ands, or buts."
- Follow a three-stage command:
  1. Take a paper in your right hand.
  2. Fold it in half.
  3. Put it on the floor.
- Read and obey the following: "Close your eyes."
- Write a sentence.
- Copy the design:

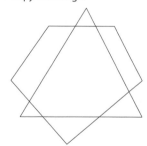

[a]Total of 30 points.

months to years, whereas the onset of delirium usually occurs over hours to days. While most dementias are irreversible, delirious states are usually reversible. This underscores the importance of a prompt and diligent workup to determine and address the underlying etiology of a perceived cognitive deficit.

Diagnostic testing is guided by findings on the history and physical examination. The workup may reveal **treatable causes** of cognitive dysfunction, such as **thyroid dysfunction** or B_{12} deficiency. **Head CT scan** or **brain MRI** should be considered in the following scenarios: **onset prior to age 65, recent onset of symptoms with rapid decline, focal neurologic examination findings, and history of head injury.**

Typical findings in irreversible major NCDs include cortical atrophy and enlarged ventricles in Alzheimer disease (Figure 47–1), preferential frontotemporal atrophy in Pick disease, and deep white-matter lacunar infarcts in vascular dementia. Lumbar puncture may be both diagnostic and therapeutic in normal pressure hydrocephalus.

NCD can often be mistaken for a depressive disorder in older individuals. Both can result in a decline in overall cognitive functioning and self-care. The level of effort put forth during cognitive examination can be revealing; NCD patients usually exert themselves fully in contrast to the amotivation seen in depressed patients.

TREATMENT

In cases where the cognitive deficits are reversible (eg, hypothyroidism, certain infections, or normal-pressure hydrocephalus), the treatment approach targets the underlying condition. Medications may slow down—but not stop—the progression of NCDs such as Alzheimer disease. In Alzheimer disease, acetylcholine is the neurotransmitter most affected. **Acetylcholinesterase inhibitors,** such as donepezil, galantamine, and rivastigmine, are used to increase the levels of acetylcholine in the central nervous system. These agents act as reversible inhibitors of acetylcholinesterase, the enzyme that catabolizes acetylcholine. Benefits are most noticeable in the mild to moderate stages of illness. Side effects include nausea, vomiting, diarrhea, and weight loss. Tacrine, the first available drug in this class, has been largely replaced because of its hepatotoxic effects and cumbersome dosing schedule. Memantine (an N-methyl-D-aspartate [NMDA] receptor antagonist) is indicated in moderate to severe Alzheimer dementia.

Other pharmacologic interventions address problematic behaviors (aggression, violence, hostility) that may present in major NCDs. A low dose of first- or second-generation antipsychotic medication can be used to manage dangerous behaviors that pose a threat to the patient or caretakers. Haloperidol and risperidone are commonly used. Patients are susceptible to the usual side effects of **extrapyramidal symptoms (EPS), orthostasis, sedation, tardive dyskinesia,** and **metabolic syndrome.** Patients with **Lewy body disease** are particularly vulnerable to developing a **dystonic reaction from first-generation antipsychotics.** Treating cognitively impaired, older patients with antipsychotics comes with an **increased risk of stroke.** Thus, these medications should **only be used after psychosocial de-escalation measures have failed. Benzodiazepines** may cause **paradoxical disinhibition, oversedation, unsteadiness, and falls in the elderly** and should, as a rule, be avoided.

Psychosocial measures for prevention of behavioral disturbances include maintenance of **natural sleep-wake cycles, adequate pain control, and regular elimination schedules.** Whenever possible, **verbal de-escalation techniques** should be employed. Use of **restraints and other tethers** (eg, IV lines, urinary catheters, or telemetry wires) should be **avoided,** as they may **precipitate or worsen agitation.**

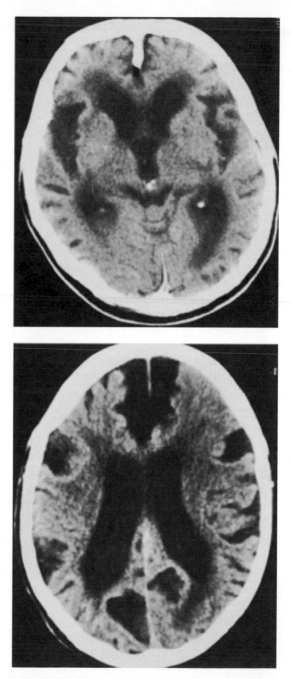

Figure 47-1. CT scan of brain of patient with dementia. Top: Alzheimer disease. Axial CT section demonstrating severe generalized cerebral cortical atrophy and moderately severe ventricular enlargement. Bottom: Pick disease. Pronounced selective atrophy of the frontal and temporal lobes. (Reproduced, with permission, from Lee SH, Rao KCVG, Zimmerman RA. Cranial MRI and CT. New York, NY: McGraw-Hill; 1992.)

CASE CORRELATION

- See also Case 13 and Case 46 for patients who may present with cognitive dysfunction. Patients with major depressive disorder may have cognitive deficits, but the pattern of them (nonspecific, more variable performance) may help distinguish them from a NCD (consistent memory and executive function deficits are typical in Alzheimer patients). Delirious patients may closely resemble patients with a vascular NCD; careful assessment of attention and arousal will help distinguish between the two.

COMPREHENSION QUESTIONS

47.1 A 75-year-old man is brought in by his daughter for a psychiatric evaluation. He has become increasingly forgetful over the past year, missing engagements with his children and grandchildren. He has gotten lost several times driving in his own neighborhood. He has no psychiatric history, but he has felt lonely since the passing of his wife 14 months ago. His medical history is significant for poorly controlled hypertension. Which of the following additional features is necessary in order to accurately diagnose a major NCD?

A. Agitation

B. Fluctuation in consciousness

C. Radiographic findings

D. Hallucinations

E. Loss of independence in IADLs

47.2 Given the above patient's feelings of sadness following the loss of his spouse, a depressive disorder (pseudodementia) is considered in the differential diagnosis of his memory issue. How would this patient be predicted to perform on cognitive testing if he has a major NCD rather than a depressive illness?

A. Reduced effort with poor insight

B. Reduced effort with good insight

C. No effort with poor insight

D. Better effort with poor insight

E. Better effort with good insight

47.3 A 73-year-old man with major NCD becomes verbally aggressive with the staff at his nursing facility. A geriatric psychiatrist is asked to evaluate the patient and provide treatment recommendations. Which of the following would be the initial step in managing the patient's behaviors?

A. Chlorpromazine

B. Donepezil

C. Lorazepam

D. Physical restraints

E. Verbal de-escalation

ANSWERS

47.1 **E.** For a diagnosis of major NCD, loss of independence in one or more IADLs must be present. Head CT scan or brain MRI may show lacunar infarcts or microvascular changes in major vascular NCD, whereas generalized cortical atrophy and ventricular enlargement are the changes seen in Alzheimer disease. Individuals with major NCDs usually remain alert, whereas those with delirium display a fluctuation in consciousness. While psychotic symptoms such as delusions and hallucinations can be seen, they are neither specific to nor necessary for the diagnosis of a major NCD.

47.2 **D.** On cognitive testing, patients with NCD generally put forth considerable effort, display poor insight into their deficits, and minimize their problems. In contrast, those with depressive disorders are often apathetic and make little effort.

47.3 **E.** The treatment approach for behavioral problems in elderly, cognitively impaired patients should normally begin with verbal de-escalation techniques. If the patient is acutely at risk of harming himself or others, treatment with a low dose of a high-potency antipsychotic such as haloperidol can decrease agitation and aggression. Lower-potency antipsychotics such as chlorpromazine should be avoided given their significant anticholinergic and orthostatic side effects. Benzodiazepines like lorazepam may cause oversedation or disinhibition in patients, potentially worsening their behavior or increasing their fall risk. Physical restraints should be avoided because they can worsen agitation. Acetylcholinesterase inhibitors such as donepezil can help to delay cognitive decline in the early and mid-stages of Alzheimer disease, but offer little benefit for treatment of behavioral disturbances.

CLINICAL PEARLS

▶ Mild and major neurocognitive disorders are characterized by a **decline in cognition.**

▶ Ability to perform **IADLs is preserved in mild NCDs.**

▶ The initial workup of cognitive impairment includes evaluation **for reversible etiologies.**

▶ **Neuropsychologic testing** is the method of choice for diagnosis and determination of severity.

▶ Patients with mild and major NCDs are at **increased risk of experiencing delirium**—this may be the initial presentation.

▶ Attempt **de-escalation techniques prior to use of chemical restraints.** Low-dose antipsychotics can be used judiciously for behavioral disturbances that threaten the safety of the individual or others around them.

▶ Patients with **Lewy body disease** are particularly **vulnerable to dystonic reactions.**

▶ **Restraints,** IV lines, urinary catheters, or telemetry wires may **precipitate or worsen agitation.**

REFERENCES

American Psychiatric Association. *Diagnostic and Statistical Manual of Mental Disorders.* 5th ed. Washington, DC: American Psychiatric Association; 2013.

Council on Geriatric Psychiatry. American Psychiatric Association. Resource document on the use of antipsychotic medications to treat behavioral disturbances in persons with dementia; 2014. http://www.psych.org/learn/library--archives/resource-documents. Accessed Sep 16, 2014.

Kaufman DM, Milstein MJ. *Kaufman's Clinical Neurology for Psychiatrists.* 7th ed. London, England: Elsevier; 2013.

Medicare Detection of Cognitive Impairment Workgroup. Alzheimer's Association. Alzheimer's Association recommendations for operationalizing the detection of cognitive impairment during the Medicare Annual Wellness Visit in a primary care setting. *Alzheimer's and Dementia.* 2013:1-10.

A 56-year-old man is referred to a psychiatrist from his primary care physician due to restricted affect and concern about possible depression. The patient denies that he is depressed or feeling stressed. He was doing well in his job as a security guard, working the night shift, until he was told that his position was being phased out and that in order to stay with the company, he would need to switch to the day shift. The patient agreed because he did not think that this would be a problem, and did not want to lose his insurance benefits and retirement plan. However, after several months in his new position he admits he is concerned that he is not doing as well in his new position. His previous position allowed him work on his own the vast majority of his work hours, while his new job requires almost constant interaction with coworkers, clients, his supervisor, and the general public, which does not agree with him as he describes himself as "not a very sociable person." The patient says that he has almost no friends, except for a cousin that he has been close to since childhood. He reports that he has never had a significant romantic relationship or sexual encounter, but does not miss not having had these experiences or not having friends. He states that he most enjoys spending hours surfing the Internet, collecting stamps, or playing computer games by himself. He has never seen a mental health professional before and has presented today only at the insistence of his primary care doctor.

On a mental status examination, the patient appears notably detached and aloof toward the examiner. He exhibits little eye contact. His mood is reported as "stressed," but his affect is not congruent with this. He appears calm, and his emotional range is flat. No other prominent symptoms are noted during the mental status examination.

▶ What is the most likely diagnosis?
▶ What is the best initial treatment?

ANSWERS TO CASE 48:

Schizoid Personality Disorder

Summary: A 56-year-old man presents to a psychiatrist due to his primary care doctor's concern of restricted affect and depression, who reports no complaints but gives a history of isolation and very limited interactions with others. The results of the patient's mental status examination are essentially normal, other than showing a restricted emotional range.

- **Most likely diagnosis:** Schizoid personality disorder.

- **Best initial treatment:** Although long-term psychotherapy might help this patient, his condition is ego-syntonic, and thus he will probably not be motivated to undergo such treatment. The best strategy for decreasing this patient's stress is for him to seek another job with a low level of interpersonal interaction.

ANALYSIS

Objectives

1. Recognize schizoid personality disorder in a patient.

2. Understand that patients with this disorder tend to do poorly in settings where a great deal of interpersonal interaction is required.

Considerations

This patient likely has schizoid personality disorder. Recent studies estimate the prevalence of schizoid personality disorder as 1% to 7.5%, with men being diagnosed twice as often as women. There is some minor association of psychotic disorders in the relatives of schizoid individuals. A personality disorder is an inflexible way of thinking about oneself or environment, causing social or occupational difficulties. The patient's life, although very socially isolated, appears adequate for the patient's needs, as he has not sought any kind of psychiatric treatment. The lack of any psychotic symptoms (hallucinations or delusions) as revealed by the patient's mental status examination is also consistent. The patient's visit to the primary care doctor is probably one of the few ways that such patients interact with medical personnel (aside from reporting other physical complaints, as in the general population).

APPROACH TO:
Schizoid Personality Disorder

DEFINITIONS

ALLOPLASTIC DEFENSES: Defenses used by patients who react to stress by attempting to change the external environment, for example, by threatening or manipulating others.

AUTOPLASTIC DEFENSES: Defenses used by patients who react to stress by changing their internal psychological processes.

EGO-DYSTONIC: Describes a character deficit perceived by a patient as objectionable, distressing, or inconsistent to the self.

EGO-SYNTONIC: Describes a character deficit perceived by the patient to be acceptable, unobjectionable, and consistent to the self. The patient tends to blame others for problems that occur. Personality disorders are ego-syntonic.

INTELLECTUALIZATION: A defense mechanism by which an individual deals with internal or external stressors by excessive use of abstract thinking or making generalizations, in order to control or minimize disturbing feelings. It is present as a component of brooding, in which events are continually rehashed in a distant, abstract, emotionally barren fashion.

PERSONALITY DISORDER: Enduring patterns of perceiving, relating to, and thinking about the environment and oneself that **are inflexible, maladaptive, and cause significant impairment in social or occupational functioning.** They are not caused by the direct physiologic effects of a substance or another general medical condition and are not the consequence of another mental disorder. They are present during the **person's stable functioning** and not only during acute stress.

PERSONALITY TRAITS: Enduring patterns of perceiving, relating to, and thinking about the environment and oneself. They are exhibited in a wide range of important social and personal contexts. Everyone has personality traits.

PROJECTION: A defense mechanism by which individuals deal with conflict by falsely attributing to another their own unacceptable feelings, impulses, or thoughts. By blaming others for their sentiments and actions, the focus is removed from the person doing the accusing. For example, a patient who is angry with his therapist suddenly accuses the therapist of being angry with him.

SCHIZOID FANTASY: A defense mechanism whereby fantasy is used as an escape and as a means of gratification so that other people are not required for emotional fulfillment. The retreat into fantasy itself acts as a means of distancing others.

PERSONALITY DISORDER CLUSTERS: Three categories into which these disorders are broadly classified: A, B, and C (Table 48–1).

Table 48–1 • CLASSIFICATION OF PERSONALITY DISORDERS				
Cluster A: "Mad"— odd and eccentric	Schizoid: Loner, detached, flat affect, restricted emotions, generally indifferent to interpersonal relationships outside of immediate family	Schizotypal: Odd, eccentric, magical thinking, paranoid, not psychotic Defense: Projection, regression, fantasy	Paranoid: Distrustful and suspicious; constricted affect Defense: Projection	
Cluster B: "Bad"— dramatic and erratic	Histrionic: Excessively emotional, attention-seeking Defense: Reaction formation	Narcissistic: Self-important, needs admiration, dismissive of the feelings of others	Antisocial: Lacks empathy toward others, acts out, aggressive, must have met criteria for conduct disorder as a child	Borderline: Impulsive, unstable relationships, affective instability Defense: Splitting, projection
Cluster C: "Sad"— anxious and timid	Obsessive-compulsive: Perfectionist, "control freak," hyperfocused on orderliness Defense: Reaction formation	Avoidant: Hypersensitive to criticism, socially uncomfortable, seeks out interpersonal relationships but with great discomfort	Dependent: Submissive, clinging, needs to be taken care of, seeks others to make decisions for him/her	

CLUSTER A: Characterized by odd or eccentric behavior. Schizoid, schizotypal, and paranoid personality disorders fall into cluster A.

CLUSTER B: Characterized by dramatic or emotional behavior. Histrionic, narcissistic, antisocial, and borderline personality disorders fall into cluster B.

CLUSTER C: Characterized by anxious or fearful behavior. Obsessive-compulsive, avoidant, and dependent personality disorders fall into cluster C.

CLINICAL PEARLS

▶ These clusters can be remembered by the words "mad" (cluster A disorders in which patients display odd or eccentric behavior), "bad" (cluster B disorders in which patients exhibit dramatic or emotional behavior), and "sad" (cluster C disorders in which patients show anxious or fearful behavior).

CLINICAL APPROACH

Diagnostic Criteria

Patients with schizoid personality disorders have a pervasive pattern of indifference to social relationships and a restricted range of emotional experience and expression.

They have difficulty in expressing hostility and are self-absorbed, detached day-dreamers. As a rule, they are indifferent to intimate personal contact. They are often functional at work, as long as it does not require a great deal of interpersonal contact. They appear somewhat indifferent to either praise or criticism.

DIFFERENTIAL DIAGNOSIS

Although patients with schizoid personality disorder may have robust fantasy lives and appear as odd, they do not evidence frank psychosis and can have successful work histories, especially if their jobs are performed in an isolated setting. Patients with schizophrenia and schizotypal personality disorder, in contrast, typically experience more difficulty functioning in a work environment or in society at large. Patients with schizotypal personality disorder often engage in quasi-delusional or magical thinking. Patients with paranoid personality disorder tend to be more verbally hostile and tend to project their feelings onto others. Although patients with obsessive-compulsive personality disorder and avoidant personality disorder can appear just as emotionally constricted, they experience loneliness as ego-dystonic. They also do not tend to have such a rich fantasy life. Patients with avoidant personality disorder strongly wish for relationships with others, but are afraid to reach out. In contrast, patients with schizoid personality disorder feel little need for relationships.

TIPS FOR INTERACTING WITH SCHIZOID PATIENTS

Patients with schizoid personality disorder need privacy and do not like interpersonal interactions. The needs of such patients should be appreciated. The physician should use a low-key, technical approach (not a "warm and fuzzy" one) when dealing with these patients.

CASE CORRELATION

- See also Case 2 and Case 50 for other patients who feel detached or uncomfortable in social situations. Individuals with mild autism may resemble patients with schizoid PD, but have more severely impaired social interactions and stereotyped behaviors. Those with avoidant PD may appear as if they are detached from social interactions, but in reality, would like to engage in them, but are too afraid of rejection or humiliation to interact socially.

COMPREHENSION QUESTIONS

48.1 A 48-year-old woman presents to a psychotherapist. The patient lives a very secluded life, largely consumed by working nights as a janitor at a department store and taking care of her elderly mother. She complains of feeling lonely and is aware that she has a great deal of difficulty relating to other people. Which of the following conditions would most distinguish her issues from a person with schizoid personality disorder?

A. Family history of a cousin with schizophrenia

B. A desire to engage in interpersonal relationships

C. Lack of hallucinations or delusional thinking

D. Her gender

E. A history of alcoholism

48.2 A patient with schizoid personality disorder comes to his primary care physician with chief complaints of polyuria and polydipsia. He is found to have insulin-dependent diabetes. Which of the following interventions by the physician is likely to be most well received by this patient?

A. Asking the patient to bring in a relative or close friend so that he can describe the treatment regimen to both of them at the same time.

B. Referring the patient to a therapist for support in dealing with a chronic illness.

C. Giving the patient detailed written information about the disease and telling him that the physician will be available to answer any questions.

D. Referring the patient to a group that helps its members learn about diabetes and to better deal with their illness.

E. Scheduling frequent appointments with the patient so that all the treatment details can be explained on a one-to-one basis.

48.3 A woman with schizoid personality disorder was involved in a motor vehicle accident in which she was rear-ended by another car. The driver of the other car refused to take responsibility for the accident and hired a lawyer to provide his defense. The woman spends hours every day thinking about the specifics of the accident, including such details as the color of the cars involved and what each party to the accident was wearing. Which of the following defense mechanisms, common to patients with schizoid personality disorder, is the woman using?

A. Sublimation

B. Undoing

C. Projection

D. Intellectualization

E. Introjection

48.4   A 20-year-old man is brought to a psychiatrist by his parents for odd thinking. He is dressed in clothes more consistent with a 1960's hippie, with long
unruly hair and marginal hygiene. He was recently fired from his job for not
showing up for his shifts and was forced to move back in with his parents.
He has artistic aspirations and is very interested in philosophy, metaphysics,
magic, and the occult. He talks about his desire for fame and wealth, given his
special talents. He has recently gotten into some legal trouble as he produced
art work of fanciful paper currency, which he attempted to use at some local
stores. However, he admits that he did not think that this was going to work
and describes this as a performance art. Which of the following is the most
likely diagnosis?

A.   Schizophrenia

B.   Schizoid personality disorder

C.   Schizotypal personality disorder

D.   Delusional disorder

E.   Bipolar disorder

ANSWERS

48.1   **B.** The hallmark of schizoid personality disorder is a detachment and disinterest in social relationships. This patient is clearly distressed by her lack of
social relationships, which would clearly steer the diagnosis away from schizoid personality disorder. Men are more frequently, though not exclusively,
diagnosed with schizoid personality disorder.

48.2   **C.** Patients with schizoid personality disorder generally prefer to keep social
interaction to a minimum. They do better with a more technical approach
with as little human interaction as possible.

48.3   **D.** Intellectualization is characterized by rehashing events over and over.

48.4   **C.** Given his odd thinking, albeit not frankly psychotic, schizotypal personality disorder is most likely. (See Case 54 for a comparison of the two diagnoses.) The lack of frank psychosis makes schizophrenia, delusional disorder, or
bipolar disorder less likely.

CLINICAL PEARLS

▶ Patients with schizoid personality disorder show a pervasive, stable pattern of disinterest in interpersonal relationships, coupled with a rich fantasy life. They appear emotionally detached.

▶ Schizoid personality disorder belongs in cluster A, the "mad" cluster.

▶ Patients with this disorder can be differentiated from patients with avoidant personality disorder by their utter lack of interest in interpersonal relationships. Patients with avoidant personality disorder wish to engage in interpersonal relationships, but find this distressing and confusing.

▶ Patients with schizoid personality disorder can be differentiated from patients with schizotypal personality disorder by the former's lack of a family history of schizophrenia, absence of magical thinking, and their often successful (if isolated) work careers. Patients with schizotypal personality disorder exhibit more flamboyantly odd behavior, such as immersion in the occult, witchcraft, and the paranormal.

▶ Physicians do well in dealing with such patients when they use a low-key, technical approach.

▶ Therapy does not tend to work well with these patients, as they are not motivated to undergo treatment. Their disorder is ego-syntonic, as are all personality disorders.

REFERENCES

Maytal G, Smallwood P. Personality disorders. *Massachusetts General Hospital Psychiatry Update & Board Preparation*. Boston, MA: MGH Psychiatry Academy Publishing; 2012:209-210.

Sadock BJ, Sadock VA, Ruiz P. *Kaplan and Sadock's Synopsis of Psychiatry: Behavioral Sciences/Clinical Psychiatry*. 11th ed. Baltimore, MD: Lippincott Williams & Wilkins; 2014.

CASE 49

A 32-year-old man is seen by a jail psychiatrist after getting into a fight with another inmate over a $5 bet. Jailed for forging bad checks, this is the patient's fourth incarceration. Previous incarcerations were for assaulting a police officer, stealing from a department store, and at age 13, stealing a car. The patient states that he fought with the other inmate because, "I was bored and felt like it." He admits that the $5 was not really his to begin with, but he shows no remorse either about trying to take the money or about getting into a physical altercation with the other inmate. The patient states that he has seen psychiatrists in the past (always reluctantly and always because of demands made either by his mother or the courts) but states, "There isn't anything wrong with me, so why should I?" He denies using drugs or alcohol while incarcerated, but admits that if he were not in jail, he would probably be using both.

A mental status examination indicates the patient is alert and oriented to person, place, and time. He cooperates with the examiner. At times, he appears open and engaging, even charming, while at other times he is rude and disrespectful. He is dressed in jail garb. His speech is normal in rate, rhythm, and tone. His mood is described as "fine," and his affect is congruent. He shows no disorders of thought processes or thought content.

▶ What is the most likely diagnosis?
▶ What other psychiatric disorders might one suspect in this patient?

ANSWERS TO CASE 49:

Antisocial Personality Disorder

Summary: A 32-year-old incarcerated man is seen by a psychiatrist after he gets into a fight with a fellow inmate. He has a long history of incarcerations and an inability to conform to societal norms, which appears to have begun at least as early as age 13. He does not seem to be remorseful about his actions.

- **Most likely diagnosis:** Antisocial personality disorder.

- **Other suspected psychiatric disorders:** High on the list of comorbid psychiatric disorders is any substance use disorder.

ANALYSIS

Objectives

1. Know the diagnostic criteria for antisocial personality disorder.

2. Understand the common comorbidities found in patients with this disorder.

Considerations

This patient presents a typical case of antisocial personality disorder. He clearly does not show any remorse for his actions, nor does he conform to societal norms (multiple arrests). He is deceitful (forging checks), impulsive (stealing cars and from department stores), and irresponsible. His behavior appears to be a lifelong pattern, beginning in his adolescence. The fact that he freely admits to drug and alcohol abuse makes it even more likely that some kind of substance abuse or dependence is comorbid in this patient.

APPROACH TO:

Antisocial Personality Disorder

DEFINITIONS

ACTING OUT: A defense mechanism in which an individual guards against uncomfortable emotional conflicts or stressors through actions rather than reflections or feelings. For example, a man who has a hard day at work and is humiliated by his boss goes out that night and starts a fight at a local bar.

PROJECTIVE IDENTIFICATION: Projective identification is a defense mechanism that helps an individual deal with emotional conflict or stressors by falsely attributing to another person the individual's own unacceptable feelings, impulses, or thoughts—just as in projection. Not infrequently, the individual induces in others the very feelings that he or she first mistakenly believed to be there, thus setting into motion a self-fulfilling prophecy. For example, a paranoid patient has uncomfortable hostile emotions and projects them onto another person, believing that the other is hostile to him. He then behaves *as if* the other person is going to be hostile to him. The other person, seeing the suspiciousness and the withdrawal of the patient, eventually acts in a frustrated (or seemingly hostile) manner toward the patient, thus completing the loop.

CLINICAL APPROACH

Diagnostic Criteria

Patients with antisocial personality disorder show a pervasive disregard for and violation of the rights of others starting by age 15. These individuals often appear to have **no conscience and no remorse about their activities.** They repeatedly perform illegal acts, lie frequently, and are impulsive and irritable. However, although antisocial personality disorder is very common in a correctional population, just a history of contact with the legal system is not pathognomic for the disorder, as individuals may resort to criminal behavior for other reasons (eg, a drug addict burglarizing homes in order to obtain money for drugs). Antisocial personality disordered patients often engage in physical fights and have an almost **reckless disregard for the safety of others.** They are consistently irresponsible as well. Although **the diagnosis is not made until the patient is older than age 18,** there must be evidence of a conduct disorder in childhood with an onset before the age of 15. The antisocial behavior cannot occur exclusively during the course of another psychiatric illness.

DIFFERENTIAL DIAGNOSIS

Patients with antisocial personality disorder must be differentiated from people who perform antisocial acts. The difference is that patients with the personality disorder lack empathy for others; have little to no remorse; and exhibit reckless, impulsive, and antisocial behavior in many areas of life. Not only do they often run afoul of the law, but they also lack stable relationships with others, and all areas of their lives are permeated by difficulties involving recklessness, impulsiveness, and irresponsibility. It can be difficult to differentiate patients with active substance abuse disorders from those with antisocial personality disorders because many individuals with antisocial personality disorder abuse substances, and many substance abusers commit antisocial acts to facilitate their addiction. However, when the antisocial behavior occurs secondary to a substance abuse disorder, antisocial personality should not be diagnosed. For example, if a person robs a convenience store to support a heroin habit, but this kind of behavior does not occur when he does not need money for drugs, a diagnosis of antisocial personality disorder should not be made.

Interviewing Tips

Patients with antisocial personality disorder can often appear colorful and seductive, or manipulative and demanding. In all instances, a firm, no-nonsense approach with firm limit setting is indicated. Clinicians should be careful not to allow themselves to become punitive because of their anger over the patient's antisocial behavior and lack of remorse.

TREATMENT

The treatment of antisocial personality disorder is **difficult** at best and is generally focused on reducing impulsive or aggressive behaviors and antisocial acts rather than on a "cure." **Selective serotonin reuptake inhibitors (SSRIs) and mood stabilizers** have shown promise in reducing aggressive symptoms. **Socially based interventions,** such as group therapy with individuals with the same diagnosis, are considered helpful because patients reduce the amount of rationalization and evasion shown by others in the group because they recognize the patterns. **Psychodynamic psychotherapy has been singularly unhelpful** in these patients.

CASE CORRELATION

- See also Case 37 and Case 38 for patients who may present with a history of antisocial acts. For patients older than age 18, a diagnosis of conduct disorder is given only if the criteria for antisocial personality disorder are not met. Substance use disordered patients may have antisocial acts as a consequence of the disorder (stealing money to use for drugs, for example) but generally do not have antisocial acts in other arenas.

COMPREHENSION QUESTIONS

49.1 A 39-year-old man is evaluated by mental health services in prison. He has a history of multiple arrests as both an adult and as a juvenile. After several interviews, a diagnosis of antisocial personality disorder is confirmed. He has a history of multiple psychiatric hospitalizations after suicide attempts and was in special education programming as a child. Which psychiatric diagnosis is most likely to have occurred comorbidly in such an individual?

    A. Attention deficit hyperactivity disorder

    B. Cocaine dependence

    C. Traumatic brain injury

    D. Major depression

    E. Conduct disorder

49.2 A 16-year-old adolescent girl is incarcerated in a juvenile detention facility. She is currently charged with theft, apparently to support her and her boyfriend's drug habit. She has had multiple involvements with child and family services for running away from home, where she apparently had been sexually abused by her mother's boyfriend. She has a diagnosis of posttraumatic stress disorder (PTSD). Prior to the onset of the abuse, she was doing extremely well in school, in an accelerated program. Which of the following factors speaks most strongly against a diagnosis of antisocial personality disorder?

A. Her concurrent diagnosis of PTSD

B. Her gender

C. Her age

D. Antisocial acts committed to support a drug habit only

E. Apparent high intelligence

49.3 A 39-year-old man with antisocial personality disorder, incarcerated for life after murdering a man, has a multitude of somatic complaints over the course of several years. Yearly physical examinations never show anything physically wrong with him, yet he complains of a variety of aches and pains, neurologic symptoms, and gastrointestinal distress. He does not enjoy the time he spends in the jail's infirmary. Which of the following is the most likely explanation for this patient's complaints?

A. He is malingering.

B. He has developed a psychotic disorder.

C. He has developed a somatic disorder.

D. He has an undiagnosed physical illness.

E. He has an undiagnosed anxiety disorder.

49.4 Which of the following scenarios is most consistent with antisocial personality **traits**?

A. A 13-year-old boy living in an extremely economically depressed area who joins a street gang to avoid being beaten by competing gangs.

B. A 38-year-old male drug addict who has been arrested seven times for retail theft.

C. A 67-year-old male CEO, who embezzles from his company, is unfaithful to his third wife, and has been involved in covering up corporate malfeasance from federal investigators.

D. A 42-year-old homeless female schizophrenic who has been arrested on misdemeanor trespassing charges five times in the past 2 years.

E. A 28-year-old woman who has a history of prostitution, drug abuse, and multiple suicide attempts with over 20 inpatient psychiatric admissions.

ANSWERS

49.1 **E.** Although all the diagnoses listed are frequently comorbid, evidence of a diagnosis of conduct disorder with onset before age 15 is *required* for a diagnosis of antisocial personality disorder. Antisocial personality disorder remains the only diagnosis in the DSM system in which an individual must have had a preceding disorder in adolescence.

49.2 **C.** Personality disorders cannot be diagnosed before 18 years of age. Antisocial personality disorder should not be overlooked in females, even though it is much more common in males. Antisocial actions committed solely during psychotic or manic episodes, or to support a drug habit, would not support a diagnosis of antisocial personality disorder.

49.3 **C.** Development of a somatic disorder becomes more common in patients with antisocial personality disorder as they grow older. There is no evidence of secondary gain here (which rules out malingering), nor is there evidence of psychotic thinking. Physical examinations have all been negative (making a physical illness less likely) and the complaints are all around somatic symptoms, making a pure anxiety disorder less likely as well.

49.4 **C.** In A, the individual is too young for any diagnosis of a personality disorder, and as also in D, appears to be resorting to antisocial acts in order to survive. In B, the individual is likely to be stealing in order to support his drug habit. In C, the individual is displaying a pattern of violating the rights of others across several settings. E is suggestive of borderline personality disorder.

CLINICAL PEARLS

▶ Patients with antisocial personality disorder show a reckless disregard for and violation of the rights of others starting in childhood or adolescence. The disorder itself cannot be diagnosed until the patient is 18 years old, although evidence of conduct disorder must be seen before the age of 15.

▶ Physicians should adopt a firm, no-nonsense, yet nonpunitive approach with these patients.

▶ Substance abuse disorders are often comorbid in patients with antisocial personality disorders. However, if the antisocial behavior occurs *only* in context of behavior designed to procure drugs and never when the patient is sober, the personality disorder should not be diagnosed.

▶ Patients with antisocial personality disorder evidence it in *all* facets of their lives, not just, for example, when robbing a store for personal gain.

  ▶ Unlawful behaviors have many other etiologies other than antisocial personality disorder.

▶ Defense mechanisms commonly used in patients with antisocial personality disorder are projective identification and acting out.

REFERENCES

American Psychiatric Association. *Diagnostic and Statistical Manual of Mental Disorders*. 5th ed. Washington, DC: American Psychiatric Publishing; 2013.

Sadock BJ, Sadock VA, Ruiz P. *Kaplan and Sadock's Synopsis of Psychiatry: Behavioral Sciences/Clinical Psychiatry*. 11th ed. Baltimore, MD: Lippincott Williams & Wilkins; 2014.

A 21-year-old woman comes to the student counseling center with complaints of being depressed and feeling anxious. She states that 2 weeks ago, while in class, she was called on by the teacher and gave the wrong answer. She says that she felt "humiliated" and has not gone back to the classroom since then. She describes a lifelong history of being painfully shy. She admits that she would like to have a boyfriend but is afraid to meet anyone because, "He'll find someone better and dump me." She describes herself as "socially retarded" and avoids going out with anyone new. She has two close friends from junior high school and does go out to dinner with them weekly, which she enjoys. She denies trouble sleeping or with her appetite, although she does admit to feeling ashamed of her social ineptitude. She is worried that she will be unable to finish college because of her problems.

▶ What is the most likely diagnosis?
▶ What is the best therapy for this patient?

ANSWERS TO CASE 50:

Avoidant Personality Disorder

Summary: A 21-year-old patient comes to the counseling center after an embarrassing interpersonal interaction in class. She has a long history of avoiding close interpersonal relationships because of her fear of being rejected. She avoids new interpersonal situations because she feels inadequate.

- **Most likely diagnosis:** Avoidant personality disorder.

- **Best therapy:** Psychodynamic or cognitive behavioral psychotherapy.

ANALYSIS

Objectives

1. Recognize avoidant personality disorder in a patient.

2. Understand the treatment that is likely to be helpful to patients with this disorder.

Considerations

This young woman presents a classic picture of avoidant personality disorder. Although she desperately desires friends and intimate relationships, she is **excruciatingly sensitive to rejection** (or even the chance of being rejected) and therefore avoids all but a few safe relationships. These patients usually view themselves as socially inept or otherwise unappealing and then assume that other people will have the same opinion. Rejections, especially in a public setting, are particularly humiliating, and patients can experience depressed and anxious moods as a result. (These moods do not, however, fit the criteria for any other psychiatric diagnosis.)

APPROACH TO:

Avoidant Personality Disorder

DEFINITIONS

DISPLACEMENT: A defense mechanism in which an individual avoids emotional conflict or stress by transferring a feeling about, or a response to, one object to another (usually a less threatening or dangerous one). For example, after being yelled at by his boss, a man comes home and lets his anger out by yelling at his children.

PROJECTION: A defense mechanism in which individuals attribute feelings they have about themselves or the world to others. For example, a man feels hostility toward his boss, so he attributes hostile motives to his supervisor's actions, even if others would see the actions as benign.

CLINICAL APPROACH

Patients with this disorder experience pervasive **social discomfort, feelings of inadequacy, and hypersensitivity to criticism and rejection.** They are often seen as very timid, and they avoid occupational or social activities because they are afraid of rejection. These patients view themselves as socially inept or inferior to others. Prevalence rates range from 0.5% to 1% in the general population.

DIFFERENTIAL DIAGNOSIS

Patients with this disorder can often be confused with patients with schizoid personality disorder because both have very few, if any, close friends or relationships. The difference lies in the reason why they lack these relationships. Patients with **avoidant personality disorder desperately wish to have close friendships** but are afraid to initiate them for fear of rejection. Patients with schizoid personality disorders do not really wish for close relationships and are happy without them. Patients with dependent personality disorder can appear similar to those with avoidant personality disorder—the difference is subtle. Patients with dependent personality disorder cling to others in their inner circle because they are afraid to function on their own. A patient with avoidant personality disorder, although appearing timid, is more afraid of rejection itself than of being able to take care of himself or herself.

Social phobia is an intense, persistent fear of being exposed to unfamiliar people or scrutiny by others because of the belief that one will be humiliated or embarrassed. When exposed to such a situation, the patient may have a situationally bound panic attack. As a result, the patient avoids feared situations even though he or she recognizes that the fear is excessive or unreasonable. In the case described, the patient is not having discrete anxiety attacks. If she was, the patient could be diagnosed with social phobia as well. Social phobia often responds to selective serotonin reuptake inhibitors (SSRIs) along with cognitive behavioral psychotherapy.

TREATMENT

Patients with this disorder are afraid of being rejected or criticized, and **so the clinician must be very tactful, accepting, and encouraging in approaching these patients.** Coercive or confrontational behavior does not work with these individuals, who can agree with the clinician at the time of the confrontation but never return.

Patients with avoidant personality disorder often have dysfunctional beliefs regarding the world. Often, they view people in general as critical and rejecting, thus they are reluctant to place their trust in people and consequently withdraw. The goal of psychotherapy is to help patients critically examine if their assumptions about themselves and other people are correct. SSRIs or beta-blockers can help reduce anxiety associated with some social situations. Benzodiazepines, with their high potential for being habit forming, should generally be avoided.

> ## CASE CORRELATION
>
> - See also Case 53 for patients who are hypersensitive to criticism and have a need for reassurance. However, the primary focus of concern in avoidant personality disordered patients is the avoidance of humiliation or rejection, while for dependent personality disordered patients, it is to be taken care of.

COMPREHENSION QUESTIONS

50.1 A 29-year-old man is sent to a counselor at his employee assistance program, upon the urging of his supervisor. The patient had been working the night shift, but was recently promoted to a position on the day shift, with new supervisory responsibilities. Subsequently, his job performance has dropped off significantly. The patient states that since his transfer, he has been so nervous at work that he has not been able to think straight. He reports that his mood at home has been good, but that he knows he will fail at the new job because, "I have always been such a dope when it comes to working with other people." After several sessions, the counselor diagnoses the patient with avoidant personality disorder. Which of the following would be the most helpful in assisting the patient to manage his anxiety regarding his new job?

A. Tell the patient that he needs to be more confident in his skills during this transition and "suck it up."

B. Engage the patient in cognitive therapy to help him deal with his distorted thinking.

C. Give the patient a beta-blocker to help him control his anxiety.

D. Prescribe a benzodiazepine.

E. Tell the patient that he is probably not ready for this job if he is this anxious.

50.2 A 24-year-old man presents to a therapist. Which of the following statements made by the patient is most consistent with avoidant personality disorder?

A. "I have a couple of close friends, but it is very hard to make friends. I'm afraid most people wouldn't want me around."

B. "I'm usually fine around people. It's just when I'm around a lot of people I've never met before that I get freaked out."

C. "I'm afraid that people are plotting against me."

D. "My mom thinks I have a problem with people. I can take them or leave them."

E. "My girlfriend thinks I have a problem with people, like with her friends. What do you think?"

50.3 Which statement best characterizes the difference between patients with avoidant personality disorders and those with schizoid personality disorders?

A. Patients with avoidant personality disorders have fewer friends than those with schizoid personality disorders.

B. Patients with avoidant personality disorders have higher self-esteem than those with schizoid personality disorders.

C. Patients with avoidant personality disorders would like to have friends more than patients with schizoid personality disorders.

D. Patients with avoidant personality disorders are better at accepting criticism than patients with schizoid personality disorders.

E. Patients with avoidant personality disorders are less anxious than are patients with schizoid personality disorders.

50.4 A 35-year-old woman is engaged in psychotherapy to address her avoidant personality disorder. In particular, she is distressed by her inability to maintain a romantic relationship with a man. During the course of treatment, the therapist learns that her father was alcoholic, and was physically abusive to the patient and her mother. Which defense mechanism best describes the patient's behavior?

A. Undoing

B. Splitting

C. Isolation of affect

D. Idealization

E. Displacement

ANSWERS

50.1 **B.** The goal of cognitive behavioral psychotherapy in such cases is to help patients critically examine if their assumptions about themselves and other people are correct. Telling the patient that he should "suck it up" or that he is not ready for his current job is unhelpful. Because the job he has taken is (hopefully) for the long term, medicating the patient with a benzodiazepine or beta-blocker would not be a first-choice therapy.

50.2 **A.** Option A is most consistent with avoidant personality disorder. The patient has some close relationships and seems to desire more, but does not feel that he can maintain such relationships. Option B is more consistent with social phobia. Option C is grossly paranoid, consistent with a psychotic disorder. Option D is highly suggestive of schizoid personality disorder, as the patient has a close relationship with his parent but has no interest in other human contact. Option E suggests dependent personality disorder.

50.3 **C.** Patients with avoidant personality disorders would desperately like to have social relationships, but they are afraid of criticism and/or rejection. Answers A, B, D, and E are not true (and neither is the converse of each sentence).

50.4 **E.** This patient can be theorized to be using displacement to assume that all men will act as punitively toward her as her father did. Displacement and projection are the two defense mechanisms most commonly utilized by patients with avoidant personality disorders. Undoing is a defense mechanism in which a person tries to "undo" an unhealthy thought or action by engaging in its opposite. Splitting is a defense mechanism (frequently used by those with borderline personality disorder) in which the person literally "splits" apart the positive and negative qualities of the self and others. For example, an individual is either all bad or all good, but never an integrated whole of both good and bad. Isolation of affect is a defense mechanism involving the creation of a gap between an unpleasant or threatening cognition, and other thoughts and feelings. Idealization is the defense mechanism in which a person attributes exaggeratedly positive qualities to the self or others.

CLINICAL PEARLS

▶ Patients with avoidant personality disorder have a pervasive hypersensitivity to criticism and rejection. They avoid interpersonal relationships in every setting because they fear criticism and rejection. Their self-esteem is low, and they usually believe that they are inferior or inadequate, especially in the social arena.

▶ Patients with avoidant personality disorder are differentiated from those with schizoid personality disorder by the fact that they desperately would like interpersonal relationships but are afraid of them. Individuals with schizoid personality disorders do not have relationships but do not miss them.

▶ Patients with avoidant personality disorder are differentiated from those with dependent personality disorder by the fact that the former are afraid of rejection and criticism in relationships. Patients with dependent personality disorder are afraid of being left alone to fend for themselves.

▶ Physicians need to be tactful, encouraging, and accepting of these patients, especially regarding their fear of rejection. Confrontation and coercion are not appropriate, as they can drive the patient away.

▶ Defense mechanisms used by patients with avoidant personality disorder include displacement and projection.

REFERENCES

American Psychiatric Association. *Diagnostic and Statistical Manual of Mental Disorders.* 5th ed. Washington, DC: American Psychiatric Publishing; 2013.

Sadock BJ, Sadock VA, Ruiz P. *Kaplan and Sadock's Synopsis of Psychiatry: Behavioral Sciences/Clinical Psychiatry.* 11th ed. Baltimore, MD: Lippincott Williams & Wilkins; 2014.

A 36-year-old man is referred to his employment assistance agency because he has trouble making timely decisions and is often late with important work. The patient has angrily complied with this request although he does not believe that anything is wrong with him. He describes himself as "so devoted to my work that I make others look bad," believing that this is why he has been singled out for attention. The patient says that he has worked at the company for 4 years and during that time has put in anywhere from 10 to 12 hours of work per day. He admits that he often misses deadlines but claims that "they are unreasonable deadlines for the quality of work that I provide." He states, "If more people in the country were like me, we would get a lot more done—there are too many lazy slobs and people who don't follow the rules." He points out that his office is always perfectly neat, and he says, "I know where every dollar I ever spent went."

On a mental status examination, the patient does not reveal any abnormalities in mood, thought processes, or thought content. His manner is notable for its rigidity and stubbornness.

▶ What is the most likely diagnosis?
▶ What other psychiatric disorder is this condition often confused with, and how does one tell them apart?

ANSWERS TO CASE 51:

Obsessive-Compulsive Personality Disorder

Summary: A 36-year-old man has a lifetime preoccupation with rules, work, order, and stinginess. Even so, he is in trouble at work because he keeps missing deadlines and has difficulty making decisions. The patient does not realize that he is the cause of his problems—rather, he blames them on others. He comes across as rigid and stubborn in manner.

- **Most likely diagnosis:** Obsessive-compulsive personality disorder.

- **Differential diagnosis:** Obsessive-compulsive disorder (OCD). When recurrent obsessions or compulsions (checking rituals, washing hands repeatedly, etc) are present, OCD rather than obsessive-compulsive personality disorder should be considered. In addition, the diagnosis of autism spectrum disorder ought to be considered as well. This is a condition that can, in addition to restricted repetitive behaviors or interests the individual has, mark impairments in the area of social relatedness.

ANALYSIS

Objectives

1. Recognize obsessive-compulsive personality disorder.

2. Understand the difference between obsessive-compulsive personality disorder and OCD itself.

Considerations

This patient's difficulties fit a personality disorder in that he is inflexible in his thinking or behavior, which causes problems in social or work settings. This man came into the employee assistance program because of problems he was having at work: rigidity, stubbornness, and difficulty in making decisions and keeping to deadlines. Typically (as in this case) the patient's disorder is ego-syntonic; that is, he does not recognize his problems as originating from within himself but rather blames them on others in the outside world. Also, he is stingy with his money, although he works many hours a week. He seems somewhat moralistic about others and about their work habits, especially when they are compared to his own. **No obsessions (intrusive, repetitive thoughts) or compulsions (ritualistic behaviors)** are noted that are typical of **OCD;** the results of his mental status examination are otherwise normal. The presence of these types of symptoms differentiates between OCD and obsessive-compulsive personality disorder.

APPROACH TO:
Obsessive-Compulsive Personality Disorder

DEFINITIONS

COMPULSION: The pathologic need to act on an impulse. If the action is not performed, anxiety results. Usually, the compulsion has no true end in itself other than to prevent some imagined disaster from occurring. For example, a patient has an obsession about being dirty, and the compulsion associated with it is ritualistic washing.

DEFENSE MECHANISM: A psychodynamic term that defines various means that an individual might use to psychologically cope with a difficult situation. These defense mechanisms range from relatively mature ones such as humor to quite immature ones such as splitting, which is often seen with borderline personality disorder. Defense mechanisms might also include mechanisms such as devaluation, idealization, projection, projective identification, and sublimation. Commonly used defense mechanisms in obsessive-compulsive personality disorder are intellectualization, rationalization, undoing, and isolation of affect.

INTELLECTUALIZATION: A defense mechanism by which an individual deals with emotional conflict or stressors by the excessive use of abstract thinking to control or minimize disturbing feelings. For example, a man is involved in a car accident that causes him to be paralyzed. He spends hours in the hospital brooding over the details of the accident and the treatment he has received in the hospital but does so in an emotionally barren manner.

ISOLATION OF AFFECT: A defense mechanism by which an individual deals with emotional conflict or stressors by separating ideas from the feelings originally associated with them. The individual loses touch with the feelings associated with the given idea (eg, the traumatic event) although remaining aware of the cognitive elements of it (eg, descriptive details). For example, a man comes home to find his wife in bed with another man. Later, describing the scene to a friend, the man can relate specific details of the scene but appears emotionally unmoved by the whole event.

OBSESSION: An intrusive, repetitive thought that comes unbidden and cannot be eliminated from consciousness by effort or logic. It is usually anxiety producing.

PERSONALITY DISORDER: An enduring pattern of inner experience and behavior that deviates markedly from the expectations of the individual's culture. It is pervasive and inflexible, has an onset in adolescence or early adulthood, is stable over time, and leads to distress or impairment.

RATIONALIZATION: A defense mechanism by which an individual deals with emotional conflict or stressors by concealing the true motivations for thoughts, actions, or feelings through the elaboration of reassuring or self-serving but incorrect explanations. For example, a woman steals a coat from a local department store although she can afford to pay for it. She tells herself, "It's okay—that department store has plenty of money, and they won't miss one coat!"

UNDOING: A defense mechanism by which an individual deals with emotional conflict or stressors with words or behavior designed to negate or to symbolically make amends for unacceptable thoughts, feelings, or actions. Undoing can be realistically or magically associated with the conflict and serves to reduce anxiety and control the underlying impulse. An example of undoing is seen in the child's game in which one avoids stepping on cracks in the sidewalk to avoid "breaking your mother's back."

CLINICAL APPROACH

Diagnostic Criteria

The essential feature of this condition is a pervasive pattern of perfectionism and inflexibility. Patients with this disorder are emotionally constricted. They are excessively orderly and stubborn and often have trouble making decisions because their perfectionism interferes. These patients usually lack spontaneity and appear very serious. They are often misers when it comes to spending and frequently cannot discard worn-out or worthless objects that have no sentimental value. They tend to be overdevoted to work to the exclusion of involvement in leisure activities and friendships.

DIFFERENTIAL DIAGNOSIS

Patients with OCD have repetitive obsessions and compulsions, whereas those with the personality disorder tend to be rigid, stubborn, and preoccupied with details. Individuals with the personality disorder can brood over imagined insults or slights, which one could interpret as being obsessive, but they do not perform the compulsory, anxiety-reducing acts, such as ritualistic hand washing, that characterize people with OCD. It is also sometimes difficult to differentiate individuals with obsessive-compulsive personality traits from those with the diagnosable disorder. The occupational or social lives of patients with the personality disorder are significantly impaired because of this condition—the question is to what degree.

The personality and personality disorders workgroup for the *DSM-5* suggested some significant changes in the diagnosis and assessment of personality disorders. However, these proposed changes received a great deal of criticism largely because of their complexity. The *DSM-5*'s most important change in personality disorders is through the loss of the multiaxial system, including Axis II which previously included personality disorders. The multiaxial system was taken out because it was not consistent with other medical diagnostic systems, and, for personality disorders especially it tended to marginalize them. Personality disorders are, however, categorized into three clusters. Obsessive-compulsive personality disorder is part of Cluster C, which includes disorders typified as anxious or dependent.

INTERVIEWING TIPS AND TREATMENT

Individuals with this disorder do best when treated with a scientific approach and should be provided with documentary evidence and details. They can be among the most compliant patients because their own thoroughness can be used to self-monitor whatever condition is being observed (eg, patients with obsessive-compulsive personality disorder and insulin-dependent diabetes can be asked to self-monitor their blood glucose level at exact times during the day, and physicians can be sure this will be done).

There are few evidence-based treatments shown effective for personality disorders such as this. However, traditionally, the definitive treatment for obsessive-compulsive personality disorder is long-term, insight-oriented psychodynamic psychotherapy, but as in all patients with personality disorders, insight and motivation are usually lacking, rendering the treatment impossible to carry out. At times, cognitive interventions can be very well received, leading to a lessening of some maladaptive behavior. For example, a patient can be confronted with a key assumption such as "I must be perfectly in control at all times," and this assumption can then be discussed and ways created to refute it.

> ## CASE CORRELATION
>
> - See also Case 22 for patients who display patterns of preoccupation with orderliness or perfectionism. However, in OCD patients, there are true obsessions and compulsions to bind the anxiety caused by the obsessions; this is not the case in obsessive-compulsive personality disorder.

COMPREHENSION QUESTIONS

51.1 A 24-year-old woman is called into the head office of the agency where she works and told that her chronic lateness in completing her assignments will result in her dismissal if she does not change her behavior. The patient really loves her job, and the news comes as a major blow. That night at home, she tells her boyfriend in great detail about each and every step of the meeting and spends the entire night thinking about her job. The boyfriend tells her that she does not "look" particularly upset. Which of the following defense mechanisms is being used by this woman?

A. Undoing

B. Displacement

C. Intellectualization

D. Rationalization

E. Splitting

51.2 A 23-year-old medical student makes lists of all the tasks that he must accomplish each day. He spends hours studying and refuses to go out with his colleagues even when there are no tests on the immediate horizon, preferring to spend his time looking at specimens in the laboratory. He keeps meticulous notes during all his classes and prefers to attend every lecture, not trusting his colleagues to take notes for him. He is doing well in school and has a girlfriend who is also a medical student. Which of the following conditions does this student most likely have?

A. Obsessive-compulsive disorder (OCD)

B. Obsessive-compulsive personality disorder

C. Obsessive-compulsive traits

D. Schizoid personality disorder

E. Paranoid personality disorder

51.3 A 26-year-old woman comes to see a psychiatrist because she has been taking showers for 6 to 7 hours every day. She explains, "It all starts when I wake up. I am sure I am covered in germs, and if I don't wash, I will get sick. If I don't wash, I get paralyzed with anxiety. Once I'm in the shower, I have to shower in a particular order. If I mess up, I have to start over, and this takes hours and hours. My skin is cracking and bleeding because I spend so much time in the water." Which of the following conditions does this patient is most likely have?

A. Obsessive-compulsive disorder

B. Obsessive-compulsive personality disorder

C. Obsessive-compulsive traits

D. Paranoid personality disorder

E. Schizoid personality disorder

51.4 A patient with obsessive-compulsive personality disorder may also be categorized in a grouping of disorders named Cluster C personality disorders. Which other personality disorder is part of Cluster C?

A. Antisocial personality disorder

B. Schizotypal personality disorder

C. Narcissistic personality disorder

D. Avoidant personality disorder

E. Borderline personality disorder

ANSWERS

51.1 **C.** Intellectualization is a defense mechanism by which an individual deals with emotional conflict or stressors with an excessive use of abstract thinking to control or minimize disturbing feelings. Because the stressors have been successfully defended against in this instance, the patient does not appear particularly distressed.

51.2 **C.** Although this student clearly demonstrates some traits of obsessive-compulsive behavior, his social and occupational functioning both are good, which rules out the personality disorder.

51.3 **A.** This patient demonstrates the classic obsessions, followed by compulsions, of OCD.

51.4 **D.** Obsessive compulsive personality disorder is considered part of Cluster C personality disorders which additionally include avoidant and dependent personality disorders. This cluster is characterized by anxious or dependent features.

CLINICAL PEARLS

▶ Patients with obsessive-compulsive personality disorder are characterized by their rigidity, stubbornness, and perfectionism such that they often have trouble meeting deadlines at work or making choices. They tend to be work centered to the exclusion of enjoying social activities and leisure time. They are often miserly with money and hoard possessions excessively. They do not exhibit frank obsessions and compulsions.

▶ Physicians can use the preoccupation with rules and order shown by these patients to teach them to self-monitor their own conditions. These individuals can be extremely adherent. They need to know the details of their condition in scientific language.

▶ Patients with OCD have prominent obsessions and compulsions that alternately create anxiety and reduce it (through the compulsive behavior).

▶ Patients with obsessive-compulsive personality traits often resemble patients with the personality disorder. The difference is one of degree and impairment of function. Individuals who are significantly impaired can exhibit symptoms that meet the requirements for the personality disorder.

▶ Defense mechanisms include rationalization, intellectualization, undoing, isolation of affect, and displacement.

REFERENCES

Black DW. Grant JE. The essential companion to the diagnostic and statistical manual of mental disorders. *DSM-5 Guidebook.* 5th ed. Arlington, VA: American Psychiatric Publishing; 2014.

Sadock BJ, Sadock VA, Ruiz P. *Kaplan and Sadock's Synopsis of Psychiatry: Behavioral Sciences/Clinical Psychiatry.* 11th ed. Baltimore, MD: Lippincott Williams & Wilkins; 2014.

A 42-year-old man comes to see a psychiatrist stating that his life is "crashing down around his ears." He explains that since his girlfriend of 2 months left him, he has been "inconsolable." He says that he is having trouble sleeping at night because he is mourning her loss. When asked to describe his girlfriend, the patient states, "She was the love of my life, just beautiful, beautiful." He is unable to provide any further details about her. He says that they had five dates, but that he simply knew that she was the one for him. He claims that he was often in the "depths of despair" in his life, but that he also felt "on top of the world." He denies any psychiatric history or any medical problems.

On a mental status examination, the patient is dressed in a bright, tropical-pattern shirt and khaki pants. He leans over repeatedly to touch the female interviewer on the arm as he speaks, and he is cooperative during the interview. He sometimes sobs for a short period of time when talking directly about his girlfriend but smiles broadly during the interview when asking the interviewer questions about herself. His speech is of normal rate, although at times somewhat loud. The patient describes his mood as "horribly depressed." His affect is euthymic the majority of the time and full range. His thought processes and thought content are all within normal limits.

▶ What is the most likely diagnosis?
▶ What is the best initial treatment for this patient?

ANSWERS TO CASE 52:

Histrionic Personality Disorder

Summary: A 42-year-old man comes to a psychiatrist with complaints of a depressed mood and difficulty sleeping. His says that his girlfriend recently left him. Although he is obviously upset about the loss of the relationship, he cannot describe her in any specific detail, and they had not been going out together for long. The patient's speech and manner appear somewhat theatrical and overblown. His affect appears euthymic and full range, and he appears to be trying to directly engage the (female) interviewer by touching her and asking her direct personal questions. In this manner, he appears to be trying to draw attention to himself by being somewhat seductive. He is shown to have normal thought processes and thought content on a mental status examination.

- **Most likely diagnosis:** Histrionic personality disorder.

- **Best initial treatment:** Supportive psychotherapy while he grieves the loss of his girlfriend. Setting strict limits on his seductive behavior needs to be implemented as well.

ANALYSIS

Objectives

1. Recognize histrionic personality disorder in a patient.

2. Be aware of other co-occurring illnesses that may present with histrionic personality disorder such as substance abuse.

3. Know the treatment recommendations for patients with this disorder who come in while experiencing some kind of psychological crisis.

Considerations

This patient provides a somewhat classic presentation of histrionic personality disorder. Newer epidemiological evidence suggests that histrionic personality disorder is more common in women than in men, affecting approximately 1.8% of Americans. Clues to making the diagnosis include his **theatrical and overblown speech and his seductive manner.** These patients are often extremely attention seeking and often exaggerate their symptoms. Other clues include the fact that although he describes himself as being deeply depressed about the loss of his girlfriend, he is unable to describe her other than superficially, and his affect appears euthymic. His case is not unusual because patients with this disorder come to psychiatrists with a depressed mood but rarely with the thought that their difficulties in functioning in daily life and work are secondary to their own maladaptive behaviors.

At one point during the development of *DSM-5* it was proposed that this personality disorder be dropped. However, after the clinician feedback stage, it was decided to keep it. Currently, histrionic personality disorder is categorized as part of the Cluster B personality disorders which also include antisocial, borderline, and narcissistic personality disorders. These four share characteristics of being dramatic, emotional, or erratic.

APPROACH TO:
Histrionic Personality Disorder

DEFINITIONS

DISSOCIATION: A defense mechanism by which an individual deals with emotional conflict or stressors with a breakdown in the usually integrated functions of consciousness, memory, perception of self or the environment, or sensory/motor behavior. For example, a woman who has just been told that her child was killed in an automobile accident suddenly feels as if she is not herself but rather is hearing the events unfold as if they are being told to "someone else."

LIMIT SETTING: An activity by which a physician clearly tells a patient what is, and what is not, appropriate behavior in a given circumstance. For example, a physician can set limits on how many times a patient can telephone the physician in a week.

REPRESSION: A defense mechanism by which individuals deal with emotional conflict or stressors by expelling disturbing wishes, thoughts, or experiences from their conscious awareness. For example, a patient is told that she has breast cancer and clearly hears what she has been told because she can repeat the information back to the physician. However, when she returns home later, she tells her husband that the visit went well but that she cannot remember what she and the physician spoke about during the appointment.

SUPPORTIVE PSYCHOTHERAPY: Therapy designed to help patients support their existing defense mechanisms so that their functioning in the real world improves. Unlike insight-oriented psychotherapy, its goal is to maintain, not improve, a patient's intrapsychic functioning.

CLINICAL APPROACH

Patients with **histrionic personality disorder** show a **pervasive pattern of excessive emotionality and attention seeking.** They are uncomfortable in settings where they are not the center of attention. Their emotions are rapidly shifting and shallow, and they often interact with others in **a seductive manner.** Their speech is impressionistic and lacks detail. They are **dramatic and theatrical and exaggerate their emotional expressions.** They often consider relationships to be much more intimate than they really are. They are suggestible to the thoughts of others as well, often adopting other's views without thinking them through.

DIFFERENTIAL DIAGNOSIS

Patients with borderline personality disorder can often appear similar to those with histrionic personality disorder, although the former make suicide attempts more often and experience more frequent (brief) episodes of psychosis. Patients who are manic can often be overly dramatic, attention seeking, and seductive, but symptoms of insomnia, euphoria, and psychosis are present as well.

INTERVIEWING TIPS AND TREATMENT

The clinician should provide emotional support for and show interest in these patients **but should be very attentive to clear professional boundaries. Tactful confrontation about seductive behavior** can help. Expressing admiration of the patient, without showing inappropriate behavior, can help in forming a therapeutic working alliance. The treatment of histrionic personality disorder is often best attempted in a group therapy setting, where such patients, particularly if there are other patients with the same diagnosis in the group, better tolerate confrontations to avoid being rejected by other group members. Most psychotherapies require insight, which these individuals lack. Dynamic psychotherapy would likely lead to tumultuous results at best. Monitoring patients for substance abuse is important, as this often co-occurs and is a poor coping skill to manage psychological issues.

CASE CORRELATION

- See also Case 55 and Case 57 for patients who may display attention-seeking behavior and excessive emotionality. Borderline personality disordered patients display a wide array of impulsive behaviors, including self-harm, as well as chronic feelings of emptiness that are not present in those with histrionic personality disorders. Those with narcissistic personality disorders may also display attention-seeking behavior, as they want to be perceived as "superior" or better than others; histrionic personality disordered patients do not mind appearing weak or fragile if this will get them the attention they crave.

COMPREHENSION QUESTIONS

52.1 A 35-year-old woman with histrionic personality disorder has seen her psychotherapist once a week for the past year. She has come in the last few visits subtly different. She appears more distracted, she is late for appointments, she reports an increased amount of arguments with her family, and she appears flushed and even sweaty. You asked about use of illicit substances and she denies it. An important next step might be which of the following?

A. Breaking confidentiality and calling a family member to discuss this change.

B. Request a urine toxicology to screen for substance use.

C. No further workup is necessary; continue with the current framework of psychotherapy and treatment.

D. Ask her to go to her primary care physician.

E. Refer her to an Alcoholics Anonymous group.

52.2 A 23-year-old woman with a diagnosis of histrionic personality disorder comes to see her physician for the chief complaint of frequent headaches. As the (male) physician is taking the patient's history, he notices that the patient is frequently reaching across the desk to touch his arm as he talks to her, as well as leaning far forward in her seat to be nearer to him. Which of the following responses is the most appropriate from the physician?

A. Tell the patient to stop touching him immediately.

B. Move his seat further from the patient so that she cannot reach him.

C. Tell the patient that she will be referred to a female physician.

D. Tell the patient that he understands her concern about her headaches, but touching him is not appropriate.

E. Tell the patient he understands her gratitude in this situation.

52.3 A 20-year-old woman comes to see a psychiatrist at the insistence of her mother, who states that her daughter just "isn't herself." The patient is spending a great deal more time alone in her bedroom, she doesn't seem to be caring for her hygiene as well as usual, and has been missing work a great deal more. She is very clingy and attention seeking with her mother. Which of the following diagnoses best fits this patient's presentation?

A. Histrionic personality disorder

B. Borderline personality disorder

C. Bipolar disorder, mania

D. Major depressive disorder

E. Delusional disorder

52.4 Which of the following personality traits is most likely seen in patients with histrionic personality disorder?

A. Callousness

B. Emotional lability

C. Recklessness

D. Cognitive dysregulation

E. Grandiosity

ANSWERS

52.1 **B.** Substance use is a common feature of Cluster B personality disorders. Significant changes in usual behavior, alienation from loved ones, and physical signs are common features. Often patients are reluctant to admit use so a urine toxicology might be the most important step to help plan an appropriate intervention.

52.2 **D.** Histrionic patients often display inappropriate or seductive behavior. This is best managed by being tactful and sympathetic to the patient, but firmly and clearly placing boundaries on such behavior.

52.3 **D.** This patient has a new onset of behavior that is unlike her usual personality. These behaviors are common in major depression. The clinician might also look into appetite problems, sleep disturbance, substance abuse, tearfulness, and thoughts of self-harm.

52.4 **B.** Patients with histrionic personality disorder most often demonstrate emotional lability. Grandiosity is seen in antisocial personalities and narcissistic personalities, cognitive dysregulation is seen in borderline and schizotypal, recklessness in antisocial and borderline, and callousness in antisocial personality disorders.

CLINICAL PEARLS

▶ Patients with histrionic personality disorder often appear very dramatic and overemotional. They do not seem to have much depth in either their emotions or their relationships with others. They are uncomfortable when they are not the center of attention.

▶ Patients with histrionic personality disorder use the defense mechanisms of dissociation and repression most commonly.

▶ In interacting with these patients, the physician should use a low-key, friendly approach but should watch interpersonal boundaries. He or she should not become caught up in personal or sexual relationships with such patients, who can be quite seductive.

▶ Patients with histrionic personality disorder can be differentiated from those with mania because the latter often develop dramatic, seductive symptoms as new-onset behavior, not as a pervasive pattern. Patients with mania commonly also have vegetative symptoms, such as a decreased need for sleep, and psychotic symptoms as well.

REFERENCES

American Psychiatric Association. *Diagnostic and Statistical Manual of Mental Disorders.* 5th ed. Washington, DC: American Psychiatric Publishing; 2013.

Sadock BJ, Sadock VA, Ruiz P. *Kaplan and Sadock's Synopsis of Psychiatry: Behavioral Sciences/Clinical Psychiatry.* 11th ed. Baltimore, MD: Lippincott Williams & Wilkins; 2014.

A 32-year-old man comes to a psychiatrist with the chief complaint of being depressed since he broke up with his girlfriend 2 weeks ago. The patient explains that although he loves his ex-girlfriend, he broke up with her because his mother did not approve of her and would not allow him to marry her. He says that he cannot go against his mother because she "has taken care of me all these years." He states he could never fend for himself without his mother and alternates between being angry with her and feeling that "maybe she knows best." He has not told her that he is angry with her, because he is worried that "she might not love me anymore." He has lived at home his entire life except for one semester away at college. He returned home at the end of the semester because he was homesick, and did not go back. The patient reports no loss of appetite, concentration, or energy.

The patient claims that he performs "adequately" at work and has no job-related problems. He works for an accounting firm in an entry-level position even though he has been there for several years. He says that he has turned down promotions in the past because he knows that he "couldn't possibly supervise anyone or make decisions for them." The patient has two close childhood friends whom he talks to on the telephone nearly every day and says he "feels lost without them." The results of his mental status examination are normal except for a depressed mood (although affect is full range).

▶ What is the most likely diagnosis?
▶ What is the best treatment?

ANSWERS TO CASE 53:

Dependent Personality Disorder

Summary: The patient is a 32-year-old man who has been depressed since he broke up with his girlfriend 2 weeks ago. He has no vegetative signs or symptoms of major depression. He is overly reliant on his mother for major decisions and still lives at home. He has difficulty expressing disagreement with his mother because he is afraid she will not support him. The patient does well at his job but has turned down any position that would require him to take responsibility for others. He seems to be very dependent on a few close friends as well.

- **Most likely diagnosis:** Dependent personality disorder.

- **Best treatment:** Insight-oriented therapies can be helpful. Behavioral therapy, assertiveness training, family therapy, and group therapy have all proven useful with selected patients. Pharmacotherapy can be used to treat specific comorbid disorders such as anxiety disorders or major depression if they arise. Patients with this diagnosis, however, rarely come into treatment, because the disorder itself is ego-syntonic.

ANALYSIS

Objectives

1. Recognize dependent personality disorder in a patient.

2. Be familiar with the treatment recommendations appropriate for these patients.

Considerations

This patient exhibits what seems to be a **pervasive pattern** of submissive and clinging behavior related to an excessive need to be taken care of. He needs others to assume responsibility for him and does not disagree with them because he fears loss of their support. He feels uncomfortable and "lost" when alone and does not believe that he could fend for himself. He lacks self-confidence and does not initiate projects. He is preoccupied with a fear of being forced to take care of himself.

APPROACH TO:
Dependent Personality Disorder

DEFINITIONS

IDEALIZATION: A defense mechanism by which an individual deals with emotional conflict or stressors by attributing exaggerated positive qualities to others. For example, a woman being abused and neglected by her husband earnestly states, "He is the best thing that ever happened to me."

REACTION FORMATION: A defense mechanism by which an individual deals with emotional conflict or stressors by substituting behavior, thoughts, or feelings that are diametrically opposed to his or her own unacceptable thoughts or feelings. For example, a woman who is very angry with her husband for having an affair cooks him a nice dinner and acts sweetly toward him.

SOMATIZATION: The expression of psychological difficulties as physical complaints. Somatization is considered a form of regression because being able to verbalize problems instead of making them physical complaints is considered a progressive step. For example, a woman who is upset about the death of her cat develops an intractable headache.

CLINICAL APPROACH

Patients with dependent personality disorder have a pervasive need to be taken care of and to rely upon others for emotional support. They are dependent and submissive and uncomfortable when alone. They are afraid of being left alone because they do not believe they can take care of themselves, and this leads to clinging behavior. They prefer to do things for others and have difficulty initiating projects on their own or disagreeing with others.

Dependence is a prominent factor in several personality disorders, including histrionic and borderline disorders. However, in these disorders, patients are generally dependent on a series of other people. Patients with dependent personality disorder tend to stick to one person, such as a parent or spouse, for the long term. Patients with this disorder also tend to be less labile and overtly manipulative than patients with histrionic or borderline personality disorders. Patients with agoraphobia can be dependent, but the dependent behavior usually does not start until the panic attacks or anxiety do—thus there is no pervasive, lifelong pattern of dependency.

Dependent personality disorder, like all personality disorders, is difficult to treat. Patients can respond to psychosocial support groups in the face of loss of their usual support systems. Long-term psychodynamic psychotherapy might eventually help, but many patients do not have either the motivation or the insight needed to successfully undergo treatment.

CASE CORRELATION

- See also Case 52 and Case 57 for other presentations of patients that fear abandonment and need high levels of reassurance and approval. Borderline personality disordered patients, however, react to fear of abandonment with rage and demands, while dependent personality disordered patients react with submissiveness. Histrionic personality disordered patients need high levels of reassurance and approval, but behave in a flamboyant manner with active demands for attention, while dependent personality disordered patients are self-effacing and docile.

COMPREHENSION QUESTIONS

53.1 A 30-year-old man comes into your clinic after being referred by his primary care doctor. He lives with his mother and relies on her to make every day decisions for him. He has never worked and depends on her for financial support. He lacks self-confidence and is uncomfortable when left alone. Since his mother's diagnosis of cancer, the patient is preoccupied with the fear of his mother dying and being left alone to care for himself. You believe he is suffering from a personality disorder. Which is the most likely disorder?

A. Avoidant personality disorder

B. Borderline personality disorder

C. Dependent personality disorder

D. Histrionic personality disorder

E. Obsessive-compulsive personality disorder

53.2 Which of the following would be the most useful psychiatric treatment for the patient in Question 53.1?

A. Antianxiety medication

B. Antidepressant medication

C. Nothing at this time because research suggests personality disorders improve over time

D. Individual psychotherapy

E. Sociotherapies

53.3 You are consulted to evaluate a 45-year-old married woman who was admitted to the surgical service 2 days ago for an appendectomy. The procedure went well, but she was found to be tearful, stating, "I wish I were dead." On obtaining further history, she is quite cooperative and talkative. She is questioned about her earlier comments, and she states that she "wanted attention, I guess." She is upset that her husband is not with her in the hospital; she has "never been away from him" for this long since they started dating when the patient was 16 years old. She feels helpless and is having a difficult time being active in her care. She feels overwhelmed regarding her postsurgical and discharge instructions, and the nursing staff has become frustrated with her constant "need for reassurance." Although at times she is tearful during the interview, she denies prior or recent pervasive depressive or neurovegetative symptoms and is not actively suicidal. Which of the following is the most appropriate approach to this patient?

A. Encourage her to learn more about her surgery and become more proactive in her care.

B. Persuade her to become less dependent on her husband.

C. Insist her husband be present at all times while his wife is hospitalized.

D. Spend regular, short periods of time with her to discuss discharge planning and aftercare.

E. Transfer her to the psychiatric unit.

ANSWERS

53.1 **C.** Other personality disorders may be confused with dependent personality disorder due to common features. Dependent personality disorder is distinguished by submissive, reactive, and clinging behavior evident in this question. Avoidant personality disorders have a strong fear of humiliation and rejection. Borderlines have a typical pattern of unstable and intense relationships. Histrionic personality disorders are characterized by flamboyance with active demands for attention. Obsessive-compulsive disorders have a pattern of preoccupation with order, perfection, and control not evident in this question.

53.2 **E.** Sociotherapies (group, family, and milieu) have demonstrated to be moderately effective treatments for these patients when faced with loss of their usual support systems. Medications for depression, anxiety, and/or psychosis would be indicated if the patient had a comorbid psychiatric illness which is not evident at this time. While it true some personality disorders improve over time, others can become worse. Intervention provides the best opportunity for a positive change in this patient.

53.3 **D.** This patient displays characteristics consistent with dependent personality disorder. The most effective approach in dealing with a patient with this disorder is to respect her need for attachment and schedule limited but regular appointments with her. Individuals with this illness wish to be taken care of, and therefore will not be proactive in their care; in circumstances such as these, it is helpful for the physician to be more active. Encouraging the patient to be less dependent in her primary relationship is not only *not* helpful, but can be damaging as she can feel rejected and become more regressed, upset, and helpless. Insisting that her husband be at the hospital at all times only continues the cycle of "being taken care of" and does not facilitate the patient's involvement in postoperative care.

CLINICAL PEARLS

▶ Patients with dependent personality disorder have a pervasive need to be taken care of by others. They are dependent and submissive and are uncomfortable when alone because they do not believe they can take care of themselves.

▶ Physicians should reassure these patients of their availability but set limits as to how often the patient can contact them. If feeling "burned out" by the patient's extreme dependence, they should be careful not to reject the patient.

▶ Dependence is a prominent factor in several personality disorders, including histrionic and borderline disorders. Patients with dependent personality disorder tend to stick to one caregiver, such as a parent or spouse, for the long term and tend to be less manipulative.

▶ Patients with agoraphobia can be dependent, but the dependent behavior usually does not start until the panic attacks or anxiety do—thus there is no lifelong pattern of dependency.

REFERENCES

American Psychiatric Association. *Diagnostic and Statistical Manual of Mental Disorders*. 5th ed. Arlington, VA: American Psychiatric Publishing; 2013.

Hales RE, Yudofsky SC, Roberts LW. *The American Psychiatric Publishing Textbook of Psychiatry*. 6th ed. Washington, DC: American Psychiatric Publishing; 2014:851-872, 886-887.

A 24-year-old woman was admitted to the obstetrical service for the delivery of a full-term baby boy. One day after the delivery, the obstetrics service requested a consultation from the psychiatrist on duty to "rule out schizophrenia."

The psychiatrist interviews the patient and finds out that the pregnancy was because of a rape the patient suffered 9 months previously. The patient is planning to give the baby up for adoption. She claims that she has never seen a psychiatrist and has never felt a need to do so. She speaks at length about how the rape was "written in the stars" for all to see; she is an avid astrologer. She denies having recurrent thoughts or nightmares about the rape itself. She states that she has very few close friends, preferring to study astrology and astral projection at home by herself. She believes strongly in reincarnation, although she knows that her family thinks this belief is strange. She admits that she has worked intermittently as a "crystal ball gazer" but has never held a steady, full-time paying job.

During the mental status examination the patient sits upright in her hospital bed dressed in three hospital gowns and a robe, which she is wearing backward. Her hair is neatly combed, although one side is in braids and the other is not. She is cooperative with the interviewer. She states that her mood is good, and her affect is congruent although constricted. She has tangential thought processes and ideas of reference but no suicidal or homicidal ideation, hallucinations, or delusions.

▶ What is the most likely diagnosis?
▶ What should your recommendations to the obstetrics service be?

ANSWERS TO CASE 54:
Schizotypal Personality Disorder

Summary: A 24-year-old immediately postpartum woman is referred to a psychiatrist by the obstetrics service because staff members believe she might be schizophrenic. The patient has odd beliefs and thinking, ideas of reference, and a constricted affect. She also dresses in a peculiar manner. She does not have close friends. Her thinking is tangential, but her thought content is within normal limits.

- **Most likely diagnosis:** Schizotypal personality disorder (SPD).

- **Recommendations to the obstetrics service:** Outpatient psychiatric follow-up. The patient does not have schizophrenia. Although transient psychotic episodes can occur in response to stress in patients with SPD, the patient is not having psychotic symptoms currently. The patient's odd beliefs and magical thinking should be conceptualized as a **nonpsychotic thought disorder or partial loss of reality testing.** If she develops an acute psychosis (hallucinations, thought disorganization, loose association), then treatment with a typical or atypical antipsychotic medication in the hospital is indicated. Otherwise, medication is not started in the hospital in the absence of acute psychosis because the patient will be unlikely to comply with medication unless she has a good therapeutic relationship with a psychiatrist.

    Ideally, the psychiatrist who will follow her as an outpatient will see her briefly before discharge to increase the likelihood that she will follow through. Once a therapeutic relationship has been developed, there is a growing body of evidence to suggest that a low-dose neuroleptic can impact the magical thinking and odd beliefs. Studies show that only 10% of patients with SPD have ever received antipsychotic medication. The same studies show that in their lifetimes, patients with SPD spend approximately 44 months involved in psychotherapy, countering the belief that these patients will not seek treatment.

ANALYSIS

Objectives

1. Recognize SPD in a patient.

2. Understand the relationship of SPD and schizophrenia.

Considerations

This patient is viewed by members of the obstetrics team as odd, but she does not see herself in this manner. Although several abnormalities are observed during her mental status examination, including ideas of reference (not delusions of reference), unusual beliefs, unconventional thinking, a constricted affect, and an odd appearance, she does not exhibit any signs of a true psychosis. **She does not have hallucinations or fixed delusions,** and therefore her symptoms do not meet the diagnostic criteria for schizophrenia. She does not appear to have any psychological sequelae resulting from the rape (no symptoms of posttraumatic stress disorder), although she does seem to have incorporated its meaning into her unusual beliefs about the world.

Currently conceptualized as being a biologically based disorder that is related to schizophrenia, SPD is a milder disorder on the schizophrenic spectrum. Family and adoptive studies suggest a greater prevalence of SPD in the relatives of patients with schizophrenia than in the general population. Interestingly, a greater prevalence of chronic schizophrenia in the relatives of patients with SPD is not consistently found. It is thought that this means that susceptibility genes for psychosis are less prevalent in families of patients with SPD than those with schizophrenia. It appears that there are at least two inherited sets of genetic factors in SPD: one related to the bizarre thinking (nonpsychotic thought disorder) and one related to the social isolation and lack of comfort with other people seen in individuals with SPD.

APPROACH TO:
Schizotypal Personality Disorder

DEFINITIONS

DENIAL: A defense mechanism in which an individual deals with emotional conflict or stressors by refusing to acknowledge some painful aspect of external reality or subjective experience that is apparent to others. The term "psychotic denial" is used when there is gross impairment in reality testing.

DEREALIZATION: A feeling that the world, or reality, has changed. The environment feels unreal or strange.

DYSPHORIA: A state of mood that is unpleasant, often sad.

IDEALIZATION: A defense mechanism in which an individual deals with emotional conflict or stressors by attributing exaggerated positive qualities to others. Use of this mechanism can alternate with devaluation, its opposite.

MAGICAL THINKING: Thinking similar to that seen in young children in which the patient's thoughts, words, or actions are seen to have power over external events. (For example: It snows in the winter because I buy sidewalk salt every fall.)

CLINICAL APPROACH

Diagnostic Criteria

Patients with SPD have deficits in their abilities to have interpersonal relationships and **peculiarities in ideation, appearance, and behavior.** There is a pattern of acute discomfort when in close relationships, cognitive or perceptual distortions, and **eccentricities in behavior.** These patients **usually do not have close friends.** A patient can experience anxiety, depression, or other dysphoric mood states and can be suspicious or paranoid. Under stress, these patients can become **transiently psychotic.** Occurring in approximately 3% of the population, SPD is frequently diagnosed in females with fragile X syndrome.

DIFFERENTIAL DIAGNOSIS

Although both schizoid and SPD patients have discomfort with interpersonal relationships, patients with SPD can be differentiated from those with schizoid personality disorder by their peculiar behavior, thinking, and speech. Individuals with paranoid personality deal with the world as a hostile place and are suspicious that others will take advantage of them, but their suspiciousness never becomes of delusional quality, and they do not have the odd behavior seen in SPD. Individuals with SPD are not frankly psychotic (ie, do not have delusions and hallucinations), except perhaps transiently when under stress, which differentiates them from those with schizophrenia. More than 50% of individuals with SPD have at least one lifetime episode of major depression, and this should be treated with antidepressants when it occurs with SPD.

TREATMENT

Although these patients often exhibit bizarre speech, behavior, or beliefs, it is important for physicians not to ridicule their beliefs or to be judgmental about them, as this disrupts any alliance that is to be built. Low-dose antipsychotic agents can be helpful if transient psychoses appear. Second-generation antipsychotics are usually well tolerated and can help reduce paranoia, anxiety, and unusual perceptual experiences. Group therapy can sometimes help alleviate the social anxiety and awkwardness common to such patients. Supportive individual psychotherapy can be beneficial.

CASE CORRELATION

- See also Case 6 and Case 48 for patients who may present with odd or detached behavior. Schizophrenic patients all must have a period of persistent psychotic symptoms (hallucinations or delusions), distinguishing themselves from schizoid personality disordered patients. Patients with schizoid personality disorder may also present with social detachment, but they do not have cognitive or perceptional distortions or marked eccentricity or oddness.

COMPREHENSION QUESTIONS

54.1 An epidemiological survey of the general public showed between 9% and 16% met criteria for one or more personality disorders. In psychiatric samples the prevalence is even higher. What percentage of personality disorders would you expect to find in an outpatient psychiatric sample?

A. 15% to 30%

B. 30% to 50%

C. 50% to 70%

D. 60% to 80%

E. 70% to 90%

54.2 Which of the following features must be present in a patient's history for schizotypal personality disorder to be diagnosed?

A. Auditory hallucinations

B. Cognitive and perceptual distortions

C. Impulsive or manipulative behaviors

D. Paranoid ideations

E. Unstable and intense relationships

54.3 A 25-year-old man with schizotypal personality disorder comes to his psychiatrist with a chief complaint of a depressed mood. He notes that since losing his job as an astrologer, he has been depressed and unable to sleep. He states that although his mood is usually fairly low (4 out of a possible 10), it has lately been a constant 2. The patient also notes problems with concentration and energy level and has experienced several crying spells. He reports he had premonitions that certain foods could heal him, so he has been mixing "magical potions" and eating "magical foods." A mental status examination reveals an oddly dressed man with constricted affect, ideas of reference, unusual beliefs, and some mild paranoia. Which of the following medications is most likely to be helpful to this patient?

A. Zolpidem (Ambien) for insomnia

B. Divalproex sodium for mood disturbance

C. Escitalopram for depressive symptoms

D. Risperidone for paranoia

E. Ziprasidone for ideas of reference

ANSWERS

54.1 **B.** Studies have shown 30% to 50% of psychiatric patient samples also have a personality disorder. The frequency and types of personality disorder differ depending on the mental disorder assessed. The percentages of persons with major depression, generalized anxiety or panic disorder have an even higher frequency of personality disorders.

54.2 **B.** The odd quality with which these patients perceive and think about the world is one of the diagnostic criteria for schizotypal personality disorder. Answers A and D are symptoms of a variety of Axis I disorders, but do not point to any particular personality disorder. Answer C and E are characteristics seen in borderline personality disorder patients.

54.3 **C.** Escitalopram is a selective serotonin reuptake inhibitor (SSRI) useful in the treatment of depression. Patients with schizotypal personality disorder who have either a depressive component to their illness or a secondary superimposed major depression (as is the case with this patient) should be treated with antidepressants. Ziprasidone (Geodon) and risperidone (Risperdal) are atypical antipsychotics that would be effective if the patient was having a transient psychotic episode, but he is not. Divalproex sodium is an antiepileptic agent used as a mood stabilizer to treat conditions such as mania.

CLINICAL PEARLS

▶ Patients with schizotypal personality disorder show a pervasive, stable pattern of social and interpersonal deficits, a reduced capacity for (and discomfort with) interpersonal relationships, cognitive or perceptual distortions, and odd behavior.

▶ Schizotypal personality disorder is currently conceptualized as being a biologically based disorder that is related to schizophrenia but is a milder disorder on the schizophrenia spectrum.

▶ Individuals with SPD can be differentiated from those with paranoid personality in that the latter deal with the world as a hostile place and are suspicious that others will take advantage of them, but their suspiciousness never becomes of delusional quality.

▶ Patients with this disorder can be differentiated from patients with schizoid personality disorder by their family history of schizophrenia, rarely successful work careers, and odd behavior, speech, and beliefs.

▶ Physicians do well in dealing with these patients when they can remain nonjudgmental about the patient's peculiar speech, beliefs, and behavior.

REFERENCES

American Psychiatric Association. *Diagnostic and Statistical Manual of Mental Disorders*. 5th ed. Arlington, VA: American Psychiatric Publishing; 2013:645-649, 655-659.

Black BW, Andreasen NC. *Introductory Textbook of Psychiatry*. 6th ed. Washington, DC: American Psychiatric Publishing; 2014:461-470, 473-474.

Hales RE, Yudofsky SC, Roberts LW. *The American Psychiatric Publishing Textbook of Psychiatry*. 6th ed. Washington, DC: American Psychiatric Publishing; 2014:873-875.

A 45-year-old man is admitted to a cardiac intensive care unit after suffering a heart attack. Twenty-four hours after admission, the consultation psychiatrist is called in to make an evaluation because the patient is trying to sign himself out against medical advice. When the psychiatrist enters the patient's hospital room, she finds him getting dressed and yelling at the top of his lungs, "I won't be treated in this manner! How dare you!" The patient does agree to sit down and speak with the psychiatrist, however. He tells the psychiatrist that staff members are simply rude and do not treat him "in the manner to which he is accustomed." He says that he is a small business owner, but that he is on the way up and "as soon as people realize my full potential, I will be a millionaire." He cannot understand why the staff will not bring food up from an outside cafeteria for him because the food in the hospital is so bad. He asks the psychiatrist whether, after the interview, she will get some food for him, and he becomes angry when she declines. He then eyes her new, expensive watch enviously. On a mental status examination, the psychiatrist finds no disorders of thought process or content, and the patient is found to be oriented to person, place, and time.

▶ What is the most likely diagnosis?
▶ What would be the most successful approach in dealing with this patient?

ANSWERS TO CASE 55:
Narcissistic Personality Disorder

Summary: A 45-year-old man is admitted to the hospital after a heart attack. Twenty-four hours later, he tries to leave the hospital against medical advice because he is angry about the way the staff has treated him. He has a grandiose sense of self-importance and feels entitled. He is interpersonally exploitative with the psychiatrist who interviews him and is obviously envious of a watch that he thinks is expensive. He shows no other abnormalities on a mental status examination.

- **Most likely diagnosis:** Narcissistic personality disorder.

- **Most successful approach:** If the psychiatrist and/or the treatment team can show validation for the patient's experience, feelings, and concerns, he will most likely calm down and agree to stay in the hospital for treatment.

ANALYSIS

Objectives

1. Know the diagnostic criteria for narcissistic personality disorder.

2. Know some strategies to employ when working with patients with this disorder.

Considerations

This patient has suffered a "narcissistic injury" at the hands of the staff in that they refuse to cater to his need for admiration and special treatment. This injury has been inflicted on top of the injury of realizing that his body is not immortal. The patient has responded by becoming arrogant, hostile, and demanding, and has tried to sign himself out against medical advice. He continues to demand attention when speaking with the psychiatrist by telling her how important he is and how he feels entitled to special treatment. He even tries to manipulate her and is angry when she does not comply. He is envious of her success as evidenced by her watch. Patients like these respond best to a show of honest admiration from another individual—it can be difficult to react in this manner because these patients often engender strong negative countertransference feelings.

APPROACH TO:
Narcissistic Personality Disorder

DEFINITIONS

DENIAL: A defense mechanism in which an individual deals with emotional conflict or stress by refusing to acknowledge some painful aspect of external reality or subjective experience that is apparent to others. For example, a patient hospitalized after a severe heart attack tells a physician he feels "as fit as a fiddle" and jumps out of bed and starts performing jumping jacks. When there is gross impairment in reality testing, the denial can be termed psychotic.

DEVALUATION: A defense mechanism in which an individual deals with emotional conflict or stress by attributing exaggerated negative qualities to themselves or to others. This behavior can alternate with idealization. For example, a patient states that her therapist is "the worst doctor in the world."

GRANDIOSITY: An exaggerated concept of one's importance, power, or fame.

IDEALIZATION: A defense mechanism in which an individual deals with emotional conflict or stress by attributing exaggerated positive qualities to themselves or to others. This behavior can alternate with devaluation. For example, a patient states that her therapist is "the most empathic person on the planet."

CLINICAL APPROACH

Diagnostic Criteria

Patients with this disorder exhibit a pervasive pattern **of grandiosity, a need for admiration, and a lack of empathy for others.** They often exaggerate their accomplishments and are jealous of the achievements or possessions of others. They believe they are special or are deserving of special treatment. They have **fantasies about obtaining unlimited power and success.** They take advantage of others and can appear haughty or arrogant. They handle criticism poorly and can become enraged quickly.

DIFFERENTIAL DIAGNOSIS

Patients with narcissistic personality disorder can often be difficult to differentiate from those with other cluster B disorders (borderline, avoidant, or histrionic personality disorders). Individuals with borderline personality disorder generally live more chaotic lives, have multiple failed relationships, and make suicidal gestures. Patients with antisocial personality disorder are often in trouble with the legal system because they have committed one or more impulsive, irresponsible, and often violent acts. Patients with histrionic personality disorder can appear to be dramatic but do not claim to be entitled to special behavior and do not appear as arrogant or haughty. The grandiosity characteristic along with the callous, needy, interactive style is the most useful feature discriminating narcissistic personality disorder from the others.

INTERVIEWING TIPS AND TREATMENT

Patients with this disorder try to appear perfect and invincible in order to protect their fragile self-esteem. When this is lost, they are especially prone to develop depression. They often denigrate their physicians in a defensive effort to maintain a sense of mastery. The clinician should be tactful and admiring if at all possible. **Treatment of these individuals is difficult because they rarely desire to change and seldom seek help.** Group therapy is helpful only if the therapist can make the inevitable confrontation by group members somehow palatable to the patient. Psychotherapy with these individuals is challenging, and the patient often terminates treatment when confrontation is attempted. Psychopharmacology can be employed to treat symptoms associated with narcissistic personality disorder (eg, lithium for the affective lability, selective serotonin reuptake inhibitors [SSRIs] for depressive symptoms).

CASE CORRELATION

- See also Case 8 and Case 52 for patients who may present with grandiose ideation or a need for attention. However, in bipolar patients there are also mood changes and functional impairments that are not seen in narcissistic personality disordered patients. Those with histrionic personality disorder have a need for attention, but it does not specifically need to be of the admiring kind, which is the case with narcissistic personality disordered patients.

COMPREHENSION QUESTIONS

55.1 A 22-year-old single graduate student with narcissistic personality disorder is admitted to a hospital after a car accident in which his right femur is fractured. A medical student has been assigned to follow the patient, but when she enters the room and introduces herself as a medical student, the patient states, "Oh, I wouldn't let a medical student touch me—I need someone with much more experience than you." Which of the following statements by the medical student is most likely to lead to a successful interview with this patient?

A. "I know this will be boring for you, but it's just one of the things that you will have to put up with in the hospital."

B. "I know you must be scared to be in the hospital, but you will be safe here."

C. "I'm told that you are a very articulate person, and so I'm hoping you'll teach me what I need to know."

D. "I understand that you think you deserve only the best, but *I* have been assigned to you."

E. "Please don't make this difficult, I have to interview you as part of my job."

55.2 The patient in Question 55.1 would be most likely to become depressed after which of the following life occurrences?

A. Aging

B. Graduation

C. Job change

D. Marriage

E. Moving to a new city

55.3 A 36-year-old man with narcissistic personality disorder calls your office asking for an appointment with the "best therapist in the clinic." One of his complaints is difficulties in his relationships with his colleagues. The patient states "They are not giving me the credit I deserve for my accomplishments at the law firm." What is the most likely reason the patient is seeking treatment?

A. Anger

B. Anxiety

C. Attempting to identify with others

D. Grandiose thinking

E. Seeking medication

55.4 The patient in Question 55.3 has now been seeing a therapist twice weekly for the last year. The therapist and the patient have a good working alliance. During one therapy session, the therapist comes to the session 4 minutes late. He apologizes to the patient, stating that he had an emergency involving another patient. During the session, the patient notes that the therapist "isn't as sharp as some of the therapists I hear on the talk shows." Which of the following defense mechanisms is the patient using?

A. Denial

B. Devaluation

C. Isolation of affect

D. Rationalization

E. Splitting

ANSWERS

55.1 **C.** Appealing to the patient's narcissism by being admiring most often de-escalates the patient as well as improves the therapeutic alliance in these cases.

55.2 **A.** Patients with narcissistic personality disorder do not handle aging well because beauty, strength, and youth are often highly valued. Any blow to their fragile (but covert) self-esteem can raise their feelings of envy and anger, and subsequently lead to depression. All the other life occurrences represent changes which may be stressful to people, but do not affect those with personality disorders any differently than the general population (other than the fact that patients with personality disorders in general do not handle **any** kind of stressors well).

55.3 **A.** Patients with narcissistic personality disorder rarely seek treatment and tend to have little insight into their grandiosity. When these individuals do present for treatment it is usually due to underlying anger or depression resulting from being belittled or not receiving the admiration to which they feel entitled.

55.4 **B.** The patient defends against his feelings of hurt and anger toward the therapist by using devaluation. Devaluation along with idealization and denial are considered primitive (lower-functioning) defense mechanisms used by patients with personality disorders such as narcissistic and borderline.

CLINICAL PEARLS

▶ Patients with narcissistic personality disorder show a pervasive sense of grandiosity and entitlement in their thoughts and behavior. They are very seldom capable of true empathy with others and often manipulate them for personal gain.

▶ Clinicians should try to maintain an admiring stance with these patients. Tact is important as well, as these individuals handle criticism poorly.

▶ Defense mechanisms in patients with narcissistic personality disorder include denial, devaluation, and idealization.

REFERENCES

American Psychiatric Association. *Diagnostic and Statistical Manual of Mental Disorders*. 5th ed. Arlington, VA: American Psychiatric Publishing; 2013:669-672.

Black BW, Andreasen NC. *Introductory Textbook of Psychiatry*. 6th ed. Washington, DC: American Psychiatric Publishing; 2014:481-483.

Hales RE, Yudofsky SC, Roberts LW. *The American Psychiatric Publishing Textbook of Psychiatry*. 6th ed. Washington, DC: American Psychiatric Publishing; 2014:883-884.

A 47-year-old man is referred to a psychiatrist at his employee assistance program because of continuing conflicts on the job. This is the third time the patient has been referred to a psychiatrist under such circumstances. He lost two previous jobs because of conflicts with coworkers. The patient states that people do not like him and would like to see him fail. He cites as an example one instance in which one of his colleagues was late in sending him some material he needed, resulting in the patient being unable to complete his assignment in a timely fashion. Although the colleague apologized for the mistake, the patient says that he knows that this man is "out to get me fired." He has since broken off all contact with this coworker and refuses to speak with him directly, preferring to use only written communication.

On a mental status examination, the patient appears somewhat angry and suspicious. He glares intently at the interviewer and sits with his back to the wall. He repeatedly requests a clarification of questions, often asking, "What will this material be used for? I bet you are going to use it against me so that I will be fired." When the interviewer's pager goes off, the patient accuses him of trying to shorten the time allotted to him by arranging to have the pager interrupt them. The patient's mood is described as "fine," but his affect is tense and he appears suspicious and ill at ease. The patient's thought processes and thought content are both within normal limits.

▶ What is the most likely diagnosis?
▶ What is the best strategy in approaching this patient?

ANSWERS TO CASE 56:
Paranoid Personality Disorder

Summary: A 47-year-old man comes to a psychiatrist because of conflicts with others at work. He appears suspicious of his colleagues and of the interviewing psychiatrist. He reads hidden meanings into benign remarks or actions (such as the pager going off). The results of his mental status examination are normal except for his paranoia, which does not reach delusional proportions.

- **Most likely diagnosis:** Paranoid personality disorder.

- **Best approach:** Form a working alliance with the patient.

ANALYSIS

Objectives

1. Recognize paranoid personality disorder.

2. Maintain a respectful alliance in working with a patient with paranoid personality disorder.

Considerations

The presentation in the case vignette is probably one of the most common for these patients, who do not normally seek out mental health treatment. Although pervasive paranoia and suspiciousness characterize this patient, the **absence of any true paranoid delusions or hallucinations make a true psychotic disorder unlikely.** The psychiatrist should take a low-key approach and not try to overcompensate by making friends with the patient. He or she should provide clear, straightforward answers to all questions and explain everything that he or she is doing or recommending. When challenged with some kind of paranoid ideation (such as the patient's response to the pager going off), the psychiatrist should provide clear, direct, reality testing. (For example, "I'm sorry the pager went off. I did not prearrange for it to go off. I will defer answering it until after we are finished talking.")

APPROACH TO:
Paranoid Personality Disorder

DEFINITIONS

DELUSIONS: Fixed, false beliefs about the world that cannot be corrected with reasoning, education, or information.

HALLUCINATIONS: False sensory perceptions not associated with any real sensory stimulus. Hallucinations can occur in all five senses (gustatory, olfactory, auditory, visual, and tactile).

IDEAS OF REFERENCE: A person's false beliefs that people are talking about him or her.

PARANOID IDEATION: Suspiciousness that is less than delusional in nature.

WORKING ALLIANCE: A therapeutic relationship formed between patients and their physicians that allows them to interact in a constructive manner.

CLINICAL APPROACH

Patients with this disorder have a pervasive tendency to interpret the actions of others as being demeaning or deliberately harmful. These patients are often preoccupied with questioning the loyalty or trustworthiness of friends, even when this is unjustified. Patients are unforgiving of mistakes or slights, and they hold grudges. They believe that the motives of others are malevolent, and they are quick to react to defend their characters. These counterattacks are almost always angry and hostile. As in all personality disorders, these symptoms cannot occur exclusively during the course of another psychiatric illness such as schizophrenia, or occur due to another medical condition or the use of a substance.

DIFFERENTIAL DIAGNOSIS

Patients with paranoid personality disorder can be differentiated from those with schizophrenia because they do not have frankly psychotic symptoms such as delusions, hallucinations, or a formal thought disorder. They can be differentiated from those with a delusional disorder by the absence of fixed delusions, as the paranoia of patients with a personality disorder never reaches delusional proportions. Although one might consider the possibility of borderline personality disorder (BPD) in a patient who displays angry outbursts toward others, patients with paranoid personality disorder typically do not have other features seen in patients with BPD, such as involvement in many short-lived, tumultuous relationships or chronic feelings of emptiness.

Interview Tips

Patients with paranoid personality disorder can become even more suspicious when a physician tries to become too friendly or close because they wonder about the motives behind this behavior. Therefore, be honest and respectful toward the patient, but use a low-key approach. Acknowledge any mistakes made and expect to explain procedures in detail. Use reality testing where necessary. For example, "No, Mr. Jones, I did not arrange to have my pager go off in the middle of our meeting. Someone from the outside simply needed to speak with me, and therefore my secretary paged me."

CASE CORRELATION

- See also Case 6 and Case 8 for patients who may also present with paranoia or paranoid behavior. In the case of both schizophrenia and bipolar disorder with psychotic features, however, there must be evidence of persistent psychotic symptoms (delusions or hallucinations).

COMPREHENSION QUESTIONS

56.1 A 36-year-old man comes to a physician's office with the chief complaint that "people are out to hurt me." Despite being reassured by his wife that this is untrue, the patient is convinced that men are observing his behavior and actions at home and at work, using telescopic lenses and taping devices. He has torn apart his office on more than one occasion looking for "bugs." The patient's wife says that this behavior is relatively new, appearing somewhat suddenly after the patient was robbed on the way to his car approximately 6 months previously. Which of the following symptoms best describes what the patient is experiencing?

A. Ideas of reference

B. Hallucinations

C. Paranoid delusions

D. Paranoid ideations

E. Thought disorder

56.2 What is the best treatment option for the patient in Question 56.1?

A. Antianxiety medication.

B. Antipsychotic medication.

C. Hospitalization.

D. Psychotherapy.

E. Reassure the patient that he is safe.

56.3   A 42-year-old woman undergoing psychotherapy storms into her therapist's office for her session and angrily accuses the therapist of "trying to undermine her intelligence." After a discussion with the therapist, it becomes clear that it is the patient who is second guessing herself, thereby "undermining" her own intelligence. Which of the following defense mechanisms is this patient using?

   A.   Denial
   B.   Identification with the aggressor
   C.   Intellectualization
   D.   Projection
   E.   Reaction formation

ANSWERS

56.1   **C.** This patient's problem is more than mere suspiciousness; he has full-blown paranoid delusions: fixed, false beliefs. Paranoid ideation is mere suspiciousness—the **worry** that harm is meant by others. People with paranoid ideation may often be consoled or reassured by a trusted friend, and they do not often act on these suspicious. By contrast, people with paranoid delusions have fixed (ie, they are not able to be reassured) and false beliefs that others mean them harm. These patients may act on these beliefs as well. For example, this patient tearing apart his office is looking for "bugs."

56.2   **B.** This patient would benefit from small dosage, short-term antipsychotic therapy to manage his delusional thinking. With a paranoid delusion, which is, by definition, a psychotic symptom, antipsychotic drugs are the therapy of choice. Because the patient is not exhibiting dangerous behavior to himself or others, hospitalization is not required. Reassurance, by definition of a delusion (fixed, false belief), will be unhelpful. Antianxiety medication is unhelpful and ineffective with a psychotic disorder, as is psychotherapy.

56.3   **D.** Projection is a defense mechanism by which individuals deal with conflict by falsely attributing to another their own unacceptable feelings, impulses, or thoughts. Blaming others for their own sentiments and actions directs the focus away from the person doing the accusing. For example, a patient who is angry with his therapist suddenly starts accusing the therapist of being angry with him.

CLINICAL PEARLS

▶ Patients with paranoid personality disorder show a pervasive distrust and suspiciousness of others, often interpreting others' motives as malevolent.

▶ Paranoid personality disorder belongs in cluster A, the "mad" cluster.

▶ Patients with paranoid disorder need to be dealt with in a low-key manner without trying to be too close or friendly, which could increase the patient's suspiciousness.

▶ The difference between a patient with paranoid personality disorder and a patient with delusional disorder is really a matter of degree, the difference between paranoid ideations and paranoid delusions.

REFERENCES

American Psychiatric Association. *Diagnostic and Statistical Manual of Mental Disorder.* 5th ed. Arlington, VA: American Psychiatric Publishing; 2013:649-652.

Black BW, Andreasen NC. *Introductory Textbook of Psychiatry.* 6th ed. Washington, DC: American Psychiatric Publishing; 2014:470-471.

Hales RE, Yudofsky SC, Roberts LW. *The American Psychiatric Publishing Textbook of Psychiatry.* 6th ed. Washington, DC: American Psychiatric Publishing; 2014:868-872.

A 23-year-old woman is admitted to the inpatient psychiatric unit after slashing both wrists when her therapist left for a week's vacation. The cuts were superficial and did not require stitches. The patient says that she is angry with her psychiatrist for "abandoning her." She claims that she is often depressed, although the depressions last "only a couple of hours." When she was first admitted to the hospital, she told the admitting psychiatrist that she heard a voice telling her that "she will never amount to anything," but she subsequently denies having heard the voice. This is the patient's fourth hospital admission, and all of them have been precipitated by someone in her life leaving, even temporarily. After 3 days in the unit, the patient's psychiatry resident gets into an argument with the nursing staff. He says that the patient has been behaving very well, responding to his therapy, and is deserving of a privilege. The nurses claim that the patient is not following unit rules, sleeping through her group meetings, and ignoring the limits set. Both parties go to the unit director complaining about the other.

► What is the most likely diagnosis?
► What defense mechanism is being employed by the patient?
► What should the hospital staff do next?

ANSWERS TO CASE 57:

Borderline Personality Disorder

Summary: A 23-year-old woman is admitted to the psychiatric unit after she superficially lacerates her wrists because she feels she was abandoned by her therapist. She was admitted on previous occasions during which she also claimed she was "abandoned." She admits to having a depressed mood that varies by the hour. On admission, she claimed that she heard a voice speaking to her, although she currently denies it. She seems to be at the center of a disagreement between the psychiatric resident and the nursing staff, who have conflicting views of her behavior in the unit.

- **Most likely diagnosis:** Borderline personality disorder (BPD).

- **Defense mechanism used:** Splitting.

- **Next step for hospital staff:** The unit director should mediate a meeting between the psychiatric resident and the staff, at which time he or she should point out that splitting is occurring. The patient should be brought to the meeting, and everyone involved should discuss whether or not she is ready for a privilege.

ANALYSIS

Objectives

1. Recognize the defense mechanism of splitting, which is commonly employed by patients with BPD.

2. Understand treatment strategies to contain splitting in an inpatient unit.

Considerations

This young woman displays several classic signs of BPD, including frantic efforts to avoid abandonment, impulsive behavior, suicidal behavior, and transient psychosis. She also uses the defense mechanism of splitting, during which she "sits calmly on the sidelines" while her treatment team splits in half over whether or not she should be allowed to go on a pass. (Each side sees very different patient behavior and reports it, believing that the other side must be misrepresenting the patient's actions because the observations on each side are so completely different.)

APPROACH TO:
Borderline Personality Disorder

DEFINITIONS

COUNTER TRANSFERENCE: A set of expectations, beliefs, and emotional responses induced in the physician (often unconsciously) through interactions with a particular patient. For example, a patient comes to a physician and is denigrating and hostile at every interaction. The physician develops a negative countertransference to the patient and finds himself avoiding the patient and forgetting their appointments.

DEFENSE MECHANISMS: A psychodynamic term which defines various means which an individual might use to psychologically cope with a difficult situation. These defense mechanisms range from relatively mature ones such as humor to quite immature ones such as often seen with BPD. Typical defense mechanisms used by persons with BPD might include devaluation, idealization, projection, projective identification, and splitting.

DIALECTICAL BEHAVIORAL THERAPY: A type of cognitive therapy specifically designed to help manage difficult BPD patients. Through individual relationships with a therapist, patients learn skills to confront and manage the volatile emotions and impulses they are feeling.

CLINICAL APPROACH

Patients with BPD demonstrate a pervasive instability of affect, interpersonal relationships, self-image, and a marked impulsivity that begins by early adulthood. It is seen in a variety of contexts. Patients are often chronically depressed and are markedly impulsive. Psychosis, including paranoid ideation, can be seen transiently under stress. Patients make frantic efforts to avoid real or perceived abandonment because they have chronic feelings of emptiness. Suicidal behavior, gestures, or threats are common.

DIFFERENTIAL DIAGNOSIS

Patients with **BPD can become psychotic**, but these episodes are **generally transient**. There is generally no thought disorder or other signs of schizophrenia, which helps rule out this diagnosis. Patients with paranoid personality disorder **can show paranoid ideation** as well, but these symptoms are generally long lasting and pervasive. Patients with BPD can appear depressed and have vegetative symptoms—if they do, overlying their pervasive behavioral patterns, a major depression can be diagnosed. As such, disorders such as impulse control disorders, substance abuse disorders, eating disorders, and sexual/identity disorders can also coexist. These diagnoses must occur as additional signs and symptoms on top of those that fulfill the BPD diagnosis for two (or more) disorders to be diagnosed.

Interviewing Tips

These patients are often extremely difficult to work with, as they have a peculiar ability to "get under the skin" of the clinician (induce countertransference). Give patients clear, nontechnical answers. Do not encourage the patient to idealize you or other members of the treatment team. Strike a balance that is not too close, but not avoidant or punitive. Set limits early and often on what behavior is acceptable.

CASE CORRELATION

- See also Case 14 and Case 52 for patients with self-destructive behavior or rapidly shifting emotions. While persistent depressive disorder may often co-occur with borderline personality disorder, they may often be distinguished by looking at the long-term patterns of behavior and age at onset of the patient in question. Histrionic personality disordered patients may have rapidly shifting emotions, but do not have the chronic feelings of deep emptiness or loneliness or the constant, angry disruptions in relationships that characterize those with borderline personality disorder.

COMPREHENSION QUESTIONS

57.1 A 24-year-old woman with BPD is admitted to a psychiatric hospital because of suicidal ideation. The physician on call tells the patient about all the rules and regulations in the unit and that "although it is a great place to get better, it is a lot of work." Which of the following is this physician attempting to do with this patient?

A. Decrease idealization of the unit and the hospitalization.

B. Discourage the patient from splitting.

C. Dissuade the patient from signing in voluntarily.

D. Encourage the patient to seek admission elsewhere.

E. Investigate the patient's motivation for desiring admission.

57.2 The patient in Question 57.1 complains to her psychiatrist that all the nurses on the floor don't know what they are doing and they are rude. She later tells her nurse she is the best nurse on the floor and wished her psychiatrist cared about her the way the nurse did. Which of the following defense mechanisms is this patient using?

A. Altruism

B. Intellectualization

C. Splitting

D. Sublimation

E. Undoing

57.3 A 24-year-old woman is seen in the emergency department after superficially cutting both her wrists. Her explanation is that she was upset because her boyfriend of 3 weeks just broke up with her. When asked about other relationships, she says that she has had numerous sexual partners, both male and female, but none of them lasted more than several weeks. Which type of psychotherapy might she be most likely to respond to?

A. Dialectical behavioral therapy

B. Interpersonal psychotherapy

C. Parent assertiveness training

D. Psychopharmacotherapy

E. Supportive psychotherapy

57.4 A 22-year-old man with BPD patient loses his job at a local restaurant, the first job he has held for longer than a month. His mother dies suddenly 3 weeks later. One month after his mother's death, the patient tells his therapist, whom he has been seeing once a week, that he has trouble sleeping, waking up at 3 AM and then unable to go back to sleep. He has lost 13 lb in 5 weeks without trying to do so. He reports low energy and a decreased interest in his usual hobbies. He states that he feels depressed but then grins and says, "But I'm always depressed, aren't I?" Based on his history, which of the following should the clinician do next?

A. Ask the patient to keep a sleep log.

B. Begin seeing the patient for daily psychotherapy.

C. Hospitalize the patient.

D. Start treating the patient with a mood stabilizer such as carbamazepine.

E. Start treating the patient with an antidepressant such as paroxetine.

ANSWERS

57.1 **A.** Decreasing idealization of the unit before admission will help decrease the devaluation that inevitably follows. Since these swings (between idealization and devaluation) are so typical in borderline personality disordered patients, it is useful to minimize them right from the time of admission. Otherwise, they can become quite disruptive on an inpatient unit, as the patient first comes to the unit believing he or she can be completely and perfectly taken care of, followed by intense anger when devaluation follows and the patient believes the inpatient unit is incompetent and useless.

57.2 **C.** Individuals with BPD often use the defense mechanism of splitting. Splitting is literally the "splitting off" a person's good and bad characteristics into two separate (and nonoverlapping) views of a person, which then alternate. Most healthy adults will be able to characterize people with their good and bad points at the same time. Borderline patients will characterize another as either all good, or all bad, depending on which side of the split the patient is currently seeing.

57.3 **A.** Dialectical behavioral therapy, a form of cognitive therapy, has been shown in controlled studies to be effective in treating BPD. This therapy attempts to help patients explore their own behavior, thoughts, and feelings in the present without delving into the patient's childhood, which tends to be regressive for these patients, resulting in increased suicidal behavior and acting out.

57.4 **E.** Comorbidity of major depression with BPD is quite common. When vegetative symptoms or other qualitative changes occur, medication for the major depression is necessary. SSRIs are the first-line psychopharmacologic treatments. This is often a difficult call to make, because borderline personality disorder patients present as "stably unstable," that is, their lives are often disruptive and chaotic and they often have severely depressed moods. Changes in sleep or appetite are often the best clues as to when a BPD patient has developed a concurrent major depression.

CLINICAL PEARLS

▶ Patients with BPD show a pervasive pattern of unstable personal relationships, self-images, and emotions. They can often be markedly impulsive, displaying sexual acting out, suicidal gestures, and substance abuse.

▶ Physicians need to set limits early and often with these patients. They need to be firm but not punitive. They must keep a constant eye on their own countertransference to these patients, as they can be extremely difficult to work with.

▶ Although patients with this disorder can become psychotic, it is transient, and they do not have signs of a thought disorder or other signs of schizophrenia.

▶ These patients can have other coexisting disorders such as eating disorders, major depression, and substance abuse. The specifics of each must be teased out of the multiple signs and symptoms presented by patients with BPD.

▶ Defense mechanisms used by these patients include splitting, projection, projective identification, devaluation, idealization, distortion, and acting out.

REFERENCES

American Psychiatric Association. *Diagnostic and Statistical Manual of Mental Disorders*. 5th ed. Arlington, VA: American Psychiatric Publishing; 2013:663-666.

American Psychiatric Association Practice Guideline for the Treatment of Patients With Borderline Personality Disorder. Accessed August 15, 2014. psychiatryonline.org/pb/assets/raw/sitewide/practice_guidelines/guidelines/bpd.pdf.

Black BW, Andreasen NC. *Introductory Textbook of Psychiatry*. 6th ed. Washington, DC: American Psychiatric Publishing; 2014:477-479.

Hales RE, Yudofsky SC, Roberts LW. *The American Psychiatric Publishing Textbook of Psychiatry*. 6th ed. Washington, DC: American Psychiatric Publishing; 2014:878-882.

A 32-year-old man and his 28-year-old wife come to a psychiatrist because of problems in their relationship. The wife states that the two have been married for 6 months and that they dated for 2 months prior to that. During all their sexual encounters, the husband insists that the wife wear very high-heeled shoes at all times. Although the wife initially thought that this behavior was sexy, she now worries that it is the shoes that the husband finds attractive and not her. She thinks the behavior is "freaky" and has asked the husband to stop, which he has refused to do. The husband states that he is unable to achieve an erection or orgasm without the presence of the shoes. He notes that for as long as he can remember, he has needed high-heeled shoes as part of his sexual play. He feels no shame or guilt about this behavior, although he is worried that it is causing problems between him and his wife.

▶ What is the most likely diagnosis for the husband?
▶ What is the course of and prognosis for this disorder?

ANSWERS TO CASE 58:

Fetishistic Disorder

Summary: A 32-year-old man insists that his wife wear very high-heeled shoes during all sexual encounters. This behavior causes problems in their marriage, and the patient has refused to stop because he is unable to achieve an erection or an orgasm without the presence of the shoes. This association with sexual arousal and orgasm has been a long-standing one for the patient. Although he feels no shame or guilt about it, he is concerned about its impact on his marriage.

- **Most likely diagnosis:** Fetishistic disorder.

- **Course of and prognosis for this disorder:** The course of this disorder is chronic, and it has a poor prognosis.

ANALYSIS

Objectives

1. Recognize the diagnostic criteria of fetishistic disorder in a patient (Table 58–1).

2. Understand the course, prognosis, and mitigating factors of this disorder.

Considerations

The patient has a long history of using high-heeled shoes to achieve erection and orgasm during intercourse. He cannot achieve either without the presence of the shoes. He does not feel guilty about his behavior but is worried that his wife now objects to it and that it is causing friction in his marriage. A poor prognosis is associated with an early age of onset, a high frequency of acts, no guilt or shame about the act, and substance abuse. (The patient has three of these factors.) The course and prognosis are better when the patient has a history of intercourse without paraphilic activity, when the patient has a strong motivation to change, and when the patient is self-referred. (This patient has none of these factors—although he was not referred for treatment by a legal agency, it can be assumed that his wife suggested the visit to the psychiatrist.) More recently, the occurrence of a behavior called autoerotic asphyxiation has been associated with fetishistic disorder. This is a behavior that primarily occurs in young adults and involves participating in sexual

Table 58–1 • DIAGNOSTIC CRITERIA FOR FETISHISTIC DISORDER
An individual has intense, recurring sexual desires or behaviors focused on inanimate objects such as shoes or female underwear, or a specific focus on a nongenital body part such as the foot; the desires must be present for at least 6 mo.
The sexual fantasies, desires, or behaviors must cause clinically significant distress
The fetish objects are not limited to articles of clothing used for cross-dressing (as in transvestic fetishism).

activity while simultaneously restricting blood flow to the brain. This in particular is a dangerous behavior and has been shown to lead to death or severe injury in some cases.

APPROACH TO:
Fetishistic Disorder

DEFINITIONS

ERECTILE DYSFUNCTION: Difficulty in obtaining and maintaining an erection can have a psychological or an organic cause. Some studies report that erectile dysfunction has an organic basis in 20% to 50% of men with this disorder. This can include a large number of diseases such as diabetes, malnutrition, cirrhosis, chronic renal failure, atherosclerosis, and a host of others. Medications can also impair male sexual functioning, and many psychiatric drugs (antidepressants, mood stabilizers, and antipsychotics), as well as antihypertensives and other drugs, can be to blame. To differentiate psychological causes from organic ones, a study of nocturnal penile tumescence (erections occurring during sleep) is often made. In patients who **have normal nocturnal erections** but erectile dysfunction during their waking hours, or with a partner, the problem is much more likely to have a **psychological cause.**

FETISHISTIC DISORDER: A paraphilia in which the individual seeks sexual gratification primarily through contact with an object, such as shoes or underwear, which is closely associated with the body. Fetishists are mostly male, and fetishism usually starts in adolescence. The individual can masturbate with the fetishistic object or incorporate it into sexual intercourse.

PARAPHILIC DISORDER: A disorder in which an individual primarily seeks sexual gratification through means considered abnormal by society. Paraphilias include fetishism, voyeurism, exhibitionism, sadism, masochism, transvestism, and pedophilia. What is considered normal sexual behavior varies greatly among different cultures. Many individuals have more than one paraphilia.

VOYEURISTIC DISORDER: A disorder that involves achieving sexual arousal by observing an unsuspecting and nonconsenting person who is undressing or unclothed, and/or engaged in sexual activity.

EXHIBITIONISM: A disorder marked by the compulsive exposure of the genitals in public.

SADISM: The deriving of sexual gratification or the tendency to derive sexual gratification from inflicting pain or emotional abuse on others.

MASOCHISM: The deriving of sexual gratification, or the tendency to derive sexual gratification, from being physically or emotionally abused.

PEDOPHILIA: A form of paraphilia in which a person either has acted on intense sexual urges toward children, or experiences recurrent sexual urges toward and fantasies about children that cause distress or interpersonal difficulty.

TRANSSEXUAL: A person who feels as if he or she is "trapped in the body of the wrong gender," for example, a man who believes that he is really a woman although genetically and functionally male.

TRANSVESTITE: A heterosexual male who dresses in female clothing.

VAGINISMUS: An involuntary muscle constriction of the outer third of the vagina that causes marked distress or interpersonal difficulty and interferes with sexual intercourse. A diagnosis of vaginismus is not made when there is an organic cause for the disorder or when it is better accounted for by another mental disorder such as somatic symptom disorder.

CLINICAL APPROACH

Differential Diagnosis

Paraphilias tend to be compound; the presence of one should prompt the clinician to inquire about others. There are few conditions in the differential diagnosis for fetishistic disorder; one is transvestism, in which fetishistic clothing is worn to produce sexual excitement.

The *DSM-5* changes in paraphilic disorders were largely confined to nomenclature. The changes were designed to better distinguish between the behaviors and the disorder. That is, someone with a fetish may or may not have the full disorder.

TREATMENT

Fetishistic disorder, **like most paraphilias, is difficult to treat.** The presence of only one paraphilia, normal intelligence, an absence of substance dependence, and stable adult relationships are all good prognostic indicators. Fetishists do not usually seek treatment voluntarily. Interventions for fetishistic disorder include cognitive behavioral therapy (CBT) and insight-oriented psychotherapy. Cognitive behavioral therapy includes sex education, social skills training, and a reevaluation of the ways in which the individual rationalizes the behavior. Treatment can involve desensitization to the fetish, relaxation techniques, and learning to avoid triggers for the fetishism. Psychodynamic psychotherapy explores the roots of the behavior and the events that caused development of the fetish in childhood or adolescence. In this particular case, given the solitary and isolated nature of the fetish, the therapist might also consider directly addressing the problems this has developed in the patient's relationship with his wife and consider whether more acceptance of this behavior within the marriage might be helpful. This is more difficult to achieve with greater numbers of paraphilias.

There have been published clinical trials and case reports on the use of pharmacologic agents in the treatment of fetishes. Those psychiatric medications used include fluoxetine, sertraline, mirtazapine, topiramate, and buspirone. However, the number of subjects in these studies has been quite small and no clear conclusions have been reached. Antiandrogen medications such as cyproterone acetate, medroxyprogesterone acetate, and leuprolide acetate have also been studied, but again, no clear conclusion or best practice can be discerned.

> **CASE CORRELATION**
>
> - It is important to distinguish the disorder from fetishistic behavior without the disorder. Use of a fetish object for sexual arousal without distress or any other adverse consequences would not meet criteria for the disorder.

COMPREHENSION QUESTIONS

58.1 A married pharmacist comes in for treatment at the insistence of his wife, who was disturbed to find that he was wearing some of her undergarments under his clothes. He admitted to her that he often masturbates when wearing her underwear and fantasizes about wearing it while having intercourse with her. Which of the following words best define this paraphilia?

A. Fetishistic disorder

B. Fetish behavior

C. Transvestic disorder

D. Transvestic behavior

E. Masochism

58.2 Which of the following is a poor prognostic indicator in the treatment of fetishists?

A. A stable adult relationship

B. Presence of another paraphilia

C. Normal intelligence

D. Self-referral for treatment

E. History of sexual relations without the paraphilia

58.3 A 23-year-old man comes to his physician asking for sexual reassignment surgery. He states that for "as long as I can remember" he has felt that he was born in the wrong body. He states that he believes that "truly I am a woman" and is disgusted by his male body habitus. He has been living as a woman since he moved out of his parents' house several years ago. He wishes to have his penis removed, and would like female breasts and genitalia. He considers himself a heterosexual because he is attracted to men. When talking with the patient, which of the following should be used to describe this man?

A. He has a paraphilic disorder.

B. He has fetishistic disorder.

C. He has gender dysphoria.

D. She has gender dysphoria.

E. He is a sadist.

58.4 A 55-year-old man complains of inability to achieve an erection. He has been worried about his health recently and takes antihypertensive medication. Which of the following would most likely differentiate between an organic and psychiatric condition?

  A. A lower-extremity myographic examination

  B. Magnetic resonance imaging of the lumbosacral spine

  C. An erection on awakening in the morning

  D. The interpretation of projective tests

  E. An electroencephalographic reading

ANSWERS

58.1 **D.** Transvestic behavior would be the best answer based on the information given. For a diagnosis of transvestic disorder, additional information would be needed such as duration or degree in which it affects his life. Fetishistic behavior is similar, but will also include objects other than clothing to develop arousal.

58.2 **B.** The presence of multiple paraphilias is a poor prognostic indicator. Self-reporting is considered indicative of good prognosis as often the legal system is involved; a stable long-term relationship is a very good sign, as is achievement of sexual gratification without paraphilias.

58.3 **D.** The individual is experiencing discomfort with assigned sex. She has felt for a long period of time that her gender is female. She has been living as a woman for more than a year. The best answer is to refer to her feelings about her conflict and to respect her desire to live as a woman by referring to her with female language.

58.4 **C.** An erection on awakening is good evidence of a nonorganic etiology. Because the imaging of the lumbosacral spine may or may not indicate the capacity for erection, these options are not as predictive.

CLINICAL PEARLS

  ▶ Fetishists rarely seek treatment and are usually very treatment resistant.

  ▶ The presence of one paraphilia should prompt the clinician to inquire about other paraphilias.

  ▶ Erectile dysfunction is a common disorder in men and has primary, acquired, organic, and nonorganic causes. Waking up with an erection is good evidence of a nonorganic etiology.

  ▶ Vaginismus is an involuntary contraction of vaginal musculature that prevents intercourse; it is best treated with behavioral therapy.

REFERENCES

American Psychiatric Association. *Diagnostic and Statistical Manual of Mental Disorders*. 5th ed. Washington, DC: American Psychiatric Publishing; 2013.

Sadock BJ, Sadock VA, Ruiz P. *Kaplan and Sadock's Synopsis of Psychiatry: Behavioral Sciences/Clinical Psychiatry*. 11th ed. Baltimore, MD: Lippincott Williams & Wilkins; 2014.

A 22-year-old man presents to the emergency room with a chief complaint of "they are making me look toward heaven." The patient admits to a past diagnosis of schizophrenia, "but God cured me of it." Review of the medical record reveals that he was, in fact, just discharged from the hospital the previous week on risperidone 4 mg at bedtime. His dose was subsequently increased to 6 mg by his outpatient psychiatrist 2 days prior to this visit. The patient believes that angels are forcing him to look up to heaven as, since this morning, he has been unable to look "down to the devil in hell." His mental status examination demonstrates a cooperative and appropriately dressed young man, alert and oriented three times. His speech is not spontaneous. His mood is "worried," but his affect is flat. His thoughts are logical without looseness. He denies suicidal or homicidal ideation but he has delusions. His insight is poor, but his judgment and impulse control are not currently impaired. His physical examination is notable for continued upward gaze of his eyes bilaterally.

▶ What is the most likely diagnosis?
▶ What is the next step in treatment?

ANSWERS TO CASE 59:

Medication-Induced Acute Dystonia (Extrapyramidal Symptoms)

Summary: A 22-year-old man with a past psychiatric history of schizophrenia, recently released from the hospital on risperidone, has had his dose of this medication increased 2 days prior to the emergency room visit. He presents to the emergency room with the acute onset of a fixed upward gaze bilaterally. The patient remains delusional regarding the cause, namely believing that angels are forcing him to look up to heaven and avoid looking down to hell. His mental status examination is significant for an anxious mood, flat affect, and the above delusions. His physical examination demonstrates a continued, upward gaze of his eyes bilaterally.

- **Most likely diagnosis:** Medication-induced acute dystonia (an extrapyramidal symptom).

- **Next step in treatment:** Benztropine 2 mg (or diphenhydramine 50 mg) intramuscularly, with a repeat dose in 30 minutes if no improvement.

ANALYSIS

Objectives

1. Recognize the distinct extrapyramidal symptoms that can occur in patients treated with antipsychotic medications.

2. List the risk factors for developing extrapyramidal symptoms.

3. List the treatments of medication-induced acute dystonia in patients treated with antipsychotic medications.

Considerations

The patient is a young man with a history of schizophrenia. He has recently been released from the hospital on risperidone, the dose of which was increased 2 days prior to the emergency room visit. He now presents with the acute onset of bilateral upward gaze of his eyes. While his explanation is delusional, his history (acute onset, recent medication increase) and physical examination (contraction of superior rectus muscles bilaterally) are consistent with an oculogyric crisis, an acute dystonic reaction caused by the patient's antipsychotic medication.

APPROACH TO:
Extrapyramidal Symptoms

DEFINITION

EXTRAPYRAMIDAL SYMPTOMS: Movement disorders such as acute dystonic reactions, parkinsonism, akathisia, neuroleptic malignant syndrome, or tardive dyskinesia caused by dopamine antagonists, usually antipsychotic medications.

CLINICAL APPROACH

The therapeutic effect of antipsychotic medications stems, in part, from their ability to block dopamine receptors in the mesolimbic and mesocortical areas of the brain. However, these same medications also bind to dopamine receptors in other areas of the brain, such as the nigrostriatal pathway, thereby causing a variety of extrapyramidal side effects. These movement disorders include **acute dystonic reactions, parkinsonism, akathisia, neuroleptic malignant syndrome**, and **tardive dyskinesia**, and they each vary in their risk factors, severity, time course, and treatment.

Acute dystonic reactions are abnormal, prolonged, and often painful contractions of the muscles of the eyes (oculogyric crisis), head, neck (torticollis or retrocollis), limbs, or trunk, developing within several hours to days of initiating or increasing the dose of antipsychotics. Risk factors include young age, male gender, and high doses of antipsychotic medications.

Neuroleptic (antipsychotic)-induced parkinsonism consists of the triad of resting ("pill-rolling") tremor, muscular (cogwheel) rigidity, and bradykinesia/akinesia. It may also include drooling, shuffling gait, and rabbit syndrome (tremors of lips and perioral muscles). This syndrome generally occurs within a few weeks after initiation or increase of an antipsychotic medication. Older age and female gender increase the risk of developing neuroleptic-induced parkinsonism.

Akathisia is the most common form of medication-induced movement disorder (incidence rates between 25% and 75%). It is often described as a subjective feeling of restlessness, which may include anxiety, pacing, or frequent sitting/standing. The time course for developing akathisia is similar to parkinsonism, but may occur within several days. Older females may be at an increased risk.

Neuroleptic malignant syndrome (NMS) is a medical emergency, consisting of muscle ("lead-pipe") rigidity, fever, autonomic instability, diaphoresis, as well as delirium, tremor, mutism, leukocytosis, and elevated (often markedly) creatinine phosphokinase. While NMS can occur at any point during treatment with antipsychotic medications, most cases develop within 30 days of initiation of antipsychotics. High potency, typical (first generation) antipsychotics appear to pose a greater risk than low-potency or atypical (second generation) antipsychotics, although all antipsychotics can cause NMS. In addition, a prior episode of NMS increases future risk.

Tardive dyskinesia is a late-onset development of involuntary, choreoathetoid movements, particularly of (but not limited to) the tongue, lower face and jaw, and extremities. It is usually irreversible. Risk factors for tardive dyskinesia include long-term treatment with antipsychotics (especially typical or first-generation), older age, and (possibly) a history of early extrapyramidal reactions to antipsychotic medications.

TREATMENT

Acute dystonic reactions need to be treated urgently, and in some cases (oculogyric crises, laryngospasm), emergently. The mainstay of treatment is anticholinergic medications such as benztropine, or antihistamines such as diphenhydramine. These can be administered orally, intramuscularly, or intravenously. Resolution is swift, but doses may need to be repeated one or more times. After the acute episode has improved, consideration should be given to possibly decreasing the dose of the antipsychotic, switching to another antipsychotic less likely to cause dystonia, or continuing oral anticholinergic agents.

CASE CORRELATION

- See also Case 6 for patients with delusions and/or hallucinations, which may present with abnormal physical symptoms as well. For example, a schizophrenic patient in a catatonic state may present with an extreme, frozen stance. Likewise, a severely psychotic patient may posture, holding difficult and/or uncomfortable poses for long periods of time in response to internal stimuli. This can make it difficult to differentiate an extrapyramidal reaction (eg, oculogyric crisis) in a psychotic patient which is best treated with anticholinergics or antihistamines (with a concomitant reduction in antipsychotic dosage) from posturing in a psychotic patient on antipsychotics who needs the antipsychotic medication increased.

COMPREHENSION QUESTIONS

For the following questions, choose the most likely diagnosis (A-E):

- A. Acute dystonic reaction
- B. Akathisia
- C. Neuroleptic malignant syndrome
- D. Parkinsonism
- E. Tardive dyskinesia

59.1 A 50-year-old woman with a schizoaffective disorder, bipolar type, complains of "nervous tics." She is currently being treated with haloperidol decanoate 100 mg intramuscularly every 4 weeks. She denies significant affective symptoms but complains of chronic auditory hallucinations of "whispers" without commands. No suicidal or homicidal ideation is present. On examination, she is noted to be sticking her tongue in and out of her mouth and to have repetitive, rhythmic movements of her hands and feet.

59.2 A 25-year-old man is admitted with the new onset of psychotic symptoms, consisting of command hallucinations to harm others, paranoid delusions, and agitation. He is begun on olanzapine 30 mg daily. After several days, he becomes calmer but more withdrawn. When approached by the nurses, he is found to be lying in bed, eyes open but not responsive. He is noted to be sweating but is resistant to being moved. His vital signs demonstrate a temperature of 101.4°F, blood pressure 182/98 mm Hg, pulse 104 beats/min, and respiration 22 breaths/min.

59.3 A 43-year-old woman with schizophrenia is being followed in an outpatient community mental health clinic after being discharged from the hospital. While hospitalized, her medications were increased to risperidone 3 mg in the morning and 4 mg in the evening. She has some paranoia and ideas of reference, but she denies auditory or visual hallucinations. Her mental status examination is significant for moderate psychomotor slowing, with little spontaneous speech, but with a coarse tremor of her hands bilaterally. Her stated mood is "fine," although her affect appears blunted, with little expression. Her gait is wide based and shuffling.

59.4 A 32-year-old male patient is admitted with the provisional diagnosis of psychotic disorder, not otherwise specified, rule-out bipolar disorder. After 10 days, he is finally stabilized on valproic acid 2000 mg daily and aripiprazole 30 mg daily. The nurses are concerned his medications need to be increased or switched as he has been recently sleeping less and is more agitated, often pacing the hallways. Upon examination, he admits to feeling "edgy," but he denies racing thoughts, increased energy, paranoia, or delusions. He states, "I just can't stop walking; I feel like I'm going crazy."

ANSWERS

59.1 **E.** This female patient with chronic schizoaffective disorder now demonstrates choreoathetoid movements of her tongue and extremities, consistent with tardive dyskinesia. She has several risk factors for development of tardive dyskinesia, including likely long-term treatment with a high-potency, typical antipsychotic.

59.2 **C.** This acutely psychotic patient has been started on an antipsychotic medication, namely olanzapine, and he has now developed acute mental status changes, diaphoresis, rigidity, and fluctuating vital signs. These are signs and symptoms consistent with neuroleptic malignant syndrome, a medical emergency. Antipsychotic medications should be discontinued immediately, and supportive measures need to be employed.

59.3 **D.** The patient is a middle-aged woman with chronic psychotic symptoms, just released from the hospital with an increase in her risperidone dose. She now demonstrates bradykinesia, shuffling gait, masked facies, and a coarse tremor, all consistent with antipsychotic-induced parkinsonism. Risk factors for the development of parkinsonism include female gender and an older age.

59.4 **B.** The patient is a young man with psychotic symptoms, rule-out bipolar disorder, stabilized on valproic acid and aripiprazole, but who recently has had worsening insomnia, anxiety, and restlessness (pacing). Given the improvement in his psychiatric symptoms, his current complaints are likely due to akathisia, a feeling of restlessness or anxiety, usually arising several weeks after treatment with antipsychotic medications. Consideration should be given to either decreasing his antipsychotic dose or adding another medication such as a beta-blocker or benzodiazepine.

CLINICAL PEARLS

▶ Extrapyramidal symptoms are movement disorders, caused by antipsychotic medications.

▶ The time course for the development of medication-induced movement disorders after administration (or increased dosage) of antipsychotics is as follows:

  ▶ Dystonic reaction: hours → days

  ▶ Parkinsonism: days → weeks

  ▶ Akathisia: days → weeks

  ▶ Tardive dyskinesia: years

  ▶ Neuroleptic malignant syndrome: *Any Time*

▶ Acute dystonia is treated with anticholinergics or antihistamines.

REFERENCES

American Psychiatric Association. *Diagnostic and Statistical Manual of Mental Disorders.* 5th ed. Arlington, VA: American Psychiatric Publishing; 2013.

Burkhard PR. Acute and subacute drug-induced movement disorders. *Parkinsonism and Related Disorders.* 2014;20S1:S108-S112.

Correll CU, Schenk EM. Tardive dyskinesia and new antipsychotics. *Curr Opin Psychiatry.* 2008;21:151.

A 19-year-old adolescent man presents to a psychiatrist insisting, "I have schizo-phrenia and need to be admitted." For the past several days, he has heard voices telling him to kill himself. He says that he is possessed by the devil. The patient denies feeling depressed, but insists he will hurt himself if he is not admitted to a hospital immediately. However, he denies having any specific suicide plan. He has no prior history of psychiatric treatment or complaints, no medical problems, and is not taking any medication. He drinks one or two beers a week and denies using drugs. At the end of the interview, he again requests hospitalization. He then adds that he is currently on leave from the Navy and is due back on his ship, which is leaving in 2 days.

On a mental status examination, the patient is initially cooperative and forth-coming but becomes increasingly irritated when asked to give more details about his symptoms. His mood and affect are euthymic and full range. His thought processes are logical, without looseness of association or thought blocking. His thought content is notable for suicidal ideation but no homicidal ideation. He reports having delusions and auditory hallucinations. His insight seems good con-sidering the severity of his symptoms.

▶ What is the most likely diagnosis?
▶ How would you approach this patient?

ANSWERS TO CASE 60:

Malingering

Summary: A 19-year-old adolescent man without a psychiatric or medical history presents with a sudden onset of hallucinations, delusions, and suicidal ideation and asks to be admitted to the hospital. His social history is notable for his upcoming deployment with the Navy. His mental status examination is relatively unremarkable except for his reported symptoms, some irritability when he is questioned, and his good level of insight.

- **Most likely diagnosis:** Malingering.

- **Best approach:** Obtain collateral information (if possible) from family and/or friends, gently confront the inconsistencies in the patient's presentation, explore and validate his feelings regarding his military duty, and refer him for an appropriate follow-up (if possible).

ANALYSIS

Objectives

1. Recognize malingering.

2. Differentiate malingering from factitious and conversion disorders.

3. Understand how to approach a patient suspected of malingering.

Considerations

This man initially presents with symptoms of a psychotic disorder. Although he admits to some criteria consistent with schizophrenia, such as hallucinations and delusions, the time course is too brief. There does not appear to be any substance use or a medical condition causing his symptoms. An important factor seems to be his upcoming military duty. His mental status examination is remarkable for the lack of a flat or inappropriate affect, loose associations, or thought blocking commonly seen in a psychotic disorder. In fact, **he displays a surprisingly high level of insight into his "illness"** considering his lack of a psychiatric history. He insists that his self-diagnosis is correct and that he needs immediate hospitalization. He becomes irritable only when pressed for more details. Although a psychotic disorder should be considered, the patient's reluctance to provide more details, a lack of objective findings on the mental status examination, and his intact insight in the context of required military duty make malingering the most likely diagnosis.

APPROACH TO:
Malingering

DEFINITIONS

MALINGERING: The intentional feigning, production, or exaggeration of psychiatric or medical signs/symptoms to obtain secondary (external) gain (eg, financial compensation or avoidance of work, a prison sentence, or military service).

THOUGHT BLOCKING: The unpleasant experience of having one's train of thought curtailed absolutely.

CLINICAL APPROACH

Diagnostic Criteria

Malingering is not a psychiatric or medical diagnosis, but in the *Diagnostic and Statistical Manual of Mental Disorders, 5th edition*, it is listed as an additional condition that can be the focus of clinical attention (a V code). Factors which should raise the index of suspicion for malingering include a medicolegal context of presentation; marked discrepancy between claimed stress, severity, or disability and objectively observable findings; lack of cooperation with appropriate evaluation and treatment, and presence of antisocial personality disorder. A necessary component is the *intentional* production of symptoms or signs in order to achieve some *tangible external gain*.

DIFFERENTIAL DIAGNOSIS

The primary, most essential, differentiation must be made between malingering and an actual psychiatric or medical diagnosis. Collateral information gathered from family or friends can be helpful in further elucidating the diagnosis. Important rule outs in the differential diagnosis for malingering include both factitious and conversion disorders. In factitious disorder, a patient *intentionally* produces a physical or psychiatric illness in order to assume the *sick role*. In conversion disorder, a patient *unconsciously* produces a physical or neurologic symptom because of an *intrapsychic conflict*. Table 60–1 illustrates these differences.

Approach to the Malingering Patient

As malingering is not a psychiatric disorder, there is no specific treatment for it. However, there are several factors that can be helpful to both the clinician and

Table 60–1 • DIFFERENTIAL DIAGNOSIS FOR MALINGERING		
Condition	Production of Symptoms or Signs	Motivation
Malingering	Conscious	External gain
Factitious disorder	Conscious	Assumption of the sick role
Conversion disorder	Unconscious	Unconscious conflict

the patient. An important issue to keep in mind is the physician's own feelings (countertransference) toward malingering. Accusations, anger, and rejection serve only to inflame the situation, promote further defensiveness, send the patient elsewhere, or perhaps provoke the individual to violence. As in all other psychiatric and medical interventions, maintenance of a therapeutic alliance is essential. Whereas gentle confrontation can be necessary, empathic exploration and understanding of the feelings and issues contributing to the feigning of illness can lead to increased trust in the clinician and truth telling by the individual. If it is practical or desired, a referral for further supportive therapy can then be made to address the underlying issues.

CASE CORRELATION

- See Case 30 for patients who might also feign medical or psychiatric illness. The differentiation between the two is the difference between primary and secondary gains. Malingering patients feign symptoms for some external gain (avoiding police arrest, trying to collect disability money) while those with factitious disorder have no obvious external gains to be made. Instead, they are seeking to assume the sick role itself.

COMPREHENSION QUESTIONS

For the following clinical questions, choose the one descriptor (A-E) that *best* describes the situation:

A. Factitious disorder

B. Malingering

C. Conversion disorder

D. Somatic symptom disorder

E. Illness anxiety disorder

60.1 A 23-year-old pregnant woman complains of an inability to feel her legs. She wonders if the fetus is grabbing her spinal cord. Although she does not appear concerned about her condition, on further questioning she admits that her pregnancy was unplanned and that it has been a source of stress for her and her husband. Her neurologic examination is unremarkable except for decreased sensation below her waist. The results of a computed tomography scan and magnetic resonance imaging of her brain and spine are normal.

60.2 A 45-year-old man complains of lower back pain and weakness in his legs after lifting heavy boxes while at work. He says that he has not been able to go to work for several days. He requests treatment and a letter excusing him from work. On examination, he is found to have significant lumbar pain without spasms. The strength in his legs is decreased because of a lack of effort. His reflexes are within normal limits.

60.3 A 38-year-old woman comes in for evaluation of an abscess on her thigh. Her chart documents frequent outpatient and hospital visits. She is admitted, her abscess is drained, and she is treated with antibiotics. Culture studies demonstrate microorganisms consistent with fecal matter, and a further physical examination reveals many old scars, presumably self-inflicted.

60.4 A 50-year-old man is referred to a physician because he has ongoing migraine headaches. His headaches are chronic and bilateral, are worse with loud noises and light, and occur without aura or vomiting. His physical examination is unremarkable except that the patient does not appear to be in significant distress. When he is presented with various options for treatment, including nonsteroidal anti-inflammatory medications, he becomes angry, demanding that Tylenol with codeine is the only thing that has ever helped him. When he is told that non-narcotic medications should be tried first, he accuses the doctor of not believing him and storms out of the clinic.

60.5 A 53-year-old man pulls a back muscle while doing his usual exercise routine. He seeks out several medical opinions with sports medicine, orthopedics, and neurology, all of which assure him that he has only experienced an unfortunate muscle strain. However, the patient exhibits high levels of anxiety, and ascribes any ache or pain to some unknown malady. He is so fearful of reinjury that he no longer exercises, always walks with a cane, and is insistent that someone be with him at all times in case he becomes debilitated.

60.6 A healthy 25-year-old man becomes preoccupied with his health after his father has a stroke. This man monitors his blood pressure several times a day, starts an aggressive cardiovascular exercise program, and becomes a vegan. He spends 2 to 3 hours per day researching the latest research in strokes and other cardiovascular disease. He attempts to make quarterly appointments with his primary care doctor, although there is no apparent reason to do so.

ANSWERS

60.1 **C.** The most likely diagnosis for this woman is conversion disorder. She presents with symptoms of a neurologic disorder without an obvious cause or trauma. She does not appear particularly concerned about her symptoms (*la belle indifference*), and there is no obvious possibility of obtaining external gain. Her motivation does not seem to be assuming the sick role but rather expressing an unconscious conflict involving her unwanted pregnancy.

60.2 **B.** In this case, the most likely diagnosis is malingering. Although this man may indeed have some minor injury, his physical examination is remarkable only in revealing tenderness without spasms. His complaints of weakness and inability to work appear exaggerated given the lack of objective findings. The patient clearly has an obvious external motivation for embellishing his symptoms, namely, avoiding work.

60.3 **A.** The most likely diagnosis for this woman is factitious disorder. She presents with a self-induced infection, as well as a history of frequent utilization of hospitalizations and other medical services. Her illnesses are consciously created, without a desire to obtain obvious external gain other than assumption of the patient role.

60.4 **B.** In this case, the most likely diagnosis is malingering. This man presents with only subjective complaints; there are no significant medical findings or apparent suffering. He is angry and defensive, and he appears to be motivated solely by a desire to obtain narcotics rather than appropriate treatment.

60.5 **D.** In this case, the most likely diagnosis is somatic symptom disorder. This man exhibits a distressing somatic symptom which disrupts his usual life routines, excessive thoughts of his physical condition, and persistent anxiety.

60.6 **E.** This man is preoccupied with acquiring a serious illness, without any somatic symptoms. He demonstrates a high level of anxiety about his health and indulges in excessive health-related behaviors. This symptom array is consistent with the diagnosis of illness anxiety disorder.

CLINICAL PEARLS

▶ Consider malingering when there is an inconsistent history or presentation, coupled with the possibility of obtaining an obvious external gain.

▶ Patients with factitious disorder also consciously produce symptoms, but their motivation is to assume the patient/sick role.

▶ Gentle confrontation can be necessary with malingerers, but an empathic stance often promotes a more effective physician–patient alliance.

▶ Referral to a mental health professional can be indicated to help a malingering individual cope with the ongoing stressors promoting the deception.

REFERENCES

American Psychiatric Association, *Diagnostic and Statistical Manual of Mental Disorders*. 5th ed. Washington, DC: American Psychiatric Publishing; 2013.

Sadock BJ, Sadock VA, Ruiz P. *Kaplan and Sadock's Synopsis of Psychiatry: Behavioral Sciences/Clinical Psychiatry*. 11th ed. Baltimore, MD: Lippincott Williams & Wilkins; 2014.

Review Questions

1. A 35-year-old man comes to his physician for his yearly checkup. He tells the physician that he is having real difficulty at his job. He has been working for 6 years at a computer company which had him sitting in his cubicle working alone, which worked just fine. Recently, because of his exemplary performance at the job, he was promoted to a position which requires far more interactions with others. He now feels overwhelmed and unhappy at his job. The man lives alone (and states he likes it that way) and has only one friend with whom he speaks to irregularly. Which of the following is the most likely diagnosis?

    A. Schizoid personality disorder

    B. Paranoid personality disorder

    C. Schizotypal personality disorder

    D. Adjustment disorder with anxiety

    E. Avoidant personality disorder

2. A 30-year-old woman comes to her physician because she is sad about the fact that she does not have any friends. She describes herself as "a loner" and spends most of her free time either at home alone or going to the movies solo. She denies problems with appetite or insomnia, and notes that none of this is new, but her feelings of sadness have grown because her one friend has told her that she is getting married next month. Which of the following is the most likely diagnosis?

    A. Schizoid personality disorder

    B. Paranoid personality disorder

    C. Schizotypal personality disorder

    D. Adjustment disorder with anxiety

    E. Avoidant personality disorder

3. An 18-year-old woman is brought to the physician by her parents because she is displaying several odd behaviors. They state that the girl takes showers for hours at a time. When questioned, the girl says she does not like to do this, but must do so to keep germs off herself. If she does not wash this way, she becomes overwhelmingly anxious. The parents also note that the girl can't leave the house without checking that the stove is off; she must do this at least a dozen times before she can leave. Which of the following is the most likely therapy for this patient?

    A. Psychotherapy alone

    B. Antipsychotic

    C. High-dose selective serotonin reuptake inhibitor (SSRI)

    D. Anxiolytic

    E. Mood stabilizer

4. A 40-year-old woman is being seen by the psychiatrist because she is "being crippled by anxiety." She notes that while she has always been a worrier, the worry is starting to get "out of hand." She worries about everything; whether the state she lives in will go broke, whether terrorist attacks will continue, whether her finances will remain secure, and whether her house will be found to have foundation cracks, among other worries. She notes increased stress at work the last few months and marital stress which preceded the additional worries. Which of the following is the best therapy for this patient?

    A. Buspirone
    B. Anxiolytic
    C. Selective serotonin reuptake inhibitor (SSRI)
    D. Cognitive behavioral therapy
    E. Zolpidem

5. A 19-year-old man is brought into the emergency department after he is picked up by police for wandering around his neighborhood naked. On examination, the patient states that he is "receiving amazing messages from the cosmosphere" and that he believes that he is destined to do something "catastrophically wonderful" for the world. He is alternately euphoric and then irritable with the examiner. He states that he wants to go home in the new car he just charged on his American Express card. He denies medical illnesses. The urine drug screen is negative. Which of the following is the most likely diagnosis for this man?

    A. Schizoaffective disorder
    B. Schizophrenia
    C. Bipolar disorder
    D. Cyclothymic disorder
    E. Narcissistic personality disorder

6. A 20-year-old woman is being seen by her physician with the chief complaint that she is having difficulty in college. During some of her courses, she is asked to present her solution to problems and is also asked to give short talks to the peers in her class. She says that during those times, her heart races and she feels short of breath. She has become to dread these moments so much that she has withdrawn from classes that require this kind of work. She states she is afraid she will make a fool of herself. She denies other symptoms and does not use alcohol or drugs. She says she does fine around very small groups of people (two to three) with no anxiety. Which of the following is the most likely diagnosis?

    A. Avoidant personality disorder
    B. Adjustment disorder with anxiety
    C. Acute stress disorder
    D. Social anxiety disorder
    E. Specific phobia

7. A 35-year-old woman is admitted to the psychiatry unit after she attempted to kill herself by swallowing an entire bottle of an antidepressant that she had at home. The patient states that she is at her wit's end because she has terrible abdominal pain that no one is willing to treat. Her medical records show that the woman has had multiple medical workups for her stomach pain, and no diagnosis has ever been found; she has also had workups for a whole variety of other medical complaints. On the inpatient unit, she is subsequently found to be injecting feces under the skin of her arms. Per family history it was discovered that the patient's mother was a nurse. There is no evidence that the patient is in trouble with the legal system or is avoiding some other external cause of trouble. Which of the following is the most likely diagnosis?

    A. Malingering
    B. Borderline personality disorder
    C. Schizophrenia
    D. Major depression with psychosis
    E. Factitious disorder

8. A 45-year-old woman comes to her physician with the chief complaint of feeling sad and tired. She notes that for the last 4 months she has been sleeping sometimes 10 hours per day, but still feels fatigued. She notes that her mood is depressed and that she "just doesn't feel like doing anything anymore." She also notes that her appetite has increased slightly, and that she has gained over 30 lb in the last 4 months. She denies feeling suicidal or any hallucinations or delusions. She drinks four to five cups of coffee per day, but denies the use of any illicit drugs. She reports no medical problems, and the evaluation of her thyroid and hormone status is normal. Which of the following is the most likely diagnosis?

    A. Major depression
    B. Substance/medication-induced mood disorder
    C. Mood disorder due to another medical condition
    D. Persistent depressive disorder
    E. Major depression with psychosis

9. A 50-year-old man repeatedly calls his physician because he is worried about having an undiagnosed cancer. The man has had several workups, looking for a gastrointestinal (GI) cancer, a central nervous system (CNS) cancer, and leukemia/lymphoma. After every workup (and a negative result) the man feels calmer and somewhat reassured, but within weeks he is worried that he has cancer again, or some other fatal disease. The man has no other complaints and denies any physical symptoms. Which of the following is the most likely diagnosis?

    A. Factitious disorder
    B. Illness anxiety disorder
    C. Generalized anxiety disorder (GAD)
    D. Conversion disorder
    E. Somatic symptom disorder

10. A 23-year-old college student comes to the physician because her room-mates are worried about her eating. She tells the physician that she regularly eats large amounts of food (in excess of 10,000 calories on occasion) and then has to "punish herself" and "get rid of it." She explains that she does this by sticking her finger down her throat, which causes her to vomit. She tried to hide this activity from her roommates, but on more than one occasion they have heard her retching in the bathroom. The patient is 5'5" tall and weighs 132 lb. Which of the following is the most likely diagnosis?

    A. Anorexia nervosa

    B. Avoidant/restrictive food intake disorder

    C. Bulimia nervosa

    D. Binge-eating disorder

    E. Pica

11. A 9-year-old boy is brought to the pediatrician by his mother because he "wants to be a girl." The mother states that the boy repeatedly is found dressed in his sister's clothes and cries when he is forced to dress as a boy. This has been happening since he was very little. He also prefers to play with dolls and dress them up in fancy clothes. He appears revolted by his own genitals and has told his mother more than once that he would like to see his penis removed. Which of the following treatments will likely be most beneficial for this boy?

    A. Psychotherapy to explore why this boy wants to be a girl

    B. Selective serotonin reuptake inhibitor (SSRI)

    C. Risperidone

    D. Mood stabilizer

    E. Supportive psychotherapy to help the boy cope with his feelings

12. A 13-year-old boy is brought to the psychiatrist by his mother because she is "at her wit's end." She explains that the boy is often irritable and angry with his family and with his peers and teachers. He argues with adults and does not follow any rules. If he is confronted about this behavior, he is not sorry for it, and in fact, becomes even more angry. He has been displaying this behavior for at least 1 year, but the mother states that it has been worsening in the last several months. He has no other medical problems. Which of the following is the most likely diagnosis?

    A. Oppositional defiant disorder

    B. Conduct disorder

    C. Antisocial personality disorder

    D. Intermittent explosive disorder

    E. Substance/medication-induced mood disorder

13. A 75-year-old man is admitted to the hospital after he fell down a flight of stairs and broke his hip. Three days after his admission, he begins screaming for the nurse to "get that stranger out of my room!" When the nurse comes into the room, she sees that the curtains at one side of the room are moving because of a slight breeze, but there is no one in the room. That evening, the man becomes agitated and tries to pull out his IV line. All the following disorders must be considered, EXCEPT which one?

A. Delirium

B. Dementia

C. Major depression

D. Alcohol withdrawal

E. Benzodiazepine withdrawal

14. A 49-year-old woman comes to her physician with the chief complaint of feeling anxious all the time. She notes that for the past several months she has noted that when she wakes up in the morning she feel nervous, though there is nothing that she can think of that makes her so. She feels anxious and jittery all day long, and has been having trouble sleeping for the past 3 months. She sometimes wakes up in the middle of the night extremely hot and then drenched with sweat; these episodes have occurred during the day as well. She takes esomeprazole magnesium (Nexium) for reflux disease, but is otherwise healthy. Which of the following is the most likely diagnosis?

A. Generalized anxiety disorder (GAD)

B. Adjustment disorder with anxious mood

C. Substance/medication-induced anxiety disorder

D. Anxiety due to another medical condition

E. Major depression with anxiety

15. A 25-year-old woman comes to her physician for help because she continues to have intrusive memories of a rape she suffered 2 weeks previously. She notes that she thought she was going to die during the rape, and she can't stop dreaming about what happened over and over. She has been unable to feel anything positive since then, even though she acknowledges that her boyfriend and parents have been very supportive. She tries to avoid going anywhere near the area of town where she was raped. She is having trouble concentrating at work and seems to get short of breath and panicky easily. Which of the following is the most likely diagnosis?

A. Posttraumatic stress disorder (PTSD)

B. Acute stress disorder

C. Adjustment disorder with depressed mood

D. Adjustment disorder with anxious mood

E. Panic disorder

ANSWERS

1. **A.** (Schizoid personality disorder). This man was doing just fine at a job that kept him isolated from others. Once promoted to a job in which he has more personal interaction, he is overwhelmed and unhappy. The fact that he lives alone, has very few friends, but likes it that way points to a schizoid personality disorder. This man exhibits no signs of paranoid—he is not worried that others are going to hurt him are or out to do him wrong, so paranoid personality disorder is unlikely. He also shows no signs of bizarre or odd thoughts, nor is there any evidence that he is otherwise odd appearing in manner or dress, ruling down schizotypal personality disorder. The fact that the patient is overwhelmed and unhappy appears to be because of the more frequent and unwelcome human interaction; there is no note of any other trauma to which the man is adjusting, ruling down an adjustment disorder. The fact that the man likes the fact that he is isolated and has no friends rules out avoidant personality disorder, in which the patient desperately wants friends, but is so afraid of rejection he/she avoids meeting them.

2. **E.** (Avoidant Personality Disorder). In contrast to the case above, this woman is saddened by the fact that she does not have many friends. The news that her friend is getting married deepens her feelings of isolation. This appears to be a lifelong issue, not something short-term, as might be seen in an adjustment disorder. She does not PREFER to spend time alone, like might be seen in a patient with schizoid personality disorder. She does not display evidence that she things others are out to hurt her or take advantage of her, which might be seen in paranoid personality disorder. There is no mention of odd or bizarre behavior, dress, or mannerisms, as would be seen in someone with schizotypal personality disorder. Her sadness about her lack of friends, which is long-term, along with an absence of vegetative symptoms as might be found in someone with a major depression, point to an avoidant personality disorder.

3. **C.** (High dose SSRI). This girl is demonstrating classic signs and symptoms of an obsessive-compulsive disorder. She has an obsession that she is germ covered, and to keep the anxiety at bay about this, she washes compulsively, sometimes for hours at a time. She also has a checking ritual regarding the stove. Treatment with an SSRI is the medication of choice; it must sometimes be pushed to a high-dosage level to be effective in this disorder. Psychotherapy alone, an anxiolytic, or a mood stabilizer would do nothing for her symptoms. While the symptoms themselves may seem bizarre, they are not signs of psychosis—an antipsychotic would be likewise ineffective.

4. **A.** This patient is showing classic signs and symptoms of generalized anxiety disorder. She worries about a number of situations—finances of the state, terrorist attacks, personal finances, house repairs, and on and on. This condition has been long term, but has been exacerbated recently by work and marital stress. For a benzodiazepine-naïve patient (and there is no evidence in the vignette to suggest the patient has been on benzodiazepines),

the drug of choice is buspirone. Although an anxiolytic is likely to help somewhat, the addiction potential of the medication and the fact that it is not as effective as buspirone makes it a second-line medication. The other three (SSRI, cognitive behavioral therapy, zolpidem) have not been proven effective in this disorder.

5.   **C.** The man is presenting with labile mood, inappropriate behavior, grandiose thoughts, and excessive spending, all hallmarks of **bipolar disorder.** Because he is clearly manic at the moment, a cyclothymic disorder, with its smaller highs than full blown mania, is unlikely. Narcissistic personality disorder does not present with frank psychosis. Schizophrenia would be unlikely to present with the labile mood and excessive spending. Schizoaffective disorder would likely present with a background of psychosis with new affective symptoms superimposed. Because we must assume there is no prior history beyond what we have been told in the scenario, bipolar disorder is the best fit.

6.   **D.** The patient presents with the classic history of **social anxiety disorder.** She is afraid of public presentations, though she does well with small groups of people. An avoidant personality disordered patient would have trouble speaking with even those small groups of people, and would have had a long history of anxiety around people before college. While the patient is clearly anxious, it is around just one form of situation—that of public speaking, making an adjustment disorder with anxiety unlikely—the patient would be anxious all the time if this were the case. This holds true for an acute stress disorder as well, and in addition, that diagnosis requires a significant trauma that the patient has either survived or observed; neither is the case here. While it can be argued that this patient has a specific phobia, that of social speaking, the diagnosis is a better match for social anxiety disorder.

7.   **E.** This patient has **factitious disorder.** She is attempting to put herself in the role of a patient (primary gain) so that she may be cared for, ostensibly trying to unconsciously recreate being cared for by a medical caregiver (her mother). Because there is no evidence of secondary gain (avoiding the law or the military, for example), it is unlikely that she is malingering. There is no evidence of a thought disorder, hallucinations, or delusions which would make one suspicious of schizophrenia, and in addition the woman is rather old to have a first break at 35. While the patient did attempt to kill herself, it is in a background of desperation about being taken care of and not having her physical symptoms (which she has produced) addressed. Likewise we have no history of other symptoms of major depression such as insomnia, anhedonia, or weight loss.

8.   **A.** This patient presents with a depressed mood and fatigue, along with hypersomnia and weight gain, making one strongly consider a major depression; while one cannot rule out a mood disorder due to a medical condition such as hypothyroidism, on this history alone, the additional work-up makes this possibility less likely. Because the patient denies the use of substances (other than coffee, which would be unlikely to cause these symptoms) and

is not on any medications (assumed because she has no medical problems), option B is unlikely. The patient has not had a depressed mood for longer than 4 months, so she does not fit the criteria for a persistent depressive disorder.

9. **B.** It is likely this man has an **illness anxiety disorder,** because he believes he is seriously medically ill repeatedly, and despite attempts to reassure him, said reassurance is short lasting. He does not have a factitious disorder, because he is not producing either mental (hallucinations/delusions) or physical symptoms (fever, abscesses, etc) other than the recurring anxiety about his health. GAD would require that the man be worried about a myriad of problems; instead he is focused on his health alone—there is no history of other worries. The man does not report physical symptoms in a variety of body areas, nor is he in pain, making the diagnosis of somatic symptom disorder unlikely.

10. **C.** This college student has the classic symptoms of **bulimia,** in which she eats huge amounts of food (binging) and then feels the need to "get rid of it" (purging). Her body mas index (BMI) is within a normal range, and therefore anorexia is ruled out. Avoidant/restrictive food intake disorder is more commonly found in children, and at any rate, this woman's food intake is anything but restrictive. Likewise, while she does binge, she also purges, making binge-eating disorder less of a good fit than bulimia. Pica is the eating of non-nutritional objects that are not meant to be consumed (eg, lead paint chips). There is no history of this given in the vignette.

11. **E.** This boy is suffering from gender dysphoria, characterized by a strong desire to be of the other gender, a strong preference for cross-dressing, and a strong dislike of his sexual anatomy. **Treatment for the disorder is centered on helping the child cope with his feelings,** not in trying to cure the feelings of being in the "wrong body." Therefore, psychotherapy to change the boy's feelings about wanting to be a girl is unhelpful, and so are medications.

12. **A.** This boy is suffering from **oppositional defiant disorder,** characterized by at least 6 months of an angry/irritable mood, argumentative/defiant behavior, and vindictiveness. Conduct disorder and oppositional defiant disorder both have problems with conduct, but those of oppositional defiant disorder are less severe in nature and do not include aggression toward people or animals, destruction of property, or theft. Conduct disorder does not have the affective symptoms (angry/irritable mood) seen in oppositional defiant disorder. Intermittent explosive disorder patients also show serious aggression toward others, not seen in oppositional defiant disorder. Antisocial personality disorder cannot be diagnosed in one younger than 18. There is no evidence in the vignette to suspect a mood disorder secondary to some substance or medication.

13. **C.** This man is displaying the illusions and agitation in the evening ("sundowning") seen in one with a delirium, and unlikely to be due to major depression. Patients with preexisting dementia are much more prone to a

delirium in these kinds of circumstances (away from familiar surroundings and people, unfamiliar routines), so dementia as a coexisting diagnosis must be considered. Likewise, the time course for the beginning of the symptoms of alcohol withdrawal is consistent with the appearance of these symptoms; it must be considered in the differential diagnosis, as must benzodiazepine withdrawal. The use of benzodiazepines in the elderly must be undertaken only very cautiously, if at all; it is possible this man became unsteady due to a benzodiazepine, fell and broke his hip, and is now in withdrawal from the drug on top of everything else. Major depression would not present so suddenly.

14.   **D.** This woman is likely suffering from **anxiety due to another medical condition.** She has symptoms suggestive of menopause (insomnia, hot flashes leading to drenching sweats), which is known to cause anxiety symptoms frequently. She does not fit criteria for GAD, as she is not worried about a whole host of topics; in fact, she feels anxious with no particular topics in mind at all. She has no history per the vignette of any major changes that might cause an adjustment disorder. There is no evidence in the vignette to point to a substance or medication-induced anxiety disorder (esomeprazole does not cause the symptoms present in this patient). She does not complain of sadness or irritability, nor does she have other vegetative symptoms found in depression except for the insomnia.

15.   **B.** This patient has classic symptoms of an **acute stress disorder** or PTSD. It is the time course (2 weeks) that makes the diagnosis acute stress disorder; PTSD cannot be diagnosed until the symptoms have persisted for 1 month or more. She has been exposed to a severe traumatic event in which she was sexually violated. She has symptoms of intrusion (recurrent memories and dreams of the rape), a negative mood, avoidance symptoms (avoidance of the area of town where she was raped), and arousal symptoms (trouble concentrating at work). The diagnosis of adjustment disorder is made when the criterion A for the diagnosis of acute stress disorder is not met (ie, the patient has not had exposure to actual or threatened death, serious injury, or sexual violence). Although spontaneous panic attacks (such as this patient reports) are common in patients suffering from acute stress disorder, panic disorder is not diagnosed unless the panic attacks are unexpected and there is fear or maladaptive changes in behavior in response to the panic attacks themselves.

Note: Page numbers followed by a *t* or *f* indicate that the entry is included in a table or figure.